THE MOLECULAR BASIS OF DEMENTIA

ANNALS OF THE NEW YORK ACADEMY OF SCIENCES
Volume 920

THE MOLECULAR BASIS OF DEMENTIA

*Edited by John H. Growdon, Richard J. Wurtman,
Suzanne Corkin, and Roger M. Nitsch*

The New York Academy of Sciences
New York, New York
2000

Library of Congress Cataloging-in-Publication Data

The molecular basis of dementia / edited by John H. Growdon ...[et al.].
    p. cm. — (Annals of the New York Academy of Sciences ; v. 920)
    Includes bibliographical references and index.
    ISBN 1-57331-283-5 (cloth : alk. paper) — ISBN 1-57331-284-3 (pbk. : alk. paper)
        1. Dementia—Molecular aspects. I. Growdon, John H. (John Herbert)
    II. Series.

    Q11.N5 vol. 920
    [RC521]
    500 s—dc21
    [616.8'3]   00-048683

GYAT / PCP
Printed in the United States of America
ISBN 1-57331-283-5 (cloth)
ISBN 1-57331-284-3 (paper)
ISSN 0077-8923

ANNALS OF THE NEW YORK ACADEMY OF SCIENCES
Volume 920
December 2000

THE MOLECULAR BASIS OF DEMENTIA

Editors and Conference Organizers
JOHN H. GROWDON, RICHARD J. WURTMAN, SUZANNE CORKIN,
AND ROGER M. NITSCH

[These papers were presented at the ninth meeting of the International Study Group on the Pharmacology of Memory Disorders Associated with Aging, held on February 18–20, 2000 in Zurich, Switzerland.]

CONTENTS

Part III. Transgenic and Knockout Approaches to Neurodegenerative Diseases

Financial assistance was received from:

Sponsors
- ALZHEIMER'S ASSOCIATION
- NATIONAL INSTITUTE ON AGING, NIH

Major Funders
- ASTRA ZENECA
- JANSSEN PHARMACEUTICA

Supporters
- BOEHRINGER INGELHEIM PHARMA AG
- CENTRE DE RECHERCHE PIERRE FABRE
- ELAN PHARMACEUTICALS
- EVOTEC NEUROSCIENCES GmbH
- FUJISAWA RESEARCH INSTITUTE OF AMERICA
- GLAXO WELLCOME, INC.
- MERCK AND COMPANY
- NOVARTIS PHARMA AG
- PFIZER PHARMACEUTICALS
- PRAECIS PHARMACEUTICALS, INC.
- SMITHKLINE BEECHAM PHARMACEUTICALS

Contributors
- BAYER AG
- KNOLL AG
- H. LUNDBECK A/S
- COLLEGE INTERNATIONAL DE RECHERCHE SEVIER
- WILLMAR SCHWABE GmbH

Preface

This volume contains the papers and poster abstracts from the ninth meeting of the International Study Group on the Pharmacology of Memory Disorders Associated with Aging (ISG), which took place in Zurich, Switzerland, on February 18–20, 2000. The ISG was founded 21 years ago in the belief that the development of effective treatments for Alzheimer's disease and other dementias would be accelerated by periodic meetings of scientists and physicians from academia and industry from around the world who are actively working on issues related to dementia. Since the last ISG meeting in 1995, tremendous progress has been made in identifying factors that are associated with the etiology and the pathogenesis of dementia. Further, many small biotechnology and large pharmaceutical companies now have drug development programs for Alzheimer's disease. These efforts have led to the approval by the Food and Drug Administration of the first drugs for the treatment of dementia and to their subsequent wide availability. Recent discoveries include information on dementias other than Alzheimer's disease, for example, Lewy body and prion diseases, and the frontotemporal dementia associated with chromosome 17. The identification of similarities and distinctive differences among these forms of dementia may suggest specific approaches for the treatment of these diseases. In parallel, technological achievements in molecular biology have made it possible to mimic, in genetically modified animals, some of the histopathological abnormalities found in the brains of demented people. These models make it possible to study the neurobiology and pathophysiology of genes and proteins associated with dementia. They also provide useful experimental systems for validating proposed treatments designed to slow—or stop—neurodegeneration associated with dementia. The overriding goal of the ISG has always been to highlight discoveries that shed light on the causes and biological mechanisms underlying Alzheimer's disease and related dementias, and to encourage the translation of such discoveries into effective treatments. The proceedings of the ninth meeting of the ISG continue this tradition and consider five major topics:

- α-Synuclein in neurodegenerative disease
- Novel mutations in dementia
- Transgenic and knockout approaches to neurodegenerative diseases
- Proteases in Alzheimer's disease
- Therapies beyond AChE inhibitors

The first section reviews the role of α-synuclein in neurodegenerative diseases associated with the formation in brain of Lewy bodies, as well as its role in cell biology. The second section deals with recently discovered mutations, including long-sought mutations of the gene encoding the tau protein. The third section reports on technical aspects and potential uses of the generation of genetically modified mice for dementia research. Speakers in this section compare recent attempts to alter expression in mouse tissues of the genes encoding α-synuclein, tau, ApoE, APP, presenilin, and the prion protein. There is growing interest in proteases as potential targets in developing drugs for dementias. The fourth section focuses on the recent discovery of some of the APP-cleaving "secretases" and on efforts to identify small molecules that modify their activities. As in most previous ISG meetings, the last section is devoted to innovative therapies for dementia. Building upon advances in APP biology, this section considers approaches other than the widely used acetyl-cholinesterase inhibitors.

In many areas of dementia research, scientists from industry and academia have contributed equally in discovering new genes, drug targets and mechanisms of neurodegeneration. The ISG fosters interactions among scientists in industry, those in academic research, and administrators in public and private agencies concerned with dementia. The ninth ISG meeting continues in this tradition by stimulating research in dementia, and by speeding the transfer of information from the basic sciences to physicians caring for persons with dementia.

— JOHN H. GROWDON
— RICHARD J. WURTMAN
— SUZANNE CORKIN
— ROGER M. NITSCH

Publications of the International Study Group on the Pharmacology of Memory Disorders Associated with Aging

CORKIN, S., K.L. DAVIS, J.H. GROWDON, E. USDIN & R.J. WURTMAN, Eds. 1982. Aging. Vol. 19. Alzheimer's Disease: A Report of Progress in Research. Raven Press. New York.

WURTMAN, R.J., S. CORKIN & J.H. GROWDON, Eds. 1984. Alzheimer's Disease: Advances in Basic Research and Therapies. Center for Brain Sciences and Metabolism Charitable Trust. Cambridge, MA.

WURTMAN, R.J., S. CORKIN & J.H. GROWDON, Eds. 1987. Topics in Basic and Clinical Science of Dementia. J. Neural Transm. Suppl. 24. Springer. New York.

WURTMAN, R.J., S. CORKIN, J.H. GROWDON & E. RITTER-WALKER, Eds. 1990. Advances in Neurology. Vol. 51. Alzheimer's Disease. Raven Press. New York.

GROWDON, J.H., S. CORKIN, E. RITTER-WALKER & R.J. WURTMAN, Eds. 1991. Aging and Alzheimer's Disease: Sensory Systems, Neuronal Growth and Neuronal Metabolism. Ann. N.Y. Acad. Sci. Vol. 640.

NITSCH, R.M., J.H. GROWDON, S. CORKIN & R.J. WURTMAN, Eds. 1993. Alzheimer's Disease: Amyloid Precursor Proteins, Signal Transduction, and Neuronal Transplantation. Ann. N.Y. Acad. Sci. Vol. 695.

WURTMAN, R.J., S. CORKIN, J.H. GROWDON & R.M. NITSCH, Eds. 1996. The Neurobiology of Alzheimer's Disease. Ann. N.Y. Acad. Sci. Vol. 777.

Clinical Lewy Body Syndromes

I.G. MCKEITH[a]

Department of Old Age Psychiatry, Institute for the Health of the Elderly, Wolfson Research Centre, Newcastle General Hospital, Newcastle upon Tyne, United Kingdom

ABSTRACT: Lewy bodies are spherical, intracytoplasmic, eosinophilic, neuronal inclusions comprising abnormally truncated and phosphorylated intermediate neurofilament proteins, α-synuclein, ubiquitin, and associated enzymes. The clinical presentation of LB disease varies according to the site of LB formation and associated neuronal loss. Three main clinicopathological syndromes have been described—movement disorder, autonomic failure, and dementia. Parkinsonism is the most common presentation of LB disease developing in middle life. In older patients, a mixture of cognitive, autonomic, and motor dysfunction is more common. Dementia with LB (DLB) is a relatively recently described clinicopathological syndrome that accounts for up to 20% of all cases of dementia in old age. Patients, typically in their seventh and eighth decades, have LB pathology in cortical neurons as well as in the brain stem. LB disease should be considered in the differential diagnosis of a wide range of clinical presentations including episodic disturbances of consciousness, syncope, sleep disorders, and unexplained delirium.

THE SPECTRUM OF LEWY BODY DISEASE

Despite early reports, Lewy bodies (LB) probably do not occur in normal aging.[1,2] Their presence indicates neurological disease, the clinical presentation varying according to the site of LB formation and associated neuronal loss. Three main clinicopathological syndromes have been described.[3]

• *Parkinson's disease (PD),* an extrapyramidal movement disorder, associated with degeneration of subcortical neurons, particularly in substantia nigra.

• *Dementia with Lewy bodies (DLB),* a dementing disorder with prominent neuropsychiatric features, associated with degeneration of cortical neurons, particularly in entorhinal anterior cingulate, insular, temporal, and frontal regions.

• *Primary autonomic failure* with syncope and orthostatic hypotension, associated with degeneration of sympathetic neurons in spinal cord and autonomic ganglia.

In clinical practice, patients often have heterogenous combinations of parkinsonism, dementia, and autonomic failure, reflecting pathological involvement at

[a]Address for correspondence: I.G. McKeith, Department of Old Age Psychiatry, Institute for the Health of the Elderly, Wolfson Research Centre, Newcastle General Hospital, Westgate Road, Newcastle upon Tyne NE4 6BE, UK. Tel.: 00 44 191 256 3018; fax: 00 44 191 219 5071.
e-mail: i.g.mckeith@ncl.ac.uk

multiple locations. Lewy body disease cases may therefore present to neurology services (movement disorder or disturbed consciousness), psychiatry (cognitive impairment, psychosis or behavioral disturbance), or internal medicine (acute confusional states or syncope).[4] The details of clinical assessment and differential diagnoses will to a large extent be shaped by these symptom and specialty biases. In all cases a detailed history from the patient and reliable informants should document the time of onset of relevant key symptoms, the nature of their progression, and their effects on social, occupational, and personal function.

Lewy bodies have also been described in association with other clinical syndromes[3] including multiple system atrophy, progressive supranuclear palsy, corticobasal degeneration, motor neuron disease, subacute sclerosing panencephalitis, Hallorvorden-Spatz disease, Down's syndrome, neuroaxonal dystrophy, sporadic and familial Alzheimer's disease (AD), and REM sleep behavior disorder.[5] Their significance in these uncommon clinical disorders is not known.

PARKINSON'S DISEASE

The population prevalence rate of PD is 100–200 per 100,000 with a 1.1:1 male predominance. Age at onset in a community-based sample ranged from 27–85 years (mean 64.4) with a mean duration of disease of 9 years (range 1–34).[6] Prevalence is highest in the seventh and eighth decades of life. Two broad clinical subtypes of PD have been described—"tremor predominant" and "akinetic" or "postural instability/gait disorder." The latter tends to be typical of older patients and may be associated with a greater risk of subsequent cognitive impairment and psychiatric features such as hallucinations. The diagnosis of PD in a typical patient with tremor, bradykinesia, and rigidity is not difficult, but diagnostic accuracy in clinical practice is surprisingly poor. Conventional clinical diagnostic criteria such as the UK Parkinson's Disease Society Brain Bank Criteria[7] (shown in TABLE 1) seem to include 20–30% of patients with alternative causes of parkinsonism.[8] A beneficial response to levodopa is a major indicator for a correct diagnosis. Up to 50% of PD patients experience marked fluctuations in motor disability (on-off phenomena) after five years of levodopa treatment.[9] Together with dyskinesia, gait disorder and falls, motor disability causes severe impairments in daily living skills and quality of life. It is, however, the onset of neuropsychiatric features in the course of PD, which are the most potent source of patient and carer distress, and the most significant risk factors for nursing home placement.[10]

DEMENTIA IN PARKINSON'S DISEASE

The precise diagnosis of a dementia syndrome in PD is problematic, particularly in the early stages. Minor performance deficits in set-shifting, retrieval of learned material, and reduced verbal fluency are very frequent. They usually do not warrant a diagnosis of dementia because, although demonstrable in up to two-thirds of PD clinic attenders by timed tests of frontal and executive function, they fail to impact substantially on the person's day-to-day functioning. These phenomena are probably

TABLE 1. UK Parkinson's Disease Society Brain Bank clinical diagnostic criteria

Step 1. Diagnosis of parkinsonian syndrome

Bradykinesia (slowness of initiation of voluntary movement with progressive reduction in speed and amplitude of repetitive actions)

And at least one of the following:

a. Muscular rigidity

b. 4–6 Hz rest tremor

c. Postural instability not caused by primary visual, vestibular, cerebellar, or proprioceptive dysfunction.

Step 2. Exclusion criteria for Parkinson's disease

History of repeated strokes with stepwise progression of parkinsonian features

History of repeated head injury

History of definite encephalitis

Oculogyric crises

Neuroleptic treatment at onset of symptoms

More than one affected relative

Sustained remission

Strictly unilateral features after 3 years

Supranuclear gaze palsy

Cerebellar signs

Early severe autonomic involvement

Early severe dementia with disturbances of memory, language, and praxis

Babinski sign

Presence of cerebral tumor or communicating hydrocephalus on CT scan

Negative response to large doses of levodopa (if malabsorption excluded)

MPTP exposure

Step 3. Supportive prospective positive criteria for Parkinson's disease

(Three or more required for diagnosis of definite Parkinson's disease)

Unilateral onset

Rest tremor present

Progressive disorder

Persistent asymmetry most affecting side of onset

Excellent response (70–100%) to levodopa

Severe levodopa-induced chorea

Levodopa response for 5 years or more

Clinical course of 10 years or more

a consequence of diminished ascending cholinergic and dopaminergic projections to neocortical regions, particularly via striatofrontal loops. The term subcortical dementia is helpful in clinical practice to describe these deficits, manifest clinically as bradyphrenia (mental slowing), memory dysfunction, dilapidation of complex mental functions, and mood and personality changes.[11]

Significant disorientation, impairment in new learning, dysphasia, and dyspraxia developing in the course of PD are indicative of more generalized cortical LB disease or other degenerative pathologies. Risk factors for developing dementia in PD include later age of onset, current age, severity of motor impairment, prior history of depression, and poor response to levodopa.[12] Levodopa-induced confusion and poor performance on verbal fluency may best be characterized as early manifestations of dementia in patients with PD rather than risk factors per se.[13]

OTHER NEUROPSYCHIATRIC FEATURES IN PARKINSON'S DISEASE

Neuropsychiatric symptoms other than cognitive impairment are also common in PD, particularly depression, hallucinations, delusions, anxiety, and apathy. Depression appears equally common in the presence or absence of dementia and may represent either a psychological reaction to disability or result from degeneration of monoaminergic neurons, particularly dopaminergic projections to mesolimbic structures and orbitofrontal cortex.[14]

Psychotic symptoms are by contrast strongly associated with cognitive impairment. Other clinical correlates of psychosis in PD are old age, advanced PD and coexistent sleep disorder including altered dream phenomena and sleep fragmentation.[15,16] Visual hallucinations and illusions of people or animals are the most common feature. Although a prevalence of 25% is generally quoted, up to 44% of PD clinic attenders may admit to visual hallucinations if directly asked.[17] Hallucinations in other modalities (auditory, tactile, kinesthetic) can occur but are uncommon. The affective response to hallucinations varies from indifference, pleasure or fear. As cognitive impairment increases and insight is lost, the patient's delusional interpretations of his experiences are more likely to occur and lead to increasingly severe behavioral disturbances.

Antiparkinsonian medications are usually held responsible for hallucinations and confusion in PD, but research findings do not support this clinical impression. Factors associated with the development of visual hallucinosis are later age of onset of PD, total duration of illness, and the presence of cognitive impairment. Hallucinators and nonhallucinators are distinguished neither by severity of motor disability nor by dosage of antiparkinsonian medication. The emergence of psychotic symptoms is not related to the dose, duration, or number of dopaminergic agents,[15] and hallucinations do not relate to plasma levels of levodopa or sudden changes in plasma levels.[18] Thus, dopaminergic agents may provide a neurochemical milieu with a high risk for psychosis in PD, but do not cause psychosis per se.

DEMENTIA WITH LEWY BODIES

Several studies in a range of settings have suggested that DLB accounts for just under 20% of all cases of dementia referred for neuropathological autopsy.[19–21] The male to female ratio in these autopsy series is 1.5:1, but it is unclear to what extent this represents increased male susceptibility or reduced survival. Age at onset ranges from 50 to 83 years and at death 68 and 92 years.[22]

The recent consensus criteria for the clinical diagnosis of DLB[23] are shown in TABLE 2. Particular emphasis needs to be given to recognizing the characteristic dementia syndrome. Attentional deficits and prominent frontosubcortical and visuospatial dysfunction are the main features. Symptoms of persistent or prominent memory impairment are not always present early in the course of illness, although they are likely to develop in most patients with disease progression. Patients with dementia with Lewy body perform better than those with AD on tests of verbal recall, but relatively worse on tests of copying and drawing.[24] With the progression of dementia, the selective pattern of cognitive deficits may be lost, making differential diagnosis based on clinical examination difficult during the later stages.

TABLE 2. Consensus criteria for the clinical diagnosis of dementia with Lewy bodies (DLB)

1. The central feature required for a diagnosis of DLB is progressive cognitive decline of sufficient magnitude to interfere with normal social or occupational function. Prominent or persistent memory impairment may not necessarily occur in the early stages, but is usually evident with progression. Deficits on tests of attention and of frontal-subcortical skills and visuospatial ability may be especially prominent.

2. Two of the following core features are essential for a diagnosis of probable DLB, and one is essential for possible DLB.
   a. Fluctuating cognition with pronounced variations in attention and alertness
   b. Recurrent visual hallucinations that are typically well formed and detailed
   c. Spontaneous motor features of parkinsonism

3. Features supportive of the diagnosis are
   a. Repeated falls
   b. Syncope
   c. Transient loss of consciousness
   d. Neuroleptic sensitivity
   e. Systematized delusions
   f. Hallucinations and other modalities

4. A diagnosis of DLB is less likely in the presence of
   a. Stroke disease, evident as focal neurologic signs or on brain imaging
   b. Evidence on physical examination and investigation of any physical illness or other brain disorder sufficient to account for the clinical picture.

Probable DLB can be diagnosed if any two of the three key symptoms (fluctuation, visual hallucinations, spontaneous motor features of parkinsonism) are present. Fluctuation is undoubtedly the most difficult symptom to establish. Some patients identify the variable cognitive state themselves, but generally the most productive approach is to interview a reliable informant. Questions such as "Are there episodes when his/her thinking seems quite clear and then becomes muddled?" may be useful probes. Substantial changes in mental state and behavior may be seen within the duration of a single interview or between consecutive examinations. Parkinsonism and visual hallucinations pose fewer problems of identification.

There are four main categories of disorder that should be considered in the differential diagnosis of DLB:

- *Other dementia syndromes.* Sixty-five percent of autopsy-confirmed DLB cases meet the NINCDS-ADRDA clinical criteria for probable or possible AD, and this is the most frequent clinical misdiagnosis of DLB patients presenting with a primary dementia syndrome.[25] This suggests DLB should routinely be excluded when making the diagnosis of AD. Up to one-third of DLB cases are additionally misclassified as vascular dementia by the Hachinski Ischemic Index by virtue of items such as fluctuating nature and course of illness.[25] Pyramidal and focal neurological signs are, however, usually absent. The development of myoclonus in patients with a rapidly progressive form of DLB may lead the clinician to suspect Creutzfeldt-Jacob disease.[23]

- *Other causes of delirium.* In patients with intermittent delirium, appropriate examination and laboratory tests should be performed during the acute phase to maximize the chances of detecting infective, metabolic, inflammatory or other etiological factors. Pharmacological causes are particularly common in elderly patients. Although the presence of any of these features makes a diagnosis of DLB less likely, co-morbidity is not unusual in elderly patients, and the diagnosis should not be excluded simply on this basis.

- *Other neurological syndromes.* In patients with a prior diagnosis of PD, the onset of visual hallucinations and fluctuating cognitive impairment may be attributed to side effects of antiparkinsonian medications, and this must be tested by dose reduction or withdrawal. Other atypical parkinsonian syndromes associated with poor levodopa response, cognitive impairment, and postural instability include progressive supranuclear palsy and multisystem atrophy. Syncopal episodes in DLB are often incorrectly attributed to transient ischemic attacks, despite an absence of focal neurological signs. Recurrent disturbances in consciousness accompanied by complex visual hallucinations may suggest complex partial seizures (temporal lobe epilepsy), and vivid dreaming with violent movements during sleep may meet criteria for REM sleep behavior disorder. Both of these conditions have been reported as uncommon presenting symptoms of autopsy-confirmed DLB.[5,26]

- *Other psychiatric disorders.* If a patient spontaneously develops parkinsonian features or cognitive decline, or shows excessive sensitivity to neuroleptic medication,[27] in the course of late onset delusional disorder, depressive psychosis or mania, DLB should be considered.[26]

DIAGNOSTIC ACCURACY

Seven studies have now reported on either the sensitivity (proportion of cases positively identified) or specificity (proportion of negative cases correctly identified) of the International Consensus criteria for DLB against neuropathological diagnosis.[28] All five that examine the issue find the criteria for probable DLB to have specificity > 0.8, a figure comparable with the best clinical criteria for AD and PD. Reported sensitivity rates for detecting probable DLB are, however, much more variable and generally lower.

AUTONOMIC FAILURE

In addition to subcortical and cortical pathologies, PD and DLB cases also show a variable degree of LB in the autonomic nervous system leading to postural hypotension and syncope.[29] Lewy bodies and LN were present in the cardiac plexuses of 7 of 7 patients with PD, in sympathetic but not parasympathetic ganglia, and were associated with significant orthostatic hypotension.[30]

SUMMARY

The majority of cases with LB disease are found at autopsy to have pathological involvement at multiple sites in the central and autonomic nervous system. In older, demented subjects, Alzheimer-type pathology and additional minor vascular changes are also common and probably contribute significantly to the clinical presentation. Autopsy cases, however, represent end-stage disease and it is unclear how the distribution of pathologies seen at that time reflects the evolution of disease and clinical symptomatology through earlier stages.

REFERENCES

1. FORNO, L.S. 1969. Concentric hyalin intraneuronal inclusions of Lewy type in the brains of elderly persons (50 incidental cases): relationship to parkinsonism. J. Am. Geriatr. Soc. **17**: 557–575.
2. PERRY, R.H., D. IRVING & B.E. TOMLINSON. 1990. Lewy body prevalence in the aging brain: relationship to neuropsychiatric disorders, Alzheimer-type pathology and catecholaminergic nuclei. J. Neurol. Sci. **100**: 223–233.
3. LOWE, J.S. et al. 1996. Pathological significance of Lewy bodies in dementia. In Dementia with Lewy Bodies. R. Perry, I. McKeith & E. Perry, Eds.: 195–203. Cambridge University Press. New York.
4. McKEITH, I.G., D. GALASKO, G.K. WILCOCK & E.J. BYRNE. 1995. Lewy body dementia—diagnosis and treatment. Br. J. Psych. **167**: 709–717.
5. BOEVE, B.F., M.H. SILBER, T.J. FERMAN, et al. 1998. REM sleep behaviour disorder and degenerative dementia: an association likely reflecting Lewy body disease. Neurology **51**: 363–370.
6. TANDBERG, E., J.P. LARSEN, E.G. NESSLER, T. RIISE & J.A. AARLI. 1995. The epidemiology of Parkinson's disease in the county of Rogaland, Norway. Movement Disord. **10**(5): 541–549.
7. GIBB, W.R.G. & A.J. LEES. 1988. The relevance of the Lewy body to the pathogenesis of idiopathic Parkinson's disease. J. Neurol. Neurosurg. Psychiatry **51**: 745–752.
8. HUGHES, A.J., S.E. DANIEL, L. KILFORD & A.J. LEES. 1993. Accuracy of clinical diagnosis of Parkinson's disease. A clinicopathological study of 100 cases. J. Neurol. Neurosurg. Psychiatry **55**: 181–184.
9. MARSDEN, C.D. et al. 1982. Fluctuations of disability in Parkinson's disease—clinical aspects. In Movement Disorders. C.D. Marsden & F. Stanley, Eds.: 96–122. Butterworths. London.
10. GOETZ, C.G. & G.T. STEBBINS. 1993. Risk factors for nursing home placement in advanced Parkinson's disease. Neurology **43**: 2227–2229.
11. CUMMINGS, J.L. 1990. Subcortical Dementia. Oxford University Press. New York.
12. MAYEUX, R. et al. 1996. Putative clinical and genetic antecedents of dementia associated with Parkinson's disease. In Dementia with Lewy Bodies. R. Perry, I. McKeith & E. Perry, Eds.: 33–45. Cambridge University Press. New York.
13. AARSLAND, D. et al. 1999. Neuropsychiatric aspects of Parkinson's disease. Curr. Psychiatr. Rep. **1**: 61–68.
14. MAYBERG, H.S. et al. 1995. Depression in Parkinson's disease: a biological and organic viewpoint. In Advances in Neurology, Vol. 65. W.J. Weiner & A.E. Lang, Eds.: 49–60. Raven Press. New York.
15. AARSLAND, D., J.P. LARSEN, J.L. CUMMINS & K. LAAKE. 1999. Prevalence and clinical correlates of psychotic symptoms in Parkinson's disease: a community-based study. Arch. Neurol. **56**: 595–601.
16. NAIMARK, D., E. JACKSON, E. ROCKWELL & D.V. JESTE. 1996. Psychotic symptoms in Parkinson's disease patients with (and without) dementia. J. Am. Geriatr. Soc. **44**: 296–299.
17. HAESKE-DEWICK, H.C. 1995. Hallucinations in Parkinson's disease: characteristics and associated clinical features. Int. J. Geriatr. Psychiatry **10**: 487–495.
18. GOETZ, C.G., E.J. PAPPERT, L.M. BLASUCCI, et al. 1998. Intravenous levodopa in hallucinating Parkinson's disease patients: high dose challenge does not precipitate hallucinations. Neurology **50**: 515–517.
19. PERRY, R.H., D. IRVING, G. BLESSED, A. FAIRBAIRN & E.K. PERRY. 1990. Senile dementia of Lewy body type. A clinically and neuropathologically distinct form of Lewy body dementia in the elderly. J. Neurol. Sci. **95**: 119–139.

20. HANSEN, L.A., D. SALMON, D. GALASKO, et al. 1990. The Lewy body variant of Alzheimer's disease: a clinical and pathologic entity. Neurology **40:** 1–8.
21. HOLMES, C., N. CAIRNS, P. LANTOS & A. MANN. 1999. Validity of current clinical criteria for Alzheimer's disease, vascular dementia and dementia with Lewy bodies. Br. J. Psychiatry **174:** 45–50.
22. MCKEITH, I.G. 1998. Dementia with Lewy bodies: clinical and pathological diagnosis. Alz. Rep. **1**(2): 83–87.
23. MCKEITH, I.G., D. GALASKO, K. KOSAKA, et al. 1996. Consensus guidelines for the clinical and pathologic diagnosis of dementia with Lewy bodies (DLB): report of the consortium on DLB international workshop. Neurology **47:** 1113–1124.
24. WALKER, Z., R.L. ALLEN, S. SHERGILL & C.L. KATONA. 1997. Neuropsychological performance in Lewy body dementia and Alzheimer's disease. Br. J. Psychiatry **170:** 156–158.
25. MCKEITH, I.G., A.F. FAIRBAIRN, R.H. PERRY & P. THOMPSON. 1994. The clinical diagnosis and misdiagnosis of senile dementia of Lewy body type (SDLT)—do the diagnostic systems need to be revised? Behav. Neurol. **7**(1): 21.
26. MCKEITH, I.G., R.H. PERRY, A.F. FAIRBAIRN, S. JABEEN & E.K. PERRY. 1992. Operational criteria for senile dementia of Lewy body type (SDLT). Psychol. Med. **22:** 911–922.
27. MCKEITH, I.G., A. FAIRBAIRN, R. PERRY, P. THOMPSON & E. PERRY. 1992. Neuroleptic sensitivity in patients with senile dementia of Lewy body type. Br. Med. J. **305:** 673–678.
28. MCKEITH, I.G., J.T. O'BRIEN & C. BALLARD. 1999. Diagnosing dementia with Lewy bodies. Lancet **354**: 1227–1228.
29. KUZUHARA, S. & M. YOSHIMURA. 1993. Clinical and neuropathological aspects of diffuse Lewy body disease in the elderly. Adv. Neurol. **60:** 464–469.
30. IWANAGA, K. et al. 1999. Lewy body-type degeneration in cardiac plexus in Parkinson's and incidental Lewy body diseases. Neurology **52:** 1269–1271.

Clinical and Neuropathological Correlates of Dementia with Lewy Bodies

E. GÓMEZ-TORTOSA, M.C. IRIZARRY, T. GÓMEZ-ISLA, AND B.T. HYMAN[a]

Alzheimer Disease Research Unit, Massachusetts General Hospital, Charlestown, Massachusetts 02129, USA

ABSTRACT: Dementia with Lewy bodies (DLB) is characterized pathologically by widespread Lewy body (LB) neuronal inclusions in the brain, but the contribution of LBs to the clinical syndrome of dementia and parkinsonism is unclear. In a clinical-pathological study of 25 cases with DLB, we examined the regional neuroanatomical distribution of Lewy-related pathology using α-synuclein immunostaining to evaluate the relationship between LBs, neuronal loss, Alzheimer-type changes, and the clinical phenotype. Compared to traditional ubiquitin immunostaining, α-synuclein immunohistochemistry was more specific and slightly more sensitive, staining about 5% more intracytoplasmic structures. There was a consistent pattern of vulnerability to LB formation across subcortical, paralimbic, limbic, and neocortical structures, which was independent of concomitant Alzheimer-type changes. There were no significant differences in regional LB densities among patients with or without cognitive fluctuations, visual hallucinations, delusions, recurrent falls or parkinsonism. Duration of disease correlated weakly with LB density. There was no neuronal loss in superior temporal sulcus or entorhinal cortex in pure DLB cases compared to nondemented controls. Thus, DLB is characterized by a specific neuroanatomical vulnerability to LB pathology, distinct from AD pathology, with a complicated relationship to clinical symptoms.

INTRODUCTION

Dementia with Lewy bodies (DLB) is a recently recognized cause of neurodegenerative dementia that overlaps in clinical, pathological, and genetic features with Alzheimer's disease (AD) and Parkinson's disease (PD). The clinical and pathological hallmarks are summarized in TABLE 1. In DLB, Lewy bodies (LBs) are widely distributed throughout limbic, paralimbic, and neocortical regions. The standard technique for identifying LBs in the cortex has been immunostaining for ubiquitin. The presynaptic protein α-synuclein was recently identified as a major component of LBs and Lewy-related neurites, and appears to be a more specific marker for these inclusions. It is not clear to what extent cortical LBs are responsible for neuronal injury and, therefore, for the clinical syndrome. Other pathological changes, including Alzheimer-type pathology, frequently coexist with the LBs and may contribute to the clinical phenotype.

[a]Address for correspondence: Dr. Bradley T. Hyman, Alzheimer Disease Research Unit, Massachusetts General Hospital—East, 149 13th Street, Charlestown, Massachusetts 02129. Tel.: (617) 726-2299; fax: (617) 726-5677.
e-mail: b_hyman@helix.mgh.harvard.edu

TABLE 1. Clinical and pathological features in dementia with Lewy bodies[20]

Clinical Features	Pathological Features
1. Central feature: progressive dementia	1. Essential for diagnosis: Lewy bodies
2. Probable (2/3)[a] or possible (1/3) if: Fluctuating cognition and alertness Recurrent visual hallucinations Spontaneous parkinsonism	2. Associated but not essential: Lewy-related neurites Amyloid plaques (all types) Neurofibrillary tangles Neuronal loss/synapse loss Spongiform change (temporal) Neurotransmitter abnormalities
3. Supportive features: repeated falls, syncopes, neuroleptic hypersensitivity, delusions, hallucinations in other modalities	

[a]Two of the three features are required for a diagnosis of probable DLB, one for possible DLB.

Our clinical and quantitative neuropathological studies of DLB had the following aims: (a) to survey the pathological spectrum and the distribution of Lewy-related inclusions in several brain regions with α-synuclein immunostaining; (b) to study the correlation between LB accumulation, neuronal loss, and Alzheimer neurofibrillary tangles and senile plaques; and (c) to examine the relationship between LB accumulation in specific brain areas with clinical symptoms.

METHODS

We studied brain specimens of 25 cases with the neuropathological diagnosis of DLB obtained from the Massachusetts Alzheimer's Disease Research Center (ADRC) Brain Bank, Boston: 19 male/6 female; age at onset, 69.3 ± 7.1 years (mean $\pm$ S.D.), age at death, 78.6 ± 5.8; disease duration, 9.4 ± 4.5.[1-3] All cases had been followed clinically at the Memory Disorders Unit of the ADRC for an average of 43.1 ± 40.2 months. Thirteen cases had almost no concomitant Alzheimer changes (Braak stage I or II), eleven cases had paralimbic tangles and met criteria for a Braak stage III or IV, and one case met criteria for a Braak stage V. We studied paraffin-embedded tissue from the following areas: substantia nigra at the level of the red nucleus, entorhinal cortex, cingulate gyrus, insula, hippocampus, medial frontal and associative occipital cortex. In selected cases, coronal frozen sections containing the whole temporal lobe at the level of the hippocampus were also studied. Sections were stained with H&E, cresyl violet, and modified Bielchowsky, and immunostained with antibodies against α-synuclein, ubiquitin, and neurofilament proteins (SMI-32, SMI-312). A computer-based image analysis system with stereological overlays (Bioquant Image Analysis System, Nashville, TN) was used to assist in the quantitation of structures. This program records the positions of each of the counted structures with x/y coordinates and provides an accurate visual image of their distribution within a given area.

RESULTS AND DISCUSSION

Lewy-related Pathology Assessed with α-Synuclein

α-Synuclein immunohistochemistry differentiated immunoreactive LBs from nonstaining globose neurofibrillary tangles, and thus was more specific than traditional ubiquitin immunostaining. α-Synuclein staining was also slightly more sensitive, identifying approximately 5% more intracytoplasmic structures. The morphology of α-synuclein immunoreactivity varied based on anatomic location. The substantia nigra showed the greatest morphological diversity of α-synuclein immunoreactive structures, with neuritic inclusions and a wide spectrum of intracytoplasmic inclusions with variable ubiquitin co-staining. These different types of inclusions may represent progressive stages of α-synuclein aggregation and LB formation. In contrast, neocortical and paralimbic α-synuclein inclusions were more homogeneous in morphology and ubiquitin staining. The cortex contained mostly α-synuclein and ubiquitin double-labeled LBs in deep layers, and a subset of cases showed dystrophic double-stained neuritic processes in superficial layers of entorhinal cortex and cingulate gyrus.[3]

Lewy neurites were observed in the CA2–3 regions, as first described by Dickson *et al.*[4] They were frequent in 16 cases, few in four, and absent in five. Double immunostaining against α-synuclein and either SMI-32 (nonphosphorylated dendritic neurofilaments) or SMI-312 (phosphorylated axonal neurofilaments) suggests that Lewy neurites derive from axonal afferents to CA2–3. The CA2–3 fields receive major inputs from monoaminergic brainstem nuclei, cholinergic septal nuclei, entorhinal cortex, and dentate gyrus. The absence of tyrosine hydroxylase immunoreactivity in the Lewy neurites suggests that they do not originate in brainstem nuclei.[5] These neurites originate in septal nuclei and/or entorhinal cortex layer III, because our preliminary data show that the severity of α-synuclein pathology in these regions is well correlated. These connections are crucial for memory and cognition, suggesting that the neuritic inclusions may disrupt hippocampal function by interfering with inputs to the CA1 field and contribute to the cognitive deficits in DLB. In fact, Churchyard and Lees have found the degree of cognitive impairment in Parkinson's disease patients to be correlated with the density of CA2 Lewy neurites.[5]

Quantitation of LB

LB density followed a consistent anatomical trend as follows: substantia nigra > entorhinal cortex > cingulate gyrus > insula > frontal cortex > hippocampus > occipital cortex (FIG. 1). This gradient was very similar in cases with (group B) or without (group A) concurrent AD pathology and supports a hierarchical vulnerability to LB formation across brain regions, independent of the presence of Alzheimer changes. A strong correlation was found between paralimbic and neocortical LB burdens ($p < 0.0001$), but neither of these correlated directly with LB density in substantia nigra, which suggests that DLB does not simply reflect severe or long-lasting PD. LBs frequently occurred in the deep cortical layers V and VI. In some cases LBs were clearly confined to deep layers, whereas in others they were more widespread through all cortical lamina. However, each individual case usually displayed the identical pattern (cortical vs. widespread) in all paralimbic and neocortical areas.[2]

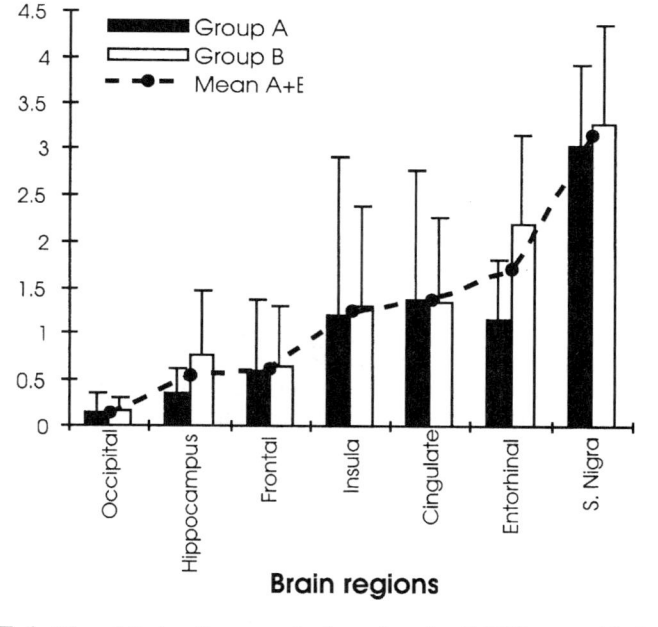

FIGURE 1. Mean LB density across brain regions in all DLB cases (*dashed line, n =* 25), in DLB cases without significant concomitant Alzheimer-type changes (*black bar—* Group A, Braak stage I or II, *n* = 13), and in DLB cases with concomitant AD changes (*white bars*—Group B, Braak stages III to V, *n* = 12); error bars = S.D. (Adapted from Gómez-Tortosa *et al.*[2])

Neuronal Loss

Two studies from our group have assessed neuronal loss in DLB. In the superior temporal sulcus region, pure DLB brains showed no significant neuronal loss in comparison with controls, whereas DLB cases with concomitant AD pathology had pronounced neuronal loss comparable to that of pure AD cases.[1] In the entorhinal cortex, seven pure DLB cases had no significant decrease in the neuronal density of layers V/VI—where the LBs are mainly found—compared to controls. The number of LBs did not correlate with neuronal loss in these studies, suggesting that they are not directly implicated in widespread neuronal death in pure DLB.

Other studies have not found significant neuronal or synaptic loss in the temporal, entorhinal or frontal cortices, or in the hippocampus of DLB compared with control brains.[7–12] These data support the conclusion that cortical neuronal loss in DLB is associated more with the concomitant Alzheimer-type pathology than with the α-synuclein inclusions.

Relationship with Alzheimer Changes

AD pathology frequently coexists with DLB. Ten to thirty percent of cases fulfilling neuropathological criteria for AD have cortical LBs, and 32 to 89% (depending on the criteria used to define AD) of the DLB cases have concomitant Alzheimer changes.[13,14] However, we have not found any correlation between LB density and the degree of neurofibrillary tangle involvement or the amount of cortical senile plaques, which suggests an independence in the formation or in the dynamic turnover of these pathological structures.[1,2] The distribution of LBs (see above) does not coincide with that of neurofibrillary tangles, which are most abundant in the hippocampus and superficial layers (II and III) of association cortex.

AD pathology likely has an additive or synergistic effect in producing the clinical phenotype of DLB, but cannot be the sole cause. In contrast to typical AD, Alzheimer changes in most DLB brains is a plaque-predominant type (diffuse or non-neuritic plaques which have little or no effect on cognition) with very few tangles. There is also a small but well-documented number of DLB cases that represent pure LB pathology.[15,16]

Clinical-Pathological Correlations

Because the pathological specimens from DLB brains were obtained from subjects who had been extensively clinically evaluated at the Massachusetts Alzheimer Disease Research Center, we were able to perform detailed clinical-pathological correlations.[2] First, we compared the LB pathology between groups of DLB patients ($n = 25$) with different *symptoms at onset*. Patients who presented with parkinsonism ($n = 7$) had higher LB density in substantia nigra, and those who started with cognitive impairment ($n = 17$) had slightly higher LB density in neocortex, but the differences were not statistically significant.

Second, we compared LB pathology in subjects with specific *clinical symptoms* during the course of the illness. All patients developed dementia, 19 developed parkinsonian signs, and 13 had visual hallucinations. Fluctuations in cognitive status and alertness—including variable cognitive performance as well as recurrent confusional, lethargic or syncopal-like episodes—were reported in 16 cases. Recurrent falls were reported in eight cases, and systematized delusions in eight cases. We hypothesized that cases with parkinsonism or recurrent falls would have higher LB burdens in substantia nigra than those without these symptoms and that clinical evidence of psychiatric symptoms or cognitive fluctuations would be related to a higher neocortical or paralimbic LB burden. However, no significant differences were found in LB density in any region when comparing patients with or without these specific clinical features. There was only a trend toward the association of visual hallucinations with a higher total LB burden, and of delusions with a higher LB density in the cingulate cortex.

Finally, the *duration of disease* correlated with a global LB burden for each case ($p = 0.02$), but did not correlate with LB density in any individual area.

Other studies have assessed the correlation between cortical LBs and dementia severity—either as a functional or as a neuropsychological score—with contradictory results. Perry *et al.*[15] and Gómez-Isla *et al.*[1] did not find any correlation. In contrast, other groups have found a significant correlation between dementia severity and neocortical LB counts.[17–19] However, in some of these studies the significance relies upon the most severely demented patients having a higher cortical LB density. The lack of correlation between LB densities and disease duration has been shown in other studies.[1–19]

CONCLUSIONS

In summary, there is a consistent pattern of vulnerability to LB formation across brain regions that is independent of the presence of Alzheimer-type changes. α-Synuclein immunoreactivity in DLB reveals a wide spectrum of structures, including the typical LBs, other intracytoplasmic inclusions and extensive neuritic processes. We analyzed the clinical and pathological features of DLB to determine associations between motor symptoms and LB densities in substantia nigra or between dementia/psychiatric symptoms and cortical LBs, but these correlations were not statistically significant. It is possible that the abnormal neurites, present in hippocampus and in other cortical regions, rather than the LBs, would play a significant role in the progression of cognitive deficits by interfering neuronal connectivity. The possibility that cortical LBs are a marker of a widespread pathological process resulting in selective neuronal loss, neuritic dysfunction in crucial pathways, and neurochemical imbalances, suggests a complex contribution of α-synuclein inclusions to the clinical syndrome in DLB.

ACKNOWLEDGMENTS

This work was supported by NIH grants P5O-AGO5134 (ADRC), AGO8487 and MGH-MIT Parkinson Center. E. Gómez-Tortosa was supported by a grant from Fundación Ramón Areces, Spain.

REFERENCES

1. GOMEZ-ISLA, T., W.B. GROWDON, M. MCNAMARA, *et al.* 1999. Clinicopathologic correlates in temporal cortex in dementia with Lewy bodies. Neurology **53:** 2003–2009.
2. GOMEZ-TORTOSA, E., K. NEWELL, M.C. IRIZARRY, M. ALBERT, J.H. GROWDON & B.T. HYMAN. 1999. Clinical and quantitative pathologic correlates of dementia with Lewy bodies. Neurology **53:** 1284–1291.
3. GOMEZ-TORTOSA, E., K. NEWELL, M.C. IRIZARRY, J.L. SANDERS & B.T. HYMAN. 1999. Alpha-synuclein immunoreactivity in dementia with Lewy bodies: morphological staging and comparison with ubiquitin immunostaining. Acta Neuropathologica. In press.
4. DICKSON, D.W., D. RUAN, H. CRYSTAL, *et al.* 1991. Hippocampal degeneration differentiates diffuse Lewy body disease (DLBD) from Alzheimer's disease: light and electron microscopic immunocytochemistry of CA2–3 neurites specific to DLBD. Neurology **41:** 1402–1409.
5. DICKSON, D.W., M.L. SCHMIDT, V.M.-Y. LEE, M.-L. ZHAO, S.-H. YEN & J.Q. TROJANOWSKI. 1994. Immunoreactivity profile of hippocampal CA2/3 neurites in diffuse Lewy body disease. Acta Neuropathologica **87:** 269–276.
6. CHURCHYARD, A. & A.J. LEES. 1997. The relationship between dementia and direct involvement of the hippocampus and amygdala in Parkinson's disease. Neurology **49:** 1570–1576.
7. WAKABAYASHI, K., L.A. HANSEN & E. MASLIAH. 1995. Cortical Lewy body-containing neurons are pyramidal cells: laser confocal imaging of double-immunolabeled sections with anti-ubiquitin and SMI32. Acta Neuropathologica **89:** 404–408.
8. LIPPA, C.F., T.W. SMITH & J.M. SWEARER. 1994. Alzheimer's disease and Lewy body disease: a comparative clinicopathological study. Ann. Neurol. **35:** 81–88.

9. LIPPA, C.F., D. PULASKI-SALO, D.W. DICKSON & T.W. SMITH. 1997. Alzheimer's disease, Lewy body disease and aging: a comparative study of the perforant pathway. J. Neurol. Sci. **147:** 161–166.
10. SAMUEL, W., M. ALFORD, C.R. HOFSTETTER & L. HANSEN. 1997. Dementia with Lewy bodies versus pure Alzheimer disease: differences in cognition, neuropathology, cholinergic dysfunction, and synapse density. J. Neuropathol. Exp. Neurol. **56:** 499–508.
11. HANSEN, L.A., S.E. DANIEL, G.K. WILCOCK & S. LOWE. 1998. Frontal cortical synaptophysin in Lewy body diseases: relation to Alzheimer's disease and dementia. J. Neurol. Neurosurg. Psychiatry **64:** 653–656.
12. INCE, P., D. IRVING, F. MACARTHUR & R.H. PERRY. 1991. Quantitative neuropathological study of Alzheimer-type pathology in the hippocampus: comparison of senile dementia of Alzheimer type, senile dementia of Lewy body type, Parkinson's disease and non-demented elderly control patients. J. Neurol. Sci. **106:** 142–152.
13. HANSEN, L.A. 1996. Tautological tangles in neuropathological criteria for dementias associated with Lewy bodies. *In* Dementia with Lewy bodies. Clinical, pathological and treatment issues. R. Perry, I. McKeith & E. Perry, Eds.: 204–211. Cambridge University Press. Cambridge, UK.
14. GOMEZ-TORTOSA, E., A.O. INGRAHAM, M.C. IRIZARRY & B.T. HYMAN. 1998. Dementia with Lewy bodies. J. Am. Geriatr. Soc. **46:** 1449–1458.
15. PERRY, R.H., D. IRVING, G. BLESSED, A. FAIRBAIRN & E.K. PERRY. 1990. Senile dementia of Lewy body type. A clinically and neuropathologically distinct form of Lewy body dementia in the elderly. J. Neurol. Sci. **95:** 119–139.
16. ARMSTRONG, R.A., N.J. CAIRNS & P.L. LANTOS. 1997. beta-Amyloid (A-beta) deposition in the medial temporal lobe of patients with dementia with Lewy bodies. Neurosci. Lett. **227:** 193–196.
17. LENNOX, G., J. LOWE, M. LANDON, E.J. BYRNE, R.J. MAYER & R.B. GODWIN-AUSTEN. 1989. Diffuse Lewy body disease: correlative neuropathology using anti-ubiquitin immunocytochemistry. J. Neurol. Neurosurg. & Psychiatry **52:** 1236–1247.
18. SAMUEL, W., D. GALASKO, E. MASLIAH & L.A. HANSEN. 1996. Neocortical Lewy body counts correlate with dementia in the Lewy body variant of Alzheimer's disease. J. Neuropathol. Exp. Neurol. **55:** 44–52.
19. MATTILA, P.M., M. ROYTTA, H. TORIKKA, D.W. DICKSON & J.O. RINNE. 1998. Cortical Lewy bodies and Alzheimer-type changes in patients with Parkinson's disease. Acta Neuropathologica **95:** 576–582.

The α-Synucleinopathies: Parkinson's Disease, Dementia with Lewy Bodies, and Multiple System Atrophy

MARIA GRAZIA SPILLANTINI[a,c] AND MICHEL GOEDERT[b]

[a]Department of Neurology and Brain Repair Centre, University of Cambridge, Cambridge, UK

[b]Medical Research Council Laboratory of Molecular Biology, Cambridge, UK

ABSTRACT: Parkinson's disease is the second most common neurodegenerative disease, after Alzheimer's disease. Neuropathologically, it is characterized by the degeneration of populations of nerve cells that develop filamentous inclusions in the form of Lewy bodies and Lewy neurites. Recent work has shown that the filamentous inclusions of Parkinson's disease are made of the protein α-synuclein and that rare, familial forms of Parkinson's disease are caused by missense mutations in the α-synuclein gene. Besides Parkinson's disease, the filamentous inclusions of two additional neurodegenerative diseases, namely, dementia with Lewy bodies and multiple system atrophy, have also been found to be made of α-synuclein. Recombinant α-synuclein has been shown to assemble into filaments with similar morphologies to those found in the human diseases and with a cross-β fiber diffraction pattern. The new work has established the α-synucleinopathies as a major class of neurodegenerative disease.

Parkinson's disease (PD) is the most common neurodegenerative movement disorder.[1] Neuropathologically, it is defined by nerve cell loss in the substantia nigra and the presence of Lewy bodies and Lewy neurites.[2,3] In many cases, Lewy bodies are also found in the dorsal motor nucleus of the vagus, the nucleus basalis of Meynert, the locus coeruleus, the raphe nuclei, the midbrain Edinger-Westphal nucleus, the cerebral cortex, the olfactory bulb, and some autonomic ganglia.[4]

Besides the substantia nigra, nerve cell loss is also found in the dorsal motor nucleus of the vagus, the locus coeruleus, and the nucleus basalis of Meynert. Ultrastructurally, Lewy bodies and Lewy neurites consist of abnormal filamentous material.[5] Lewy bodies and Lewy neurites also constitute the defining neuropathological characteristics of dementia with Lewy bodies (DLB), a common late-life dementia that exists in a pure form or overlaps with the neuropathological characteristics of Alzheimer's disease (AD).[6-9]

[c]Address for correspondence: M.G. Spillantini, Department of Neurology and Brain Repair Centre, University of Cambridge, Cambridge, UK. Tel.: 44-1223-331145; fax: 44-1223-331174.
  e-mail: mgs11@cam.ac.uk

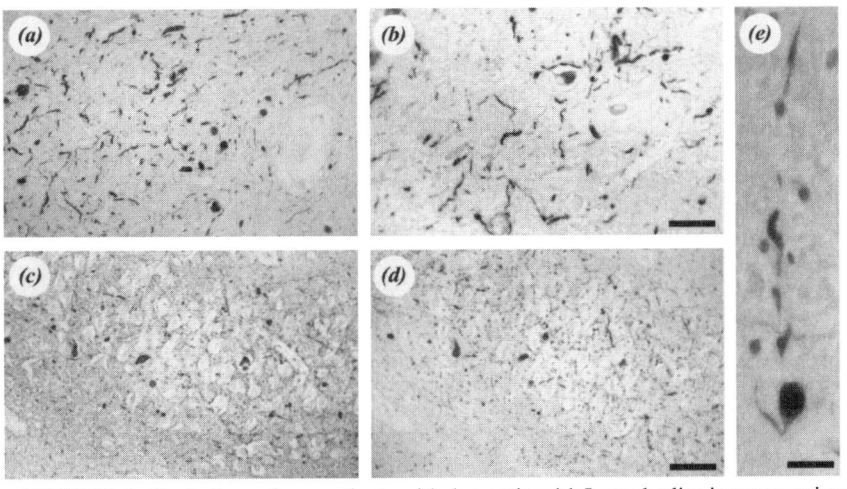

FIGURE 1. Brain tissue from patients with dementia with Lewy bodies immunostained for α-synuclein. (**a,b**) α-Synuclein-positive Lewy bodies and Lewy neurites in substantia nigra stained with antibodies recognizing the amino-terminal (**a**) or the carboxy-terminal (**b**) region of α-synuclein. Scale bar in **b**, 100 μm (for **a** and **b**). (**c,d**) α-Synuclein-positive Lewy neurites in serial sections of hippocampus stained with antibodies recognizing the amino-terminal (**c**) or the carboxy-terminal (**d**) region of α-synuclein. Scale bar in **d**, 80 μm (for **c** and **d**). (**e**) α-Synuclein-positive intraneuritic Lewy body in a Lewy neurite in substantia nigra stained with an antibody recognizing the carboxy-terminal region of α-synuclein. Scale bar, 40 μm.

Unlike PD, DLB is characterized by large numbers of Lewy bodies in cortical brain areas, such as the entorhinal and cingulate cortices. However, Lewy bodies and Lewy neurites are also present in substantia nigra in DLB, whereas hippocampal Lewy neurites are found in a proportion of individuals with PD with a severe cognitive impairment. Disorders with Lewy bodies and Lewy neurites thus present as a clinical and neuropathological spectrum. Classical PD with minor cognitive impairment and minimal cortical pathology is at one end of the spectrum, whereas severe dementia, with or without antecedent parkinsonism, but with a severe Lewy body and Lewy neurite pathology, is at the other end of the spectrum. Despite the fact that the Lewy body was first described in 1912, its biochemical composition remained unknown until the middle of 1997.

The discovery of a point mutation in the α-synuclein gene as a rare cause of familial PD has led us to the finding that α-synuclein is the major component of Lewy bodies and Lewy neurites in idiopathic PD and DLB (FIG. 1).[10–12] The Lewy body pathology that is sometimes associated with other neurodegenerative diseases, such as sporadic and familial Alzheimer's disease, Down's syndrome, and neurodegeneration with brain iron accumulation type 1 (Hallervorden-Spatz syndrome), has also been shown to be α-synuclein-positive.[12–18] Moreover, the filamentous glial and neuronal inclusions of multiple system atrophy (MSA) have been found to be made of α-synuclein (FIG. 2).[16,19–22] Taken together, this work has shown that PD, DLB, and MSA are α-synucleinopathies.

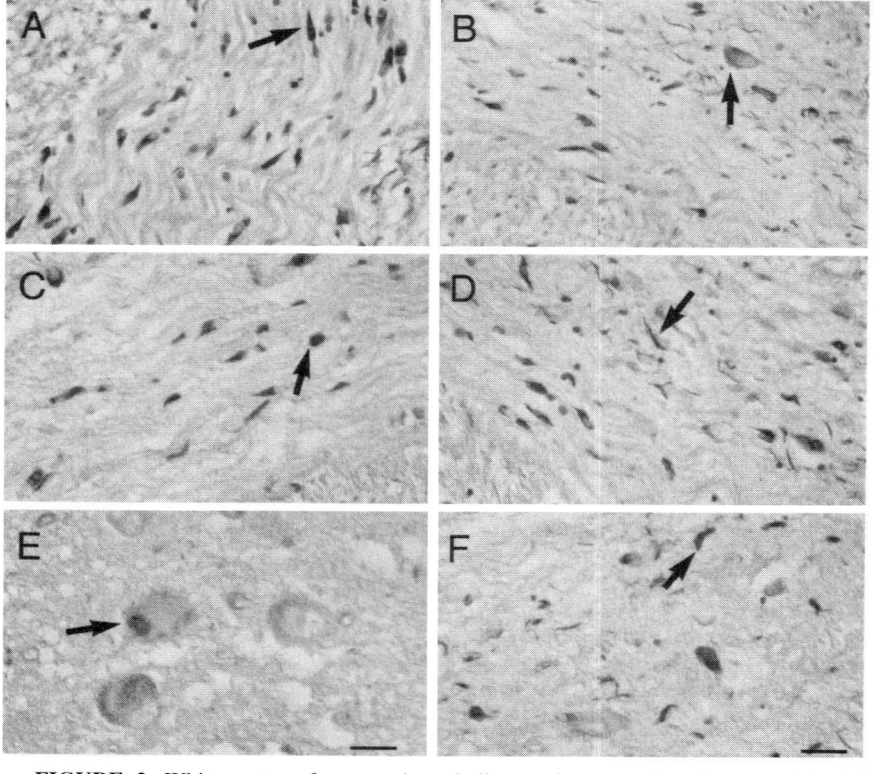

FIGURE 2. White matter of pons and cerebellum and grey matter of pons and frontal cortex from patients with multiple system atrophy immunostained for α-synuclein. (**A–D**) α-Synuclein-immunoreactive oligodendrocytes and nerve cells in white matter of pons (**A,B,D**) and cerebellum (**C**) identified with antibodies recognizing the amino-terminal (**A,C**) or the carboxy-terminal (**B,D**) region of α-synuclein (**E,F**). α-Synuclein-immunoreactive oligodendrocytes and nerve cells in grey matter of pons (**E**) and frontal cortex (**F**) identified with antibodies recognizing the amino-terminal (**E**) or the carboxy-terminal (**F**) region of α-synuclein. Arrows identify representative examples of each of the characteristic lesions stained for α-synuclein: cytoplasmic oligodendroglial inclusions (in **A** and **F**), cytoplasmic nerve cell inclusion (in **B**), nuclear oligodendroglial inclusion (in **C**), neuropil threads (in **D**), nuclear nerve cell inclusion (in **E**). Scale bars, 33 μm in **E**; 50 μm in **F** (for **A–D,F**).

THE SYNUCLEIN FAMILY

The first synuclein nucleotide and amino acid sequences were reported in 1988 by Maroteaux *et al.* from the electric organ of the Pacific electric ray (*Torpedo californica*).[23] The protein was named synuclein because of its apparent localization in presynaptic nerve terminals and portions of the nuclear envelope. All subsequent studies have shown the presence of synucleins in nerve terminals, but have failed to confirm a nuclear localization. Nonetheless, for historical reasons, the original name has survived.

In 1991, Maroteaux *et al.* reported cDNA sequences from rat brain that were homologous to the synuclein sequence from *T. californica*.[24] In 1992, Tobe *et al.* reported the amino acid sequence of an abundant protein from rat brain that they called phosphoneuroprotein-14.[25] In 1993, Uéda *et al.* reported the amino acid sequence of a protein from human brain that they named non-amyloid-β component precursor (NACP), because of the apparent localization of a portion of this protein in some amyloid plaques from Alzheimer's disease brain.[26] However, more recent studies using new antibodies have been unable to reproduce the original finding which may have resulted from antibody cross-reactivity with the β-amyloid protein Ab.[27,28] In 1994, Jakes *et al.* reported the amino acid sequences of two homologous proteins from human brain that were identified because they reacted with an antibody raised against paired helical filament preparations from Alzheimer's disease brain.[29] The first protein was identical to NACP, whereas the second protein was the human homologue of rat phosphoneuroprotein-14. We noticed that both proteins were similar to each other and to synuclein from *T. californica* and consequently named them α-synuclein and β-synuclein, respectively. Human α-synuclein is 140 amino acids in length, whereas β-synuclein is 134 amino acids long. In 1995, George *et al.* reported the amino acid sequence of a protein from zebra finch brain that they called synelfin.[30] Synelfin is the zebra finch homologue of α-synuclein.

Human α- and β-synucleins are 62% identical in amino acid sequence and share a similar domain organization. The amino-terminal half of each protein is taken up by imperfect amino acid repeats, with the consensus sequence KTKEGV. Individual repeats are separated by an inter-repeat region of 5–8 amino acids. Depending on the alignment, α-synuclein has 5–7 repeats, whereas β-synuclein has five repeats. The repeats are followed by a hydrophobic middle region and a negatively charged carboxy-terminal region, although both proteins have an identical carboxy-terminus. The human α-synuclein gene maps to chromosome 4q21, whereas the β-synuclein gene maps to chromosome 5q35.[31–35] Their genes are composed of five coding exons of similar sizes, with the overall organization of these genes being well conserved. Alternative mRNA splicing has been observed for exons 4 and 6 of the human α-synuclein gene.[36] Similarly, the rat cDNAs SYN1, SYN2, and SYN3 appear to be splice variants of the same synuclein gene.[24] However, at the protein level, there is no evidence to suggest the existence of multiple α-synuclein isoforms. So far, no splice variants have been described for β-synuclein. The α- and β-synuclein sequences from several vertebrate species are very similar. No synuclein homologues have been identified in *Saccharomyces cerevisiae* and *Caenorhabditis elegans*, suggesting that the presence of synucleins may be limited to vertebrates.

By Northern blotting, α-synuclein and β-synuclein mRNAs are expressed at highest levels in the nervous system, with lower transcript levels in other tissues.[26,29] By immunohistochemistry, both proteins are concentrated in nerve terminals, with little staining of nerve cell bodies and dendrites. Ultrastructurally, they are found in nerve terminals, in close proximity to synaptic vesicles.[24–29] The physiological functions of α-synuclein and β-synuclein are unknown. Both are abundant brain proteins, and it has been estimated that they make up 0.1–0.2% of total brain protein. Biophysical studies have shown that α-synuclein is monomeric, has little secondary structure, and is natively unfolded, in keeping with its heat-stability.[37] As a result, α-synuclein and β-synuclein have an apparent molecular mass of 19 kDa on SDS-PAGE, with α-synuclein running slightly faster than β-synuclein. It appears likely that α-synuclein is normally bound to cellular constituents through its repeats and that it becomes structured as a result. Experimental studies have shown that α-synuclein can bind to lipid membranes through its amino-terminal repeats, suggesting that it may be a lipid-binding protein.[38,39] Both synucleins have been shown to selectively inhibit phospholipase D2.[40] This isoform of phospholipase D localizes to the plasma membrane, where it may play a role in signal-induced cytoskeletal regulation and endocytosis.[41] It is therefore possible that α- and β-synuclein regulate vesicular transport processes. Little is known about post-translational modifications of synucleins in brain. In transfected cells, α-synuclein becomes constitutively phosphorylated at serine residues 87 and 129.[42]

In 1997, Ji *et al.* reported the amino acid sequence of a 127 amino acid protein that they named breast cancer-specific gene-1 (BCSG1) protein, because of its presence in large amounts in human breast cancer tissue.[43] BCSG1 shares 55% sequence identity with human α-synuclein and has therefore been renamed γ-synuclein.[44] It was independently discovered by Buchman *et al.* who named it persyn.[45] The synuclein that was originally identified in *T. californica*[23] was probably a γ-synuclein homologue. γ-Synuclein has the same general domain organization as α-synuclein and β-synuclein and is also encoded by five exons.[46,47] The human γ-synuclein gene maps to chromosome 10q23. By Northern blotting, γ-synuclein mRNA is expressed at highest levels in the nervous system and the heart, with lower transcript levels in other tissues. By immunohistochemistry, it appears to be present throughout nerve cells, unlike α-synuclein and β-synuclein which are concentrated in presynaptic nerve terminals. γ-Synuclein is heat-stable and runs with an apparent molecular mass of 18 kDa on SDS-PAGE, ahead of both α- and β-synuclein. In 1999, Surguchov *et al.* reported the sequence of a 127 amino acid protein that they named synoretin because of its expression in the retina.[48] At the amino acid level, synoretin is 87% identical to γ-synuclein. By Northern blotting, it shows the same tissue distribution as γ-synuclein mRNA. A curious feature of the synoretin sequence is that its 5′ untranslated region is identical to that of γ-synuclein. Future experiments will tell whether synoretin is a *bona fide* synuclein.

α-SYNUCLEIN IN PARKINSON'S DISEASE AND DEMENTIA WITH LEWY BODIES

In 1912, Friederich Lewy described serpentine or elongated intracytoplasmic bodies in the dorsal motor nucleus of the vagus nerve and in the substantia innominata from patients with PD.[2] Trétiakoff first described the presence of "corps de Lewy" in the substantia nigra in 1919 and proposed that they constitute a form of nigral pathology that is specific to PD.[3]

The light microscopic appearance of the Lewy body is characteristic. Classical brainstem Lewy bodies appear as intracytoplasmic circular inclusions, 5–25 μm in diameter, with a dense eosinophilic core and a clearer surrounding halo.[4] Lewy bodies can extend into nerve cell processes or lie free in the neuropil (extracellular Lewy bodies). The ultrastructure of the brainstem Lewy body is also characteristic in that it is composed of a dense core of filamentous and granular material that is surrounded by radially orientated filaments of 10–20 nm in diameter.[5] The term cortical Lewy body refers to the less well-defined spherical inclusion seen in cortical areas.[6,7] It lacks a distinctive core and halo, but is made of filaments with similar morphologies to those from brainstem Lewy bodies. The Lewy neurites constitute an important part of the pathology of PD and DLB. They correspond to abnormal neurites that have the same immunohistochemical staining profile as Lewy bodies and contain abnormal filaments similar to those found in Lewy bodies.

The Lewy body constitutes the second most common nerve cell pathology, after the neurofibrillary lesions of AD. Until recently, our understanding of the biochemical composition of the Lewy body filaments was at the same stage as was our understanding of the composition of the paired helical filaments of AD some 15 years ago. Immunohistochemical studies had shown that Lewy bodies stain to various extents with ubiquitin and neurofilament antibodies. Moreover, antibodies against some 30 different proteins had been reported to stain the halo of brainstem Lewy bodies. However, purification of Lewy body filaments to homogeneity had not been achieved. In PD and DLB the density of Lewy bodies and Lewy neurites is much lower than that of neurofibrillary lesions in AD. This renders purification and chemical analysis of the insoluble filaments a daunting task.

Most cases of PD are idiopathic, without an obvious family history. However, a small percentage of cases is familial and inherited in an autosomal-dominant manner. In 1995, Polymeropoulos *et al.* established genetic linkage of levodopa-responsive parkinsonism with autopsy-confirmed Lewy bodies in a large Italian-American kindred (the Contursi family) to chromosome 4q21-23.[49,50] This was followed in 1997 by the discovery of a point mutation in the α-synuclein gene in this family and in three Greek families that share a common founder with the Contursi family.[10,51] The mutation lies in exon 4 and consists of a G to A transition at position 157 of the coding region of α-synuclein, which changes alanine residue 53 to threonine (A53T); it lies in the linker region between repeats 4 and 5 of α-synuclein. β-Synuclein also carries an alanine at this position, whereas γ-synuclein has a threonine at the equivalent position. To date, there is no evidence suggesting an involvement of β-synuclein or γ-synuclein in the etiology of familial PD.[52–54]

Somewhat surprisingly, rodent and zebra finch α-synucleins carry a threonine residue at position 53, like the mutated human protein.[24,30] This, together with the common founder effect of the A53T mutation,[51] led some to propose that the A53T change may be nothing more than a rare, benign polymorphism. However, the discovery of a second mutation in the α-synuclein gene in a family with PD of German descent has settled this controversy in favor of the relevance of α-synuclein for the etiology and pathogenesis of at least some familial cases of PD.[55] The second mutation lies in exon 3 and consists of a G to C transversion at position 88 of the coding region of α-synuclein, which changes alanine residue 30 to proline (A30P); it lies in the linker region between repeats 2 and 3 of α-synuclein. Unlike residue 53 which, depending on the species, is alanine or threonine, residue 30 of α-synuclein is an alanine in all species examined. β-Synuclein and γ-synuclein also have alanine at this position.

Although the A53T mutation in α-synuclein accounts for only a small percentage of familial cases of PD, its identification was quickly followed by the discovery that α-synuclein is the major component of Lewy bodies and Lewy neurites in all cases of PD and DLB (FIG. 1).[11] Full-length, or close to full-length, α-synuclein has been found in Lewy bodies and Lewy neurites, with both the core and the corona of the Lewy body being stained. Staining for α-synuclein has been found to be more extensive than staining for ubiquitin, which was until then the most sensitive marker for Lewy bodies and Lewy neurites.[12] In transfected cells, α-synuclein is degraded by the proteasome-ubiquitin pathway, with the A53T mutation conferring a longer half-life to the transfected protein.[56] The Lewy body pathology does not stain for β-synuclein or γ-synuclein.[11,12] Thus, of the three brain synucleins, only α-synuclein is of relevance in the context of PD and DLB. The original finding that α-synuclein is present in Lewy bodies and Lewy neurites[11] was rapidly confirmed and extended.[12–18,57–65]

This work suggested, but did not prove, that α-synuclein is the major component of the abnormal filaments that make up Lewy bodies and Lewy neurites. In DLB, the pathological changes are particularly numerous in cingulate cortex, facilitating the extraction of filaments. Isolated filaments were strongly labeled along their entire lengths, demonstrating that they contain α-synuclein as a major component.[12] Filament morphologies and staining characteristics with several antibodies have led to the suggestion that α-synuclein molecules might run parallel to the filament axis and that the filaments are polar structures. Moreover, under the electron microscope, some filaments and granular material in partially purified Lewy bodies appeared to be labeled by α-synuclein antibodies.[59] Immunoelectron microscopy has shown decoration of Lewy body filaments in tissue sections from brain of individuals with PD and DLB.[66,67]

α-SYNUCLEIN IN MULTIPLE SYSTEM ATROPHY

MSA is largely a sporadic neurodegenerative disorder that comprises cases of olivopontocerebellar atrophy, striatonigral degeneration, and Shy-Drager syndrome.[68] Clinically, it is characterized by a combination of cerebellar, extrapyramidal, and autonomic symptoms. Neuropathologically, glial cytoplasmic inclusions (GCIs), which consist of filamentous aggregates, are the defining feature of MSA.[69] They are found mostly in the cytoplasm and, to a lesser extent, the nucleus of oligodendrocytes. Inclusions are also observed in the cytoplasm and nucleus of some nerve cells, as well as in neuropil threads. They consist of straight and twisted filaments, with reported diameters of 10–30 nm.[70] At the light microscopic level, GCIs are immunoreactive for ubiquitin and, to a lesser extent, for cytoskeletal proteins such as tau and tubulin. However, until recently, the biochemical composition of GCI filaments was unknown.

This has changed with the discovery that GCIs are strongly immunoreactive for α-synuclein (FIG. 2) and that filaments isolated from the brains of patients with MSA are labeled by α-synuclein antibodies.[16,19–22] Moreover, in tissue sections, GCI filaments are decorated by α-synuclein antibodies, as are filaments from partially purified GCIs.[65,71,72] The morphologies of isolated filaments and their staining characteristics were found to be very similar to those of filaments extracted from cingulate cortex of patients with DLB.[21] As for the latter, staining for α-synuclein was far more extensive than staining for ubiquitin, until then the most sensitive immunohistochemical marker of GCIs.[21] The number of α-synuclein filaments extracted from MSA brain is higher than that extracted from DLB brain, in keeping with the larger number of inclusions in MSA.[73] To date, there is no genetic evidence implicating α-synuclein in MSA.[74] Taken together, this work has demonstrated that α-synuclein is the major component of the GCI filaments and has revealed an unexpected molecular link between MSA and the Lewy body disorders PD and DLB.

SYNTHETIC α-SYNUCLEIN FILAMENTS

The discovery of α-synuclein filaments in Lewy body diseases and MSA has led to attempts aimed at producing synthetic α-synuclein filaments under physiological conditions. A first study reported that removal of the carboxy-terminal 20–30 residues of α-synuclein leads to spontaneous assembly into filaments within 24–48 h at 37°C, with morphologies and staining characteristics indistinguishable from those of Lewy body filaments.[75] This indicates that the packing of α-synuclein molecules in the filaments *in vitro* is very similar to that of filaments extracted from brain. A proportion of α-synuclein extracted from partially purified Lewy bodies and GCI filaments has been found to be truncated.[59,72] Two subsequent studies reported filament assembly from full-length α-synuclein after incubations ranging from one week to three months at 37°C.[76,77] The A53T mutation was shown to increase the rate of filament assembly.[77] However, based on the evidence presented, one could not exclude the possibility that the recombinant α-synuclein became truncated during the long incubation times.

More recently, improved methods requiring only 1–2 day incubations have shown unambigously that full-length α-synuclein assembles into filaments.[78–81] The synthetic filaments were decorated by an antibody that recognizes the carboxy-terminal 10 amino acids of α-synuclein, as were filaments extracted from DLB and MSA brains.[81] These experiments have also shown that the A53T mutation and carboxy-terminal truncation, as in α-synuclein(1–87) and α-synuclein(1–120), produce markedly increased rates of filament assembly. α-Synuclein thus assembles through its repeat-containing amino-terminal half. Earlier work had shown that a synthetic peptide comprising amino acids 61–95 of human α-synuclein readily assembles into filaments.[82] Interestingly, residues 66–73 of α-synuclein (VGGAVVTG) resemble residues 36–42 of amyloid Aβ (VGGVVIAT) and residues 117–124 of the prion protein (AAGAVVGG).

Depending on the study, the effect of the A30P mutation on the rate of filament assembly was either small[79] or absent.[81] Increased fibrillogenesis of mutant α-synuclein may therefore not be a feature shared by the two familial PD mutations. Unlike recombinant α-synuclein with the A53T mutation, α-synuclein with the A30P mutation has been shown to be devoid of significant vesicle-binding activity, suggesting that this may be its primary effect.[39] Rodent and zebra finch α-synuclein readily assembled into filaments, consistent with the presence of a threonine residue at position 53.[81] Based on X-ray and electron fiber diffraction patterns and circular dichroism spectroscopy, the various synthetic α-synuclein filaments showed a cross-β conformation characteristic of amyloid.[81] Under identical conditions, β-synuclein and γ-synuclein failed to assemble into filaments, in keeping with the finding that antibodies directed against β-synuclein and γ-synuclein do not stain the filamentous inclusions of PD, DLB, and MSA.[11,12]

REFERENCES

1. PARKINSON, J. 1817. An Essay on the Shaking Palsy. Sherwood, Neely, and Jones. London.
2. LEWY, F.H. 1912. Paralysis agitans. I. Pathologische Anatomie. In Handbuch der Neurologie, vol. 3. M. Lewandowsky & G. Abelsdorff, Eds.: 920–933. Springer. Berlin.
3. TRETIAKOFF, M.C. 1919. M.D. thesis, University of Paris. Paris.
4. FORNO, L.S. 1996. Neuropathology of Parkinson's disease. J. Neuropathol. Exp. Neurol. **55:** 259–272.
5. DUFFY, P.E. & V.M. TENNYSON. 1965. Phase and electron microscopic observations on Lewy bodies and melanin granules in the substantia nigra and locus coeruleus in Parkinson's disease. J. Neuropathol. Exp. Neurol. **24:** 398–414.
6. OKAZAKI, H., L.E. LIPKIN & S.M. ARONSON. 1961. Diffuse intracytoplasmic ganglionic inclusions (Lewy type) associated with progressive dementia and quadriparesis in flexion. J. Neuropathol. Exp. Neurol. **21:** 442–449.
7. KOSAKA, K. 1978. Lewy bodies in cerebral cortex. Report of three cases. Acta Neuropathol. **42:** 127–134.
8. HANSEN, L.A., D. SALMON, D. GALASKO, et al. 1990. The Lewy body variant of Alzheimer's disease: a clinical and pathological entity. Neurology **40:** 1–8.
9. PERRY, R.H., D. IRVING, G. BLESSED, A. FAIRBAIRN & E.K. PERRY. 1990. Senile dementia of the Lewy body type. A clinically and neuropathologically distinct form of Lewy body dementia in the elderly. J. Neurol. Sci. **85:** 119–139.
10. POLYMEROPOULOS, M.H., C. LAVEDAN, E. LEROY, et al. 1997. Mutation in the α-synuclein gene identified in families with Parkinson's disease. Science **276:** 2045–2047.
11. SPILLANTINI, M.G., M.L. SCHMIDT, V.M. LEE, J.Q. TROJANOWSKI, R. JAKES & M. GOEDERT. 1997. α-Synuclein in Lewy bodies. Nature **388:** 839–840.
12. SPILLANTINI, M.G., R.A. CROWTHER, R. JAKES, M. HASEGAWA & M. GOEDERT. 1998. α-Synuclein in filamentous inclusions of Lewy bodies from Parkinson's disease and dementia with Lewy bodies. Proc. Natl. Acad. Sci. USA **95:** 6469–6473.
13. LIPPA, C.F., H. JUJIWARA, D.M. MANN, et al. 1998. Lewy bodies contain altered α-synuclein in brains of many familial Alzheimer's disease patients with mutations in presenilin and amyloid precursor protein genes. Am. J. Pathol. **153:** 1365–1370.
14. LIPPA, C.F., M.L. SCHMIDT, V.M.-Y. LEE & J.Q. TROJANOWSKI. 1999. Antibodies to α-synuclein detect Lewy bodies in many Down's syndrome brains with Alzheimer's disease. Ann. Neurol. **45:** 353–357.
15. SPILLANTINI, M.G., M. TOLNAY, S. LOVE & M. GOEDERT. 1999. Microtubule-associated protein tau, heparan sulphate and α-synuclein in several neurodegenerative diseases with dementia. Acta Neuropathol. **97:** 585–594.
16. TU, P.-H., J.E. GALVIN, M. BABA, et al. 1998. Glial cytoplasmic inclusions in white matter oligodendrocytes of multiple system atrophy brains contain insoluble α-synuclein. Ann. Neurol. **44:** 415–422.
17. ARAWAKA, S., Y. SAITO, S. MURAYAMA & H. MORI. 1998. Lewy body in neurodegeneration with brain iron accumulation type 1 is immunoreactive for α-synuclein. Neurology **51:** 887–889.
18. WAKABAYASHI, K., M. YOSHIMOTO, T. FUKUSHIMA, et al. 1999. Widespread occurrence of α-synuclein/NACP-immunoreactive neuronal inclusions in juvenile and adult-onset Hallervorden-Spatz disease with Lewy bodies. Neuropathol. Appl. Neurobiol. **25:** 363–368.
19. WAKABAYASHI, K., M. YOSHIMOTO, S. TSUJI & H. TAKAHASHI. 1998. α-Synuclein immunoreactivity in glial cytoplasmic inclusions in multiple system atrophy. Neurosci. Lett. **249:** 180–182.
20. MEZEY, E., A. DEHEJIA, G. HARTA, et al. 1998. Alpha synuclein in neurodegenerative disorders: murderer or accomplice? Nature Med. **4:** 755–757.
21. SPILLANTINI, M.G., R.A. CROWTHER, R. JAKES, N.J. CAIRNS, P.L. LANTOS & M. GOEDERT. 1998. Filamentous α-synuclein inclusions link multiple system atrophy with Parkinson's disease and dementia with Lewy bodies. Neurosci. Lett. **251:** 205–208.
22. GAI, W.P., J.H.T. POWER, P.C. BLUMBERGS & W.W. BLESSING. 1998. Multiple system atrophy: a new α-synuclein disease? Lancet **352:** 547–548.

23. MAROTEAUX, L., J.T. CAMPANELLI & R.H. SCHELLER. 1988. Synuclein: a neuron-specific protein localized to the nucleus and presynaptic nerve terminal. J. Neurosci. **8:** 2804–2815.
24. MAROTEAUX, L. & R.H. SCHELLER. 1991. The rat brain synucleins; family of proteins transiently associated with neuronal membrane. Mol. Brain Res. **11:** 335–343.
25. TOBE, T., S. NAKAJO, A. TANAKA, *et al.* 1992 Cloning and characterization of the cDNA encoding a novel specific 14-kDa protein. J. Neurochem. **59:** 1624–1629.
26. UEDA, K., H. FUKUSHIMA, E. MASLIAH, *et al.* 1993. Molecular cloning of cDNA encoding an unrecognized component of amyloid in Alzheimer disease. Proc. Natl. Acad. Sci. USA **90:** 11282–11286.
27. BAYER, T.A. P. JAKALA, T. HARTMANN, *et al.* 1999. α-Synuclein accumulates in Lewy bodies in Parkinson's disease and dementia with Lewy bodies but not in Alzheimer's disease β-amyloid cores. Neurosci. Lett. **266:** 213–216.
28. CULVENOR, J.G., C.A. MCLEAN, S. CUTT, *et al.* 1999. Non-Aβ component of Alzheimer's disease amyloid (NAC) revisited. NAC and α-synuclein are not associated with Aβ amyloid. Am. J. Pathol. **155:** 1173–1181.
29. JAKES, R., M.G. SPILLANTINI & M. GOEDERT. 1994. Identification of two distinct synucleins from human brain. FEBS Lett. **345:** 27–32.
30. GEORGE, J.M., H. JIN, W.S. WOODS & D.F. CLAYTON. 1995. Characterization of a novel protein regulated during the critical period for song learning in the zebra finch. Neuron **15:** 361–372.
31. CAMPION, D., C. MARTIN, R. HEILIG, *et al.* 1995. The NACP/α-synuclein gene: chromosomal assignment and screening for alterations in Alzheimer disease. Genomics **26:** 254–257.
32. CHEN, X., H.A. DE SILVA, M.J. PETTENATI, *et al.* 1995. The human NACP/α-synuclein gene: chromosome assignment to 4q21.3-q22 and *TaqI* RFLP analysis. Genomics **26:** 425–427.
33. SPILLANTINI, M.G., A. DIVANE & M. GOEDERT. 1995. Assignment of human α-synuclein (SNCA) and β-synuclein (SNCB) genes to chromosomes 4q21 and 5q35. Genomics **27:** 379–381.
34. SHIBASAKI, Y., D.A.M. BAILLIE, D. ST. CLAIR & A.J. BROOKES. 1995. High-resolution mapping of SNCA encoding α-synuclein, the non-Aβ component of Alzheimer's disease precursor, to human chromosome 4q21.3-q22 by fluorescence *in situ* hybridization. Cytogenet. Cell. Genet. **71:** 54–55.
35. LAVEDAN, C., E. LEROY, R. TORRES, *et al.* 1998. Genomic organization and expression of the human β-synuclein gene (SNCB). Genomics **54:** 173–175.
36. UEDA, K., T. SAITOH & H. MORI. 1994. Tissue-dependent alternative splicing of mRNA for NACP, the precursor of non-Aβ component of Alzheimer's disease amyloid. Biochem. Biophys. Res. Commun. **205:** 1366–1372.
37. WEINREB, P.H., W. ZHEN, A.W. POON, K.A. CONWAY & P.T. LANSBURY. 1996. NACP, a protein implicated in Alzheimer's disease and learning, is natively unfolded. Biochemistry **35:** 13709–13715.
38. DAVIDSON, W.S., A. JONAS, D.F. CLAYTON & J.M. GEORGE. 1998. Stabilization of α-synuclein secondary structure upon binding to synthetic membranes. J. Biol. Chem. **273:** 9443–9449.
39. JENSEN, P.H., M.H. NIELSEN, R. JAKES, C.G. DOTTI & M. GOEDERT. 1998. Binding of α-synuclein to rat brain vesicles is abolished by familial Parkinson's disease mutation. J. Biol. Chem. **273:** 26292–26294.
40. JENCO, J.M., A. RAWLINGSON, B. DANIELS & A.J. MORRIS. 1998. Regulation of phospholipase D2: selective inhibition of mammalian phospholipase D isoenzymes by α- and β-synucleins. Biochemistry **37:** 4901–4909.
41. COLLEY, W.C., T.C. SUNG, R. ROLL, *et al.* 1997. Phospholipase D2, a distinct phospholipase D isoform with novel regulatory properties that provokes cytoskeletal reorganization. Curr. Biol. **7:** 191–201.
42. OKOCHI, M., J. WALTER, A. KOYAMA, *et al.* 2000 Constitutive phosphorylation of the Parkinson's disease-associated α-synuclein. J. Biol. Chem. **275:** 390–397.
43. JI, H., Y.E. LIU, T. JIA, *et al.* 1997. Identification of a breast cancer-specific gene, *BCSG1*, by direct differential cDNA sequencing. Cancer Res. **57:** 759–764.

44. GOEDERT, M., R. JAKES & M.G. SPILLANTINI. 1998. Alpha-synuclein and the Lewy body. NeuroSci. News **1**: 47–52.
45. BUCHMAN, V.L., H.J. HUNTER, L.G. PINON, *et al.* 1998. Persyn, a member of the synuclein family, has a distinct pattern of expression in the developing nervous system. J. Neurosci. **18**: 9335–9341.
46. LAVEDAN, C., E. LEROY, A. DEHEJIA, *et al.* 1998. Identification, localization and characterization of the human γ-synuclein gene. Hum. Genet. **103**: 106–112.
47. NINKINA, N.N., M.V. ALIMOVA-KOST, J.W. PATERSON, *et al.* 1998. Organization, expression and polymorphism of the human *persyn* gene. Hum. Mol. Genet. **7**: 1417–1424.
48. SURGUCHOV, A., I. SURGUCHEVA, E. SOLESSIO & W. BAEHR. 1999. Synoretin—a new protein belonging to the synuclein family. Mol. Cell. Neurosci. **13**: 95–103.
49. GOLBE, L.I., G. DI IORIO, V. BONAVITA, D.C. MILLER & R.C. DUVOISIN. 1990. A large kindred with autosomal dominant Parkinson's disease. Ann. Neurol. **27**: 276–282.
50. POLYMEROPOULOS, M.H., J.J. HIGGINS, L.I. GOLBE, *et al.* 1996. Mapping of a gene for Parkinson's disease to chromosome 4q21-q23. Science **274**: 1197–1199.
51. ATHANASSIADOU, A., G. VOUTSINAS, L. PSIOURI, *et al.* 1999. Genetic analysis of families with Parkinson disease that carry the Ala53thr mutation in the gene encoding α-synuclein. Am. J. Hum. Genet. **65**: 555–558.
52. LINCOLN, S., K. GWINN-HARDY, J. GOUDREAU, *et al.* 1999. No pathogenic mutations in the persyn gene in Parkinson's disease. Neurosci. Lett. **259**: 65–66.
53. LINCOLN, S., R. CROOK, J.C. CHARTIER-HARLIN, *et al.* 1999. No pathogenic mutations in the β-synuclein gene in Parkinson's disease. Neurosci. Lett. **269**: 107–109.
54. FLOWERS, J.M., P.N. LEIGH, A.M. DAVIES, *et al.* 1999. Mutations in the gene encoding human persyn are not associated with amyotrophic lateral sclerosis or familial Parkinson's disease. Neurosci. Lett. **274**: 21–24.
55. KRÜGER, R., W. KUHN, T. MÜLLER, *et al.* 1998. Ala30Pro mutation in the gene encoding α-synuclein in Parkinson's disease. Nature Genet. **18**: 106–108.
56. BENNETT, M.C., J.F. BISHOP, Y. LENG, *et al.* 1999. Degradation of α-synuclein by proteasome. J. Biol. Chem. **274**: 33855–33858.
57. WAKABAYASHI, K., K. MATSUMOTO, K. TAKAYAMA, M. YOSHIMOTO & H. TAKAHASHI. 1997. NACP, a presynaptic protein, immunoreactivity in Lewy bodies in Parkinson's disease. Neurosci. Lett. **239**: 45–48.
58. TAKEDA, A., M. MALLORY, M. SUNDSMO, W. HONER, L. HANSEN & E. MASLIAH. 1998. Abnormal accumulation of NACP/α-synuclein in neurodegenerative disorders. Am. J. Pathol. **152**: 367–372.
59. BABA, M., S. NAKAJO, P.H. TU, *et al.* 1998. Aggregation of α-synuclein in Lewy bodies of sporadic Parkinson's disease and dementia with Lewy bodies. Am. J. Pathol. **152**: 879–884.
60. IRIZARRY, M.C., W. GROWDON, T. GOMEZ-ISLA, *et al.* 1998. Nigral and cortical Lewy bodies and dystrophic nigral neurites in Parkinson's disease and cortical Lewy body disease contain α-synuclein immunoreactivity. J. Neuropathol. Exp. Neurol. **57**: 334–337.
61. MEZEY, E., A.M. DEHEJIA, G. HARTA, *et al.* 1998. Alpha synuclein is present in Lewy bodies in sporadic Parkinson's disease. Mol. Psychiatr. **3**: 493–499.
62. ARAI, T., K. UEDA, K. IKEDA, *et al.* 1999. Argyrophilic glial inclusions in the midbrain of patients with Parkinson's disease and diffuse Lewy body disease are immunopositive for NACP/α-synuclein. Neurosci. Lett. **259**: 83–86.
63. BRAAK, H., D. SANDMANN-KEIL, W.P. GAI & E. BRAAK. 1999. Extensive axonal Lewy neurites in Parkinson's disease: a novel pathological feature revealed by α-synuclein immunocytochemistry. Neurosci. Lett. **265**: 67–69.
64. JAKES, R., R.A. CROWTHER, V.M. LEE, J.Q. TROJANOWSKI, T. IWATSUBO & M. GOEDERT. 1999. Epitope mapping of LB509, a monoclonal antibody directed against human α-synuclein. Neurosci. Lett. **269**: 13–16.
65. GIASSON, B.I., R. JAKES, M. GOEDERT, *et al.* 2000. A panel of epitope-specific antibodies detects protein domains distributed throughout human α-synuclein in Lewy bodies of Parkinson's disease. J. Neurosci. Res. **59**: 528–533.
66. WAKABAYASHI, K., S. HAYASHI, A. KAKITA, *et al.* 1998. Accumulation of α-synuclein/NACP is a cytopathological feature common to Lewy body disease and multiple system atrophy. Acta Neuropathol. **96**: 445–452.

67. ARIMA, K., K. UEDA, N. SUNOHARA, *et al.* 1998. Immunoelectron-microscopic demonstration of NACP/α-synuclein-epitopes on the filamentous component of Lewy bodies in Parkinson's disease and in dementia with Lewy bodies. Brain Res. **808:** 93–100.
68. GRAHAM, J.C. & D.R. OPPENHEIMER. 1969. Orthostatic hypotension and nicotine sensitivity in a case of multiple system atrophy. J. Neurol. Neurosurg. Psychiatry **32:** 28–34.
69. PAPP, M.I., J.E. KAHN & P.L. LANTOS. 1989. Glial cytoplasmic inclusions in the CNS of patients with multiple system atrophy. J. Neurol. Sci. **94:** 79–100.
70. KATO, S. & H. NAKAMURA. 1990. Cytoplasmic argyrophilic inclusions in neurons of pontine nuclei in patients with olivopontocerebellar atrophy: immunohistochemical and ultrastructural studies. Acta Neuropathol. **79:** 584–594.
71. ARIMA, K., K. UEDA, N. SUNOHARA, *et al.* 1998. NACP/α-synuclein immunoreactivity in fibrillary components of neuronal and oligodendroglial cytoplasmic inclusions in the pontine nuclei in multiple system atrophy. Acta Neuropathol. **96:** 439–444.
72. GAI, W.P., J.H.T. POWER, P.C. BLUMBERGS, J.G. CULVENOR & P.H. JENSEN. 1999. α-Synuclein immunoisolation of glial inclusions from multiple system atrophy brain reveals multiprotein components. J. Neurochem. **73:** 2093–2100.
73. DICKSON, D.W., W. LIU, J. HARDY, *et al.* 1999. Widespread alterations of α-synuclein in multiple system atrophy. Am. J. Pathol. **155:** 1241–1251.
74. OZAWA, T., H. TAKANO, O. ONODERA, *et al.* 1999. No mutation in the entire coding region of the α-synuclein gene in pathologically confirmed cases of multiple system atrophy. Neurosci. Lett. **270:** 110–112.
75. CROWTHER, R.A., R. JAKES, M.G. SPILLANTINI & M. GOEDERT. 1998. Synthetic filaments assembled from C-terminally truncated α-synuclein. FEBS Lett. **436:** 309–312.
76. EL-AGNAF, O.M.A., R. JAKES, M.D. CURRAN & A. WALLACE. 1998. Effects of the mutations Ala30 to Pro and Ala53 to Thr on the physical and morphological properties of α-synuclein protein implicated in Parkinson's disease. FEBS Lett. **440:** 67–70.
77. CONWAY, K.A., J.D. HARPER & P.T. LANSBURY. 1998. Accelerated *in vitro* fibril formation by a mutant α-synuclein linked to early-onset Parkinson disease. Nature Med. **4:** 1318–1320.
78. GIASSON, B.I., K. URYU, J.Q. TROJANOWSKI & V.M.-Y. LEE. 1999. Mutant and wild type human α-synucleins assemble into elongated filaments with distinct morphologies *in vitro*. J. Biol. Chem. **274:** 7619–7622.
79. NARHI, L., S.J. WOOD, S. STEAVENSON, *et al.* 1999. Both familial Parkinson's disease mutations accelerate α-synuclein aggregation. J. Biol. Chem. **274:** 9843–9846.
80. WOOD, S.J, J. WYPYCH, S. STEAVENSON, J.C. LOUIS, M. CITRON & A.L. BIERE. 1999. α-Synuclein fibrillogenesis is nucleation-dependent. J. Biol. Chem. **274:** 19509–19512.
81. SERPELL, L.C., J. BERRIMAN, R. JAKES, M. GOEDERT & R.A. CROWTHER. 2000. Fiber diffraction of synthetic α-synuclein filaments shows amyloid-like cross-β conformation. Proc. Natl. Acad. Sci. USA **97:** 4897–4902.
82. HAN, H., P.H. WEINREB & P.T. LANSBURY. 1995. The core of Alzheimer's peptide NAC forms amyloid fibrils which seed and are seeded by β-amyloid: Is NAC a common trigger or target in neurodegenerative disease? Chem. Biol. **2:** 163–169.

Genetics of Parkinson's Disease

MIHAEL H. POLYMEROPOULOS[a]

Novartis Pharmaceuticals, Gaithersburg, Maryland 20878, USA

ABSTRACT: Several genetic factors have been recently recognized as related to the etiology of Parkinson's disease. Mutations in the genes coding for α-synuclein and ubiquitin carboxy-terminal hydrolase have been identified in families with autosomal dominant Parkinson's disease. Mutations in the Parkin gene are responsible for autosomal recessive parkinsonism. These first pieces of the molecular puzzle of Parkinson's disease offer novel insights into the pathophysiology of the illness.

Parkinson's disease is the second most common neurodegenerative disease of man. The incidence of the disorder is estimated to be between 1:100–1:500 individuals.[1] First described by James Parkinson in his "Essay on Shaking Palsy," Parkinson's is a movement disorder with peak mean onset in the sixth decade of life, characterized by bradykinesia, resting tremor, and impaired postural reflexes as cardinal clinical features.[2] In the beginning of this century, Dr. Lewy observed characteristic alterations in the brains of patients with Parkinson's disease. He observed destruction of the substantia nigra accompanied by the presence of large eosinophilic inclusions and ballooning of neuronal processes, which are now referred to as Lewy bodies and Lewy neurites, respectively. It has come to be appreciated that this pathologic hallmark is also found in diffuse Lewy body dementia, a disorder with mixed movement disorder and dementia as clinical features.[3] Patients with Parkinson's disease show beneficial response to dopamine replacement therapy. The observation that the contaminant of illicit drugs, MPTP, can cause parkinsonism rapidly led investigators to the search of environmental agents that could be etiologically related to Parkinson's disease.[4,5]

Although many factors have been postulated for the development of the disease, besides age the most significant risk factor appears to be a positive family history for the disease. Only a few large pedigrees have been described in the literature with a distinct autosomal dominant mode of inheritance. This may reflect the low penetrance of the responsible gene or genes and/or the late onset of the disorder. In 1996 we applied genetic linkage strategies in a large Italian family with early onset Parkinson's disease.[6] This family was originally collected in the U.S., and the investigators were able to trace back the family in the small village of Contursi, in southern Italy.[6]

[a]Address for correspondence: Mihael H. Polymeropoulos, Novartis Pharmaceuticals Corporation, Pharmacogenetics Department, 9 West Watkins, Gaithersburg, MD 20878. Tel.: (301) 330-3101; fax: (301) 330-2108.
e-mail: mihael.polymeropoulos@pharma.novartis.com

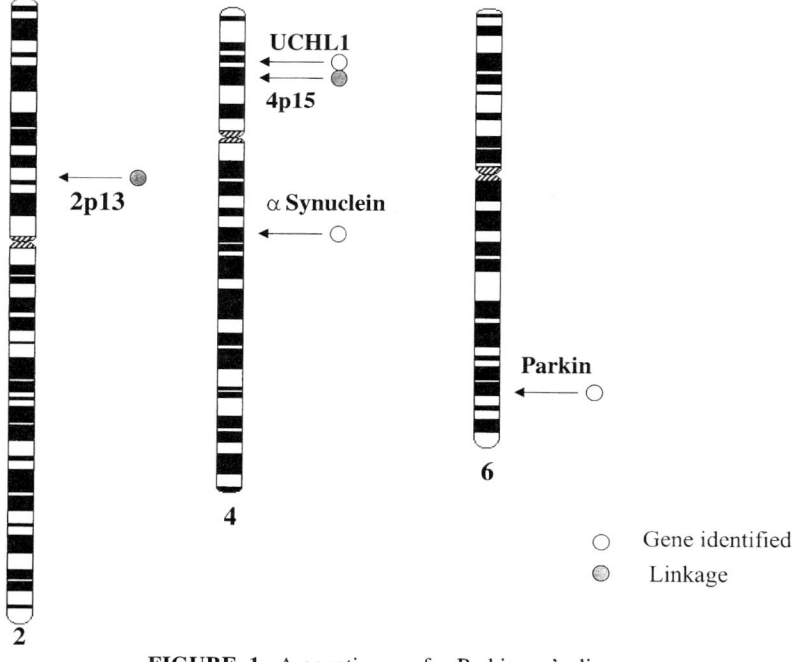

FIGURE 1. A genetic map for Parkinson's disease.

Parkinson's disease in this family appeared to be typical in symptoms, progression, pathology, and response to L-dopa. The characteristic difference, however, from sporadic cases of the disease appeared to be a rather early onset with average age of onset of 46 years, almost a whole decade younger than average age of onset.[6] Studying 11 affected individuals from the Contursi kindred with whole genome genetic linkage analysis, we located the susceptibility gene on the long arm of human chromosome 4q21-q23.[6] Positional cloning efforts identified a missense mutation in the α-synuclein gene at position 53, changing an Ala to Thr (FIG. 1).[7]

The same mutation was also found in two and subsequently six Parkinson's pedigrees from Greece.[7] The Greek families shared the early onset of the disease and a disease progression similar to the one seen in the Italian kindred.[7] Haplotype analysis of the Greek and Italian kindreds demonstrated that the affected individuals shared approximately 800 kb of sequence around the α-synuclein gene, suggesting that they had inherited a common ancestral allele.[7] The geographical proximity of the two countries makes the common ancestral theory plausible especially because in the 9th century B.C. southern Italy was colonized by the ancient Greeks.

It soon became obvious that mutations in the α-synuclein gene—very much as is the case for the presenilin mutations in Alzheimer's disease—represent only a small fraction of familial Parkinson's disease. In 1998, a new mutation was reported in the α-synuclein gene, an Ala to Pro change at position 30.[8] This mutation appeared to have a lower degree of penetrance and a later onset of disease compared to the Ala53Thr change.[8]

Despite the rarity with which it is mutated in Parkinson's disease, α-synuclein took center stage with the discovery that it is a key player in the pathology of the disorder. Immunoreactivity for α-synuclein has been identified in Lewy bodies and Lewy neurite structure in the brains of all Parkinson's disease patients studied.[9–13] This observation suggested that although infrequently mutated, other cellular processes that could lead to accumulation of this protein might play an etiologic role in Parkinson's disease.

We hypothesized that aberrations in the ubiquitin-proteasome pathway may lead to the aggregation of abnormal proteins in neurons leading to the pathology seen in Parkinson's disease. The ubiquitin-proteasome pathway is the main cellular machinery for disposal of abnormal proteins.[14] Misfolded, irreparable proteins are tagged by ubiquitin chains and targeted to the proteasome for destruction.[14] The 26S proteasome is a barrel-shaped structure with several ATPase subunits at either end. Proteins captured by this system are fragmented in small oligopepetides, 3–5 amino acids in length, which are rapidly hydrolyzed in the cytoplasm.[15]

A key enzyme in the processing of newly synthesized ubiquitin chains is the ubiquitin carboxy-terminal hydrolase L1. UCHL1 is abundant in brain and peripheral neurons accounting for approximately 2% of the protein weight of the human brain.[16–17] In 1998, mutation analysis of this gene in probands of patients with the disorder revealed one mutation in two affected siblings in a German family.[18] The mutation, an Ile to Met change at the conserved position 93, also impaired the enzymatic activity of the protein on synthetic substrates.[18] Most recently, in 1999, homozygous truncating mutations were identified in the UCHL1 gene in the GAD mouse, which exhibits a neurodegenerative phenotype.[19] These two observations suggest that aberrations in the cellular machinery responsible for protein destruction can cause neurodegenerative phenotypes.

Accumulations of abnormal proteins in neurons and supporting cells are not an observation exclusive to Parkinson's disease. We and others have shown that accumulations of α-synuclein are present in other neurodegenerative conditions as well, including diffuse Lewy body dementia, amyotrophic lateral sclerosis, and multiple systems atrophy.[9–13]

α-Synuclein, a member of at least a three-member family, is highly expressed in brain and has been shown to have a perinuclear and perisynaptic localization, hence its name.[20] Although the function of the molecule remains unknown, α-synuclein has been implicated to play a role in neuronal plasticity in the song-learning processes in the canary.[21] Most recently, α- and β-synuclein proteins were identified to inhibit phospholipase D2, a key enzyme responsible for the production of phosphatidic acid, a potent second messenger.[22] Moreover, *in vitro* experiments have confirmed that the synuclein mutants are more prone to misfolding and aggregation compared to the wild-type synuclein. Fibrils purified from the brains of patients with Parkinson's disease have been shown to consist of synuclein filaments.[11] *In vitro* aggregation experiments have long suggested that even wild-type synuclein is prone to aggregation resulting in the formation of Congo red positive structures.

While the role of α-synuclein in neurodegenerative disorders is slowly emerging, the search for additional genetic factors in Parkinson's disease is continuing. In 1998, a second locus for autosomal dominant Parkinson's disease was identified in families from southern Denmark and Northern Germany on 2p13;[23] however, this gene has not yet been identified. Similarly, in a large family with Parkinson's disease and essential tremor, a locus was identified on chromosome 4p, and the search for the mutant gene is ongoing.[24]

Besides autosomal dominant Parkinson's disease, a recessive form of the disease has also been described. This form of parkinsonism is of early onset, with initially mild symptoms, slow progression, a sleep benefit, and absence of Lewy bodies.[25] The gene was located on 6q27, and mutations were reported in 1998 in Japanese families.[25] The mutated gene, Parkin, is a large gene with a ubiquitin-like domain at the N-terminal end of the protein and a cysteine ring structure at the C-terminal end.[25] The cysteine ring domain has extensive homology with the BRCA1 gene, which is mutated in some patients with breast cancer. The majority of the mutations of the Parkin gene are deletions of one or more exons. Mutations of this gene are not restricted to Japanese families only. We have identified a three-exon deletion in a Greek family with similar clinical features, and similar findings have been reported in different ethnic groups.[26] Although this form of the disease is rare, mutations in the Parkin gene account for the majority of autosomal recessive cases.

Although all the pieces of the genetics puzzle of Parkinson's disease are not together, the role of abnormally folded proteins in the production of the disease pathology merits additional investigations. The emerging pattern suggests that mutations in abundant brain proteins that lead to their misfolding or, alternatively, mutations in the cellular processes for repairing or removing abnormally folded proteins may be contributing to the genetic risk factors for the development of Parkinson's disease. The observation of intracellular inclusions in trinucleotide repeat disorders, including the spinocerebellar ataxias and Huntington's disease point to a potentially common theme of conformational protein changes and neurodegenerative disease.

REFERENCES

1. SCHAPIRA, A.H. 1995. Nuclear and mitochondrial genetics in Parkinson's disease. J. Med. Genet. **32:** 411–414.
2. PARKINSON, J. 1817. An Essay on the Shaking Palsy. Sherwood, Neely, and Jones. London.
3. KOSAKA, K. & E. ISEKI. 1996. Dementia with Lewy bodies. Curr. Opin. Neurol. **9:** 271–275.
4. DAVIS, G.C., A.C. WILLIAMS, S.P. MARKEY, M.H. EBERT, E.D. CAINE, C.M. REICHERT & I.J. KOPIN. 1979. Chronic parkinsonism secondary to intravenous injection of meperidine analogues. Psychiatry Res. **1:** 249–254.
5. LANGSTON, J.W., P. BALLARD, J.W. TETRUD & I. IRWIN. 1983. Chronic parkinsonism in humans due to a product of meperidine-analog synthesis. Science **219:** 979–980.
6. POLYMEROPOULOS, M.H., J.J. HIGGINS, L.I. GOLBE, W.G. JOHNSON, S.E. IDE, G. DI IORIO, G. SANGES, E.S. STENROOS, L.T. PHO, A.A. SCHAFFER, A.M. LAZZARINI, R.L. NUSSBAUM & R.C. DUVOISIN. 1996. Mapping of a gene for Parkinson's disease to chromosome 4q21-q23. Science **274:** 1197–1199.
7. POLYMEROPOULOS, M.H., C. LAVEDAN, E. LEROY, S.E. IDE, A. DEHEJIA, A. DUTRA, B. PIKE, H. ROOT, J. RUBENSTEIN, R. BOYER, E.S. STENROOS, S. CHANDRASEKHARAPPA, A. ATHANASSIADOU, T. PAPAPETROPOULOS, W.G. JOHNSON, A.M. LAZZARINI, R.C. DUVOISIN, G. DI IORIO, L.I. GOLBE & R.L. NUSSBAUM. 1997. Mutation in the alpha-synuclein gene identified in families with Parkinson's disease. Science **276:** 2045–2047.
8. KRUGER, R., W. KUHN, T. MULLER, D. WOITALLA, M. GRAEBER, S. KOSEL, H. PRZUNTEK, J.T. EPPLEN, L. SCHOLS & O. RIESS. 1998. Ala30Pro mutation in the gene encoding alpha-synuclein in Parkinson's disease [letter]. Nat. Genet. **18:** 106–108.
9. SPILLANTINI, M.G., M.L. SCHMIDT, V.M. LEE, J.Q. TROJANOWSKI, R. JAKES & M. GOEDERT. 1997. Alpha-synuclein in Lewy bodies [letter]. Nature **388:** 839–840.

10. TROJANOWSKI, J.Q. & V.M. LEE. 1998. Aggregation of neurofilament and alpha-synuclein proteins in Lewy bodies: implications for the pathogenesis of Parkinson disease and Lewy body dementia. Arch. Neurol. **55:** 151–152.
11. SPILLANTINI, M.G., R.A. CROWTHER, R. JAKES, M. HASEGAWA & M. GOEDERT. 1998. Alpha-synuclein in filamentous inclusions of Lewy bodies from Parkinson's disease and dementia with Lewy bodies. Proc. Natl. Acad. Sci. USA **95:** 6469–6473.
12. WAKABAYASHI, K., M. YOSHIMOTO, S. TSUJI & H. TAKAHASHI. 1998. Alpha-synuclein immunoreactivity in glial cytoplasmic inclusions in multiple system atrophy. Neurosci. Lett. **249:** 180–182.
13. MEZEY, E., A. DEHEJIA, G. HARTA, M.I. PAPP, M.H.. POLYMEROPOULOS & M.J. BROWNSTEIN. 1998. Alpha synuclein in neurodegenerative disorders: murderer or accomplice? [In Process Citation]. Nat. Med. **4:** 755–757.
14. LARSEN, C.N., B.A. KRANTZ & K.D. WILKINSON. 1998. Substrate specificity of deubiquitinating enzymes: ubiquitin C-terminal hydrolases. Biochemistry **37:** 3358–3368.
15. MATTHEWS, W., J. DRISCOLL, TANAKA, A. ICHIHARA & A.L. GOLDBERG. 1989. Involvement of the proteasome in various degradative processes in mammalian cells [published erratum appears in Proc. Natl. Acad. Sci. USA 1989 Jul; **86**(14): 5350]. Proc. Natl. Acad. Sci. USA **86:** 2597–2601.
16. WILKINSON, K.D., K.M. LEE, S. DESHPANDE, P. DUERKSEN-HUGHES, J.M. BOSS & J. POHL. 1989. The neuron-specific protein PGP 9.5 is a ubiquitin carboxyl-terminal hydrolase. Science **246:** 670–673.
17. WILKINSON, K.D., S. DESHPANDE & C.N. LARSEN. 1992. Comparisons of neuronal (PGP 9.5) and non-neuronal ubiquitin C-terminal hydrolases. Biochem. Soc. Trans. **20:** 631–637.
18. LEROY, E., R. BOYER, G. AUBURGER, B. LEUBE, G. ULM, E. MEZEY, G. HARTA, M. J. BROWNSTEIN, S. JONNALAGADA, T. CHERNOVA, A. DEHEJIA, C. LAVEDAN, T. GASSER, P.J. STEINBACH, K.D. WILKINSON & M.H. POLYMEROPOULOS. 1998. The ubiquitin pathway in Parkinson's disease [letter]. Nature **395:** 451–452.
19. SAIGOH, K., Y.L. WANG, J.G. SUH, T. YAMANISHI, Y. SAKAI, H. KIYOSAWA, T. HARADA, N. ICHIHARA, S. WAKANA, T. KIKUCHI & K. WADA. 1999. Intragenic deletion in the gene encoding ubiquitin carboxy-terminal hydrolase in gad mice. Nat. Genet. **23:** 47–51.
20. UEDA, K., H. FUKUSHIMA, E. MASLIAH, Y. XIA, A. IWAI, M. YOSHIMOTO, D.A. OTERO, J. KONDO, Y. IHARA & T. SAITOH. 1993. Molecular cloning of cDNA encoding an unrecognized component of amyloid in Alzheimer disease. Proc. Natl. Acad. Sci. USA **90:** 11282–11286.
21. GEORGE, J.M., H. JIN, W.S. WOODS & D.F. CLAYTON. 1995. Characterization of a novel protein regulated during the critical period for song learning in the zebra finch. Neuron **15:** 361–372.
22. JENCO, J.M., A. RAWLINGSON, B. DANIELS & A.J. MORRIS. 1998. Regulation of phospholipase D2: selective inhibition of mammalian phospholipase D isoenzymes by alpha- and beta-synucleins. Biochemistry **37:** 4901–4909.
23. GASSER, T., B. MULLER-MYHSOK, Z.K. WSZOLEK, R. OEHLMANN, D.B. CALNE, V. BONIFATI, B. BEREZNAI, E. FABRIZIO, P. VIEREGGE & R.D. HORSTMANN. 1998. A susceptibility locus for Parkinson's disease maps to chromosome 2p13. Nat. Genet. **18:** 262–265.
24. FARRER, M., K. GWINN-HARDY, M. MUENTER, F.W. DEVRIEZE, R. CROOK, J. PEREZ-TUR, S. LINCOLN, D. MARAGANORE, C. ADLER, S. NEWMAN, K. MACELWEE, P. MCCARTHY, C. MILLER, C. WATERS & J. HARDY. 1999. A chromosome 4p haplotype segregating with Parkinson's disease and postural tremor. Hum. Mol. Genet. **8:** 81–85.
25. MATSUMINE, H., Y. YAMAMURA, T. KOBAYASHI, S. NAKAMURA, S. KUZUHARA & Y. MIZUNO. 1998. Early onset parkinsonism with diurnal fluctuation maps to a locus for juvenile parkinsonism. Neurology **50:** 1340–1345.
26. LEROY, E., D. ANASTASOPOULOS, S. KONITSIOTIS, C. LAVEDAN & M.H. POLYMEROPOULOS. 1998. Deletions in the Parkin gene and genetic heterogeneity in a Greek family with early onset Parkinson's disease. Hum. Genet. **103:** 424–427.

Physiology and Pathophysiology of α-Synuclein

Cell Culture and Transgenic Animal Models Based on a Parkinson's Disease-associated Protein

PHILIPP J. KAHLE,[a,d] MANUELA NEUMANN,[b] LAURENCE OZMEN,[c] AND CHRISTIAN HAASS[a,d]

[a]*Adolf Butenandt Institute, Department of Biochemistry, Ludwig Maximilians University, 80336 Munich, Germany*

[b]*Institute of Neuropathology, University of Göttingen, 37075 Göttingen, Germany*

[c]*Pharma Research, Gene Technology, F. Hoffmann–La Roche Ltd, 4070 Basel, Switzerland*

ABSTRACT: The 15–20 kDa synuclein (SYN) phosphoproteins are abundantly expressed in nervous tissue. Members of the family include α- and β-SYN, and the more distantly related γ-SYN and synoretin. SYN genes have been identified in Torpedo, canary, and several mammalian species, indicating an evolutionary conserved role. Expression of α-SYN was found to be modulated in situations of neuronal remodeling, namely, songbird learning and after target ablation of dopaminergic striatonigral neurons in the rat. The presynaptic localization of α-SYN is further supportive of a direct physiological role in neuronal plasticity. The extensive synaptic co-localization of α- and β-SYN might indicate functional redundancy of these highly homologous synucleins. However, α-SYN was the only family member identified in Lewy bodies and cytoplasmic inclusions characteristic for multiple system atrophy. Moreover, α-SYN was genetically linked to familial Parkinson's disease. The two Parkinson's disease-associated mutations accelerated the intrinsic aggregation property of α-SYN *in vitro*. Post-translational modifications, such as phosphorylation and proteolysis, and/or interaction with other proteins, might regulate α-SYN fibril formation *in vivo*. Cytoskeletal elements and signal transduction intermediates have been recently identified as binding partners for α-SYN. Preliminary data available from transgenic mice suggest that (over)expressed human α-SYN proteins are less efficiently cleared from the neuronal cytosol. Thus, Parkinson's disease-associated mutations might perturb axonal transport, leading to somal accumulation of α-SYN and eventually Lewy body formation.

THE SYNUCLEIN PROTEIN FAMILY

Synuclein (SYN) was originally isolated with an antiserum against purified cholinergic synaptic vesicles from Torpedo's electric organ.[1] Today, Torpedo synuclein is recognized as the homologue of mammalian γ-SYN, while the concomitantly

[d]Address for correspondence: Christian Haass or Philipp Kahle, Adolf Butenandt Institute, Department of Biochemistry, Ludwig Maximilians University, Schillerstrasse 44, 80336 Munich, Germany. Tel: (+49-89) 5996-471; fax: (+49- 89) 5996-415.

e-mail: chaass@pbm.med.uni-muenchen.de or pkahle@pbm.med.uni-muenchen.de identified rat synucleins[1,2] are isoforms of α-SYN (FIG. 1). β-SYN was first isolated from bovine brain and termed phosphoneuroprotein 14.[3,4] Human α-SYN was originally isolated as the precursor protein of a so-called non-amyloid β-protein (Aβ) component (NAC) of Alzheimer's disease plaques.[5] In an independent effort, human α-SYN and β-SYN were isolated from brain and identified as members of a protein family.[6] Splice variants of human α-SYN distinct from those in the rat have been found.[7,8] The relevance of these rare isoforms is unknown.

Mammalian γ-SYN proteins were independently identified as a product of the human breast cancer susceptibility gene 1,[9] and by subtractive cloning of developing rat ("synuclein-like") and mouse ("persyn") peripheral ganglia mRNA.[10,11] Finally, the predominantly retinal synoretin was found in a two-hybrid screen of proteins interacting with phototransduction intermediates.[12] Thus, the synucleins comprise an evolutionary conserved protein family (FIG. 1) with two split branches (α-SYN/β-SYN and γ-SYN/synoretin[12]). However, there is no close synuclein homologue in the completely sequenced genome of an invertebrate organism, *Caenorhabditis elegans*.

Two missense mutations in the human α-SYN gene (*SNCA*, chromosome 4q21.3-q22) have been linked to familial Parkinson's disease (PD). A G→A transversion at position 209 causes mutation to [A53T]α-SYN in an Italian-Greek kindred,[13] and a G→C transversion at position 88 causes mutation to [A30P]α-SYN in a German kindred.[14] Although these mutations are a very rare cause of PD, and at least two more loci (*PARKIN*, chromosome 6q25.2-q27; and *PARK3*, chromosome 2p13) have been genetically linked to PD,[15] a causative role for α-SYN in the etiology of PD is likely (see below). No genetic link to PD was found for the genes encoding β-SYN (*SNCB*, chromosome 5q35) and γ-SYN (*SNCG*, chromosome 10q23.2-q23.3).[16,17] There are polymorphisms in the human breast cancer susceptibility gene 1/γ-SYN, but there was no genetic link to breast cancer.[18]

A multitude of antibodies have been generated, which have provided invaluable tools to study the physiology and pathophysiology of synucleins.[6,11,12,19–25] The C-termini of synucleins were good immunogens for family member-specific antibodies. Despite the great degree of interspecies homology, several human-specific α-SYN antibodies could be raised. Interestingly, these were all directed against a juxta-NAC domain of α-SYN (amino acids 115–130).[6,25a,26] It appears that the limited number of amino acid substitutions between human and nonhuman α-SYN proteins in this region has a marked effect on antibody recognition. Human-specific antibodies are indispensable in the study of transgenic animals expressing human α-SYN over a background of endogenous α-SYN (see below).

EXPRESSION OF SYNUCLEINS IN BRAIN

The function of synucleins is presently unknown. However, some insight has been gained from the study of their spatiotemporal expression pattern. The predominantly CNS neuronal expression of α-SYN and β-SYN was recognized early on.[1,3,6,19,20] α-SYN and β-SYN were localized to presynaptic terminals in immunohistochemical studies.[2,6,19,20] Extensive synaptic co-localization of α- and β-SYN was directly demonstrated by double-labeled confocal microscopy.[25a] Synaptosomal conserved, N-terminal repeats | NAC domain | variable, acidic C-terminus

                                    30P   53T   68K   109E   106S

α-Synucleins

PD mutations |---| |-----------------| |------------------|

Hum (NACP126)   MDVFMKGLSKAKEGVVAAAEKTKQGVAEA.

Hum (NACP140)   MDVFMKGLSKAKEGVVAAAEKTKQGVVHGVATVAEKTKEQVTNVGGAVVTGVTAVAQKTVEGAGSIAAATGFVKKDQLGK.NEEGAPQEGILEDMP..VDPDN.EAYEMPSEEGYQDYEPEA

Hum   ..VAEKTKEQVTNVGGAVVTGVTAVAQKTVEGAGSIAAATGFVKKDQLGK...EGYQDVEPEA

Hum (NACP112)   GKTKEGVLV..

Rat (SYN-1)   MDVFMKGLSKAKEGVVAAAEKTKQGVAEA.......GKTKEGVLYVGSKTKEGVVHGVATVAEKTKEQVTNVGGAVVTGVTAVAQKTVEGAGSIAAATGFVKKDQMKK.GEEGYPQEGILEDMP..VDPSS.EAYEMPSEEGYQDYEPEA

Rat (SYN-2)   MDVFMKGLSKAKEGVVAAAEKTKQGVAEA.......GKTKEGVLYVGSKTKEGVVHGVTTVAEKTKEQVTNVGGAVVTGVTAVAQKTVEGAGSIAAATGFVKKDQMKK.GEEGYPQEGILEDMP..VDPSS.EAYEMPSEEGYQDYEPEA

Rat (SYN-3)   MDVFMKGLSKAKEGVVAAAEKTKQGVAEA.......GKTKEGVLYVGSKTKEGVVHGVTTVAEKTKEQVTNVGGAVVTGVTAVAQKTVEGAGSIAAATGFVKKDQMKK.GYPMSECTNHFPRLIRVKSRYEHSWRPKQLSLACVVMDFPLPT

Mus   GKTKEGVLYVGSKTKEGVVHGVATVAEKTKEQ...

Can   MDVFMKGLSKAKEGVVAAAEKTKQGVAEA.......GKTKEGVLYVGSRTKEGVVHGVTTVAEKTKEQVSNVGGAVVTGVTAVAQKTVEGAGNIAAATGFVKKDQLGK..EAYEMPEEEYQDVEPEA

β-Synucleins

Hum   MDVFMKGLSMAKEGVVAAAEKTKQGVTEA......EKTKEGVLYVGSKTKEGVVQGVASVAEKTKEQASHLGGAVFS......GAGNIAAATGLVKREEFPTDLKPEEVAQEAAEEPLIEPLMEPEGESYEDPPQEEYQEEYQEPEA

Bov   MDVFMKGLSMAKEGVVAAAEKTKQGVTEA......EKTKEGVLYVGSKTKEGVVQGVASVAEKTKEQASHLGGAVFS......GAGNIAAATGLVKKEEFPTDLKPEEVAQEAAEEPLIEPLMEPEGESYEEQPQEEYQEEYQEVEPEA

Rat   MDVFMKGLSMAKEGVVAAAEKTKQGVTEA......EKTKEGVLYVGSKTKEGVVQGVASVAEKTKEQASHLGGAVFS......GAGNIAAATGLVKKEEFPTDLKPEEVAQEAAEEPLIEPLMEPEGESYEDSPQEEYQEEYEPEAKGP

Mus   MDVFMKGLSMAKEGVVAAAEKTKQGVTEA......EKTKEGVLYVGSKTKEGVVQGVASVAEKTKEQASHLGGAVFS......GAGNIAAATGLVKKEEFPTDLKPEEVAQEAAEEPLIEPLMEPEGESYEDSPQEEYQEEYEPEAKGP

γ-Synucleins

BCSG1 polymorphisms

Hum   MDVFKKGFSIAKEGVVGAVEKTKQGVTEA......EKTKEGVMYVGAKTKENVVQSVTSVAEKTKEQANAVSEAVVSSVNTVATKTVEEAENIAVTSGVVHKEAL...RPSAPQQEGVASKEKEEVAEEAQSGGD

Rat   MDVFKKGFSIAKEGVVGAVEKTKQGVTEA......EKTKEGVMYVGAKTKEGTGTSTSVAEKTKEQANAVSEAVVSSVNTVATEEVEEAENIAVTSGVVRKEDL...EPPA.QDQEA..KEQEE.GEEAKSGGD

Mus   MDVFKKGFSIAKEGVVGAVEKTKQGVTEA......EKTKEGVMYVGAKTKEDVVQSVTSVAEKTKEQANAVSEAVVSSVNTVAEEVEEAENIVVTSGVVRKEDL...EPPA.QDQEA..KEQEE.NEEAKSGED

Tor   MDVLKKGFSIAKEGVVAAAEKTKQGVVQTKEGVVQSVNTVTEKTKEGVVQSVNTVASKTVEGVENVAAASGVKLDEHGREIPAEQVAGRKQTTQEPLVEATEETGK

Synoretins

polymorphism

Hum   MDVFKKGFSTAKEGVVGAVEKFKPVTEAA......EKTKEGVMYVGAKTKEDVVQSVTSVAEKTKEQANAVSEAVVSSVNTVATKTVEEYENIAVTSGVVHKEAL...KQPVPQEDVAAAEEQVAEETKSGGD

Bov   MDVFKKGFSTAKEGVVGAVEKKFRVTEAA......EKTKEGVMYVGAKTKEDVVQSVTSVAEKTKEQANAVSEAVVSSVNTVATKTVEEYENIAVSGVVHKEAL...KQPVPSQEDVAAAEEQVAEETKSGGD

FIGURE 1. Sequence alignment of synuclein proteins. Synucleins contain three domains, indicated on the top line. Individual N-terminal repeats are underlined. Splice variants of human and rat α-SYN are shown with respective abbreviations. Sequence polymorphisms are typed in bold, the substituted amino acid above in italics. See text for original references and illustration.

localization of α- and β-SYN was confirmed biochemically by subcellular fractionation. α-SYN and β-SYN were recovered in the soluble fraction after lysis of rapidly processed brain synaptosomes.[2,11,20,27,28] Thus, if synucleins are bound to synaptic vesicles, as visualized by the punctate immunostaining of neuronal cultures (see below) and demonstrated by the *in vitro* interaction of α-SYN with synthetic membranes and a crude vesicle preparation,[29,30] the interaction is reversible.

Synuclein expression was greatly upregulated in the CNS during the first postnatal weeks.[28,31–33] While massive onset of persyn/γ-SYN expression in the PNS occurred at early developmental stages concomitantly with ganglionic differentiation,[11] embryonic expression of α-SYN and β-SYN was low.[28,32,34] Interestingly, early α-SYN expression was confined to proliferating neuronal precursors, raising the possibility of a nonsynaptic function.[32,34]

α-SYN expression peaked in a songbird learning center just in the phase of song acquisition.[20] In the rat substantia nigra, α-SYN was stably expressed between postnatal days 4–30 in dopaminergic neurons spared from naturally occurring cell death.[35] Upon partial striatal target ablation by quinolinic acid injection, α-SYN was transiently upregulated in those dopaminergic neurons which survived and remained functional into adulthood.[35] In contrast, complete striatal lesion using the neurotoxin 6-hydroxydopamine eliminated α-SYN expression as dopaminergic neurons died.[36] Thus, α-SYN is upregulated in situations of synaptic remodeling. Since α-SYN is present in presynaptic terminals, possibly in contact with synaptic vesicles, it may actively influence synaptic plasticity. α-SYN could perform its function directly or in conjunction with binding proteins (see below). It remains to be shown whether α-SYN regulates neurotransmitter release and/or other events during the synaptic vesicle cycle, including axonal transport. It is of further interest whether the co-localized α- and β-SYN are functionally redundant.

The predominantly neuronal localization of α-SYN in mature brain raises the question of origin of glial cytoplasmic inclusions in multiple system atrophy (MSA). It is not known whether α-SYN is aberrantly induced and aggregates because of ectopic expression in oligodendrocytes, or whether glia takes up α-SYN fibrils released from certain axons affected in MSA.

MUTANT α-SYNUCLEINOPATHIES: *IN VITRO* AGGREGATION

Early studies suggested a seeding effect of α-SYN on Aβ aggregation.[37] α-SYN and β-SYN were both effective in this regard.[38] It became clear that α-SYN was capable of self-oligomerization in the presence and absence of Aβ.[38–40] However, self-aggregation of α-SYN was characterized by a long lag time, which was shortened in PD-linked mutant α-SYN.[41,42] Adding microaggregates of mutant α-SYN to a sub-critical solution of wild-type α-SYN caused rapid aggregation.[43] Thus, α-SYN can seed the formation of β-pleated sheets of Aβ and α-SYN. Ferric and cuprous ions stimulated α-SYN self-aggregation.[44,45] Iron-catalyzed oxidative reactions might be particularly relevant given the known iron mismetabolism and appreciable level of oxidative stress in PD brain. *In vitro* assembled α-SYN fibrils were morphologically similar to those isolated from Lewy bodies.[41,42,46]

MUTANT α-SYNUCLEINOPATHIES: CELL CULTURE

In primary neuron cultures, α-SYN and β-SYN localized to cell bodies and processes.[2,28,47] The punctate staining pattern was reminiscent of synaptic vesicles. In developing hippocampal neurons, axonal staining of synapsin preceded that of synelfin/α-SYN until a nearly complete overlap was reached in terminally differentiated neurons.[47] Thus, the expression of α-SYN in terminally differentiated synapses *in vitro* and *in vivo* is compatible with a role in synaptic plasticity (see above).

Few groups have presented cell line models for α-SYN. In stably transfected human embryonic kidney 293 cells, Flag-tagged α-SYN was shown to be a very stable protein.[22] Its half-life was ~48 h, as estimated from [^{35}S]methionine pulse chase experiments. By comparison, the half-life of Flag-α-SYN in stably transfected rat pheochromocytoma PC12 cells was slightly shorter, if at all. In transiently transfected human neuroblastoma SY5Y cells, His-tagged α-SYN was rapidly degraded in the proteasome.[48] In this system, the half-life of [A53T]α-SYN was ~50% longer compared with that of wild-type α-SYN, potentially providing a kinetic basis for intracellular accumulation. It remains to be shown whether α-SYN *in vivo* follows a rapid degradation pathway as it was reported for transiently transfected cells. Also, the reported effect of transient transfection of α-SYN on cellular viability[49] awaits confirmation *in vivo*.

We have recently found that α-SYN was constitutively phosphorylated in stably transfected 293 cells and PC12 cells.[22] The major phosphoacceptor site was Ser-129, and casein kinase I and II were likely responsible phosphotransferases. All mammalian synucleins bear a C-terminal serine flanked by acidic residues: Ser-129 in α-SYN, Ser-118 in β-SYN, Ser-124 in γ-SYN and synoretin. However, β-SYN was not phosphorylated by casein kinases.[4] Ca^{2+}/calmodulin-dependent protein kinase II strongly phosphorylated β-SYN,[4] whereas it phosphorylated α-SYN only moderately.[22] It will be interesting to determine which kinase(s) phosphorylates each synuclein *in vivo*. Moreover, the study on implications of synuclein phosphorylation on properties such as affinity for synaptic vesicles, interaction with binding proteins, and self-aggregation promises to be an interesting area of future research.

A number of α-SYN binding proteins have been presented. α-SYN was isolated as inhibitor protein of phospholipase D2.[50] Recombinant α- and β-SYN inhibited phospholipase D2 activity equally well. It is of note that another naturally unfolded protein, the microtubule-associated protein tau, inhibited phospholipase C-γ.[51,52] A direct interaction between tau and α-SYN was found, thereby regulating tau phosphorylation by protein kinase A.[53] A more general resemblance of α-SYN with the 14-3-3 family of molecular chaperones was proposed. Indeed, α-SYN was found to dimerize with 14-3-3 proteins, and to co-immunoprecipitate with some 14-3-3 binding proteins, namely, protein kinase C, extracellular signal-regulated protein kinase, and BAD.[49] Thus, α-SYN may belong to the class of naturally unfolded proteins that regulate intracellular signal transduction via lipid second messengers and phosphorylation cascades.

A two-hybrid screen of α-SYN binding protein revealed a novel interacting partner, termed synphilin-1.[54] This protein co-immunoprecipitated with α-SYN from brain. α-SYN and β-SYN interacted with synphilin-1 equally well. Ankyrin-like repeats and a coiled-coil domain could provide additional protein-protein contact, pos-

sibly with cytoskeletal elements. Moreover, synphilin-1 contains a predicted ATP/
GTP-binding domain. Excitingly, co-transfection of 293 cells with synphilin-1, and
the NAC fragment led to the formation of cytoplasmic eosinophilic inclusions. However, neither full-length nor wild-type nor [A53T]α-SYN were deposited in this system. Investigation of the synuclein-synphilin interactions may provide important
clues to the physiology and pathophysiology of synucleins.

MUTANT α-SYNUCLEINOPATHIES: TRANSGENIC MICE

The neuropathology of α-SYN in Lewy body diseases and MSA has been reviewed recently[55,56] and in adjacent sections of this compendium. Moreover, abnormal α-SYN-immunoreactive profiles were found in neuroaxonal dystrophies,
including Hallervorden-Spatz syndrome.[57–59]

Patients heterozygous for the A30P mutation in the *SNCA* gene developed an aggressive, early-onset form of PD.[14] [A30P]α-SYN associated less efficiently with
cellular vesicles *in vitro*, suggesting a deficiency in axonal transport for mutant α-
SYN.[30] To study the properties of [A30P]α-SYN in brain, we generated transgenic
mice. Strong expression of transgenic human [A30P]α-SYN mRNA and protein in
neurons throughout the brain was achieved with the Thy-1 promoter. Some
[A30P]α-SYN was found in synaptosomal compartments, indicating that anterograde transport of α-SYN was not completely abolished by the A30P mutation.
However, a perturbance of axonal transport was indicated by the accumulation of
[A30P]α-SYN in neuronal cell bodies and neurites (FIG. 2). Accumulation of α-
SYN in neurons of transgenic mice was also observed by other groups.[60,61] It will
be critical to determine how α-SYN accumulations turn into Lewy bodies.

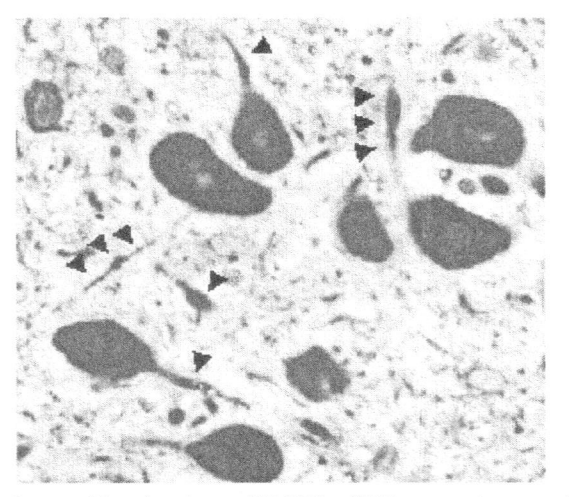

FIGURE 2. Immunohistochemistry of [A30P]α-SYN transgenic mouse brain. A section
of nucleus dentatus was incubated with human-specific α-SYN antibody and immunoreactivity developed with alkaline-phosphatase anti-alkaline phosphatase. Abnormal accumulation of
[A30P]α-SYN was detected in cell bodies and bulbous neurites (*arrowheads*).

REFERENCES

1. MAROTEAUX, L., J.T. CAMPANELLI & R.H. SCHELLER. 1988. Synuclein: a neuron-specific protein localized to the nucleus and presynaptic nerve terminal. J. Neurosci. **8:** 2804–2815.
2. MAROTEAUX, L. & R.H. SCHELLER. 1991. The rat brain synucleins; family of proteins transiently associated with neuronal membrane. Mol. Brain Res. **11:** 335–343.
3. NAKAJO, S., K. OMATA, T. AIUCHI *et al.* 1990. Purification and characterization of a novel brain-specific 14-kDa protein. J. Neurochem. **55:** 2031–2038.
4. NAKAJO, S., K. TSUKADA, K. OMATA, Y. NAKAMURA & K. NAKAYA. 1993. A new brain-specific 14-kDa protein is a phosphoprotein. Its complete amino acid sequence and evidence for phosphorylation. Eur. J. Biochem. **217:** 1057–1063.
5. UÉDA, K., H. FUKUSHIMA, E. MASLIAH, *et al.* 1993. Molecular cloning of cDNA encoding an unrecognized component of amyloid in Alzheimer disease. Proc. Natl. Acad. Sci. USA **90:** 11282–11286.
6. JAKES, R., M.G. SPILLANTINI & M. GOEDERT. 1994. Identification of two distinct synucleins from human brain. FEBS Lett. **345:** 27–32.
7. CAMPION, D., C. MARTIN, R. HEILIG, *et al.* 1995. The NACP/synuclein gene: chromosomal assignment and screening for alterations in Alzheimer disease. Genomics **26:** 254–257.
8. UÉDA, K., T. SAITOH & H. MORI. 1994. Tissue-dependent alternative splicing of mRNA for NACP, the precursor of non-Ab component of Alzheimer's disease amyloid. Biochem. Biophys. Res. Commun. **205:** 1366–1372.
9. JI, H., Y.E. LIU, T. JIA, *et al.* 1997. Identification of a breast cancer-specific gene, BCSG1, by direct differential cDNA sequencing. Cancer Res. **57:** 759–764.
10. AKOPIAN, A.N. & J.N. WOOD. 1995. Peripheral nervous system-specific genes identified by subtractive cDNA cloning. J. Biol. Chem. **270:** 21264–21270.
11. BUCHMAN, V.L., H.J. HUNTER, L.G. PINON, *et al.* 1998. Persyn, a member of the synuclein family, has a distinct pattern of expression in the developing nervous system. J. Neurosci. **18:** 9335–9341.
12. SURGUCHOV, A., I. SURGUCHEVA, E. SOLESSIO & W. BAEHR. 1999. Synoretin—a new protein belonging to the synuclein family. Mol. Cell. Neurosci. **13:** 95–103.
13. POLYMEROPOULOS, M.H., C. LAVEDAN, E. LEROY, *et al.* 1997. Mutation in the α-synuclein gene identified in families with Parkinson's disease. Science **276:** 2045–2047.
14. KRÜGER, R., W. KUHN, T. MULLER, *et al.* 1998. Ala30Pro mutation in the gene encoding α-synuclein in Parkinson's disease. Nat. Genet. **18:** 106–108.
15. GASSER, T. 1998. Genetics of Parkinson's disease. Clin. Genet. **54:** 259–265.
16. LINCOLN, S., R. CROOK, M.C. CHARTIER-HARLIN, *et al.* 1999. No pathogenic mutations in the β-synuclein gene in Parkinson's disease. Neurosci. Lett. **269:** 107–109.
17. LINCOLN, S., K. GWINN-HARDY, J. GOUDREAU, *et al.* 1999. No pathogenic mutations in the persyn gene in Parkinson's disease. Neurosci. Lett. **259:** 65–66.
18. NINKINA, N.N., M.V. ALIMOVA-KOST, J.W. PATERSON, *et al.* 1998. Organization, expression and polymorphism of the human *persyn* gene. Hum. Mol. Genet. **7:** 1417–1424.
19. IWAI, A., E. MASLIAH, M. YOSHIMOTO, *et al.* 1995. The precursor protein of non-Ab component of Alzheimer's disease amyloid is a presynaptic protein of the central nervous system. Neuron **14:** 467–475.
20. GEORGE, J.M., H. JIN, W.S. WOODS & D.F. CLAYTON. 1995. Characterization of a novel protein regulated during the critical period for song learning in the zebra finch. Neuron **15:** 361–372.
21. ARIMA, K., K. UEDA, N. SUNOHARA, *et al.* 1998. Immunoelectron-microscopic demonstration of NACP/α-synuclein-epitopes on the filamentous component of Lewy bodies in Parkinson's disease and in dementia with Lewy bodies. Brain Res. **808:** 93–100.
22. OKOCHI, M., J. WALTER, A. KOYAMA, *et al.* 2000. Constitutive phosphorylation of the Parkinson's disease associated α-synuclein. J. Biol. Chem. **275:** 390–397.
23. TU, P.-H., J.E. GALVIN, M. BABA, *et al.* 1998. Glial cytoplasmic inclusions in white matter oligodendrocytes of multiple system atrophy brains contain insoluble α-synuclein. Ann. Neurol. **44:** 415–422.

24. CULVENOR, J.G., C.A. MCLEAN, S. CUTT, *et al.* 1999. Non-Aβ component of Alzheimer's disease amyloid (NAC) revisited: NAC and α-synuclein are not associated with Aβ amyloid. Am. J. Pathol. **155:** 1173–1181.
25. WAKABAYASHI, K., K. MATSUMOTO, K. TAKAYAMA, M. YOSHIMOTO & H. TAKAHASHI. 1997. NACP, a presynaptic protein, immunoreactivity in Lewy bodies in Parkinson's disease. Neurosci. Lett. **239:** 45–48.
25a. KAHLE, P.J., M. NEUMANN, L. OZMEN, *et al.* 2000. Subcellular localization of wild-type and Parkinson's disease-associated mutant α-synuclein in human and transgenic mouse brain. J. Neurosci. **20:** 6365–6373.
26. JAKES, R. *et al.* 1999. Epitope mapping of LB509, a monoclonal antibody directed against human α-synuclein. Neurosci. Lett. **269:** 13–16.
27. IRIZARRY, M.C., T.W. KIM, M. MCNAMARA, *et al.* 1996. Characterization of the precursor protein of the non-Ab component of senile plaques (NACP) in the human central nervous system. J. Neuropathol. Exp. Neurol. **55:** 889–895.
28. SHIBAYAMA-IMAZU, T., I. OKAHASHI, K. OMATA, *et al.* 1993. Cell and tissue distribution and developmental change of neuron specific 14 kDa protein (phosphoneuroprotein 14). Brain Res. **622:** 17–25.
29. DAVIDSON, W.S., A. JONAS, D.F. CLAYTON & J.M. GEORGE. 1998. Stabilization of alpha-synuclein secondary structure upon binding to synthetic membranes. J. Biol. Chem. **273:** 9443–9449.
30. JENSEN, P.H., M.S. NIELSEN, R. JAKES, C.G. DOTTI & M. GOEDERT. 1998. Binding of α-synuclein to brain vesicles is abolished by familial Parkinson's disease mutation. J. Biol. Chem. **273:** 26292–26294.
31. BUCHMAN, V.L., J. ADU, L. G.P. PIÑON, N.N. NINKINA & A.M. DAVIES. 1998. Persyn, a member of the synuclein family, influences neurofilament network integrity. Nat. Neurosci. **1:** 101–103.
32. HSU, L.J., M. MALLORY, Y. XIA, *et al.* 1998. Expression pattern of synucleins (non-Aβ component of Alzheimer's disease amyloid precursor protein/α-synuclein) during murine brain development. J. Neurochem. **71:** 338–344.
33. PETERSEN, K., O.F. OLESEN & J.D. MIKKELSEN. 1999. Developmental expression of α-synuclein in rat hippocampus and cerebral cortex. Neuroscience **91:** 651–659.
34. BAYER, T.A., P. JAKALA, T. HARTMANN, *et al.* 1999. Neural expression profile of α-synuclein in developing human cortex. Neuroreport **10:** 2799–2803.
35. KHOLODILOV, N.G., M. NEYSTAT, T.F. OO, *et al.* 1999. Increased expression of rat synuclein in the substantia nigra pars compacta identified by mRNA differential display in a model of developmental target injury. J. Neurochem. **73:** 2586–2599.
36. KHOLODILOV, N.G., T.F. OO & R.E. BURKE. 1999. Synuclein expression is decreased in rat substantia nigra following induction of apoptosis by intrastriatal 6-hydroxydopamine. Neurosci. Lett. **275:** 105–108.
37. YOSHIMOTO, M., A. IWAI, D. KANG, D.A. OTERO, Y. XIA & T. SAITOH. 1995. NACP, the precursor protein of the non-amyloid β/A4 protein (Aβ) component of Alzheimer disease amyloid, binds Aβ and stimulates Aβ aggregation. Proc. Natl. Acad. Sci. USA **92:** 9141–9145.
38. JENSEN, P.H., P. HOJRUP, H. HAGER, *et al.* 1997. Binding of Aβ to α- and β-synucleins: identification of segments in α-synuclein/NAC precursor that bind Aβ and NAC. Biochem. J. **323:** 539–546.
39. HASHIMOTO, M., L.J. HSU, A. SISK, *et al.* 1998. Human recombinant NACP/α-synuclein is aggregated and fibrillated *in vitro*: relevance for Lewy body disease. Brain Res. **799:** 301–306.
40. PAIK, S.R., J.-H. LEE, D.-H. KIM, C.-S. CHANG & Y.-S. KIM. 1998. Self-oligomerization of NACP, the precursor protein of the non-amyloid β/A4 protein (Aβ) component of Alzheimer's disease amyloid, observed in the presence of a C-terminal Aβ fragment (residues 25–35). FEBS Lett. **421:** 73–76.
41. NARHI, L., S.J. WOOD, S. STEAVENSON, *et al.* 1999. Both familial Parkinson's disease mutations accelerate α-synuclein aggregation. J. Biol. Chem. **274:** 9843–9846.
42. CONWAY, K.A., J.D. HARPER & P.T. LANSBURY. 1998. Accelerated *in vitro* fibril formation by a mutant α-synuclein linked to early-onset Parkinson disease. Nat. Med. **4:** 1318–1320.

43. WOOD, S.J., J. WYPYCH, S. STEAVENSON, J.C. LOUIS, M. CITRON & A.L. BIERE. 1999. α-Synuclein fibrillogenesis is nucleation-dependent. Implications for the pathogenesis of Parkinson's disease. J. Biol. Chem. **274:** 19509–19512.
44. PAIK, S.R., H.-J. SHIN, J.-H. LEE, C.-S. CHANG & J. KIM. 1999. Copper(II)-induced self-oligomerization of α-synuclein. Biochem. J. **340:** 821–828.
45. HASHIMOTO, M., L.J. HSU, Y. XIA, *et al.* 1999. Oxidative stress induces amyloid-like aggregate formation of NACP/α-synuclein *in vitro*. Neuroreport **10:** 717–721.
46. GIASSON, B.I., K. URYU, J.Q. TROJANOWSKI & V.M.-Y. LEE. 1999. Mutant and wild-type human α-synucleins assemble into elongated filaments with distinct morphologies *in vitro*. J. Biol. Chem. **274:** 7619–7622.
47. WITHERS, G.S., J.M. GEORGE, G.A. BANKER & D.F. CLAYTON. 1997. Delayed localization of synelfin (synuclein, NACP) to presynaptic terminals in cultured rat hippocampal neurons. Dev. Brain. Res. **99:** 87–94.
48. BENNETT, M.C., J.F. BISHOP, Y. LENG, P.B. CHOCK, T.N. CHASE & M.M. MOURADIAN. 1999. Degradation of α-synuclein by proteasome. J. Biol. Chem. **274:** 33855–33858.
49. OSTREROVA, N., L. PETRUCELLI, M. FARRER, *et al.* 1999. α-Synuclein shares physical and functional homology with 14-3-3 proteins. J. Neurosci. **19:** 5782–5791.
50. JENCO, J.M., A. RAWLINGSON, B. DANIELS & A.J. MORRIS. 1998. Regulation of phospholipase D2: selective inhibition of mammalian phospholipase D isoenzymes by α- and β-synucleins. Biochemistry **37:** 4901–4909.
51. JENKINS, S.M. & G.V.W. JOHNSON. 1998. Tau complexes with phospholipase C-γ *in situ*. Neuroreport **9:** 67–71.
52. HWANG, S.C., D.-Y. JHON, Y.S. BAE, J.H. KIM & S.G. RHEE. 1996. Activation of phospholipase C-γ by the concerted action of tau proteins and arachidonic acid. J. Biol. Chem. **271:** 18342–18349.
53. JENSEN, P.H., H. HAGER, M.S. NIELSEN, P. HOJRUP, J. GLIEMANN & R. JAKES. 1999. α-Synuclein binds to tau and stimulates the protein kinase A-catalyzed tau phosphorylation of serine residues 262 and 356. J. Biol. Chem. **274:** 25481–25489.
54. ENGELENDER, S., Z. KAMINSKY, X. GUO, *et al.* 1999. Synphilin-1 associates with α-synuclein and promotes the formation of cytosolic inclusions. Nat. Genet. **22:** 110–114.
55. HASHIMOTO, M. & E. MASLIAH. 1999. Alpha-synuclein in Lewy body disease and Alzheimer's disease. Brain Pathol. **9:** 707–720.
56. DICKSON, D.W., W. LIN, W.K. LIU & S.H. YEN. 1999. Multiple system atrophy: a sporadic synucleinopathy. Brain Pathol. **9:** 721–732.
57. ARAWAKA, S., Y. SAITO, S. MURAYAMA & H. MORI. 1998. Lewy body in neurodegeneration with brain iron accumulation type 1 is immunoreactive for α-synuclein. Neurology **51:** 887–889.
58. NEWELL, K.L., P. BOYER, E. GOMEZ-TORTOSA, *et al.* 1999. α-Synuclein immunoreactivity is present in axonal swellings in neuroaxonal dystrophy and acute traumatic brain injury. J. Neuropathol. Exp. Neurol. **58:** 1263–1268.
59. WAKABAYASHI, K., M. YOSHIMOTO, T. FUKUSHIMA, *et al.* 1999. Widespread occurrence of α-synuclein/NACP-immunoreactive neuronal inclusions in juvenile and adult-onset Hallervorden-Spatz disease with Lewy bodies. Neuropathol. Appl. Neurobiol. **25:** 363–368.
60. LEE, M.K. *et al.* 1999. Overexpression of wild type and familial Parkinson's disease linked mutant human α-synuclein in transgenic mice. Soc. Neurosci. Abstr. **25:** 49.
61. MASLIAH, E., E. ROCKENSTEIN, I. VEINBERGS, *et al.* 2000. Dopaminergic loss and inclusion body formation in alpha-synuclein mice: implications for neurodegenerative disorders. Science **287:**1265–1269.

Accelerated Oligomerization by Parkinson's Disease Linked α-Synuclein Mutants

K.A. CONWAY, S.-J. LEE, J.-C. ROCHET, T.T. DING, J.D. HARPER,
R.E. WILLIAMSON, AND P.T. LANSBURY, JR.[a]

*Center for Neurologic Diseases, Brigham and Women's Hospital and
Department of Neurology, Harvard Medical School, Boston, Massachusetts 02115, USA*

Two mutations, Ala53Thr (A53T) and Ala30Pro (A30P), in the protein α-synuclein were identified in families with early-onset familial Parkinson's disease (PD).[1,2] Subsequent to this discovery, α-synuclein was identified as a component of Lewy bodies in idiopathic PD and dementia with Lewy bodies (DLB) by immunohistochemical[3] and, in the case of DLB, by biochemical methods.[4] Also, fibrils extracted and partially purified from DLB brain were shown by immunogold electron microscopy to contain α-synuclein.[5]

We and others have demonstrated that recombinant α-synuclein forms fibrils *in vitro* that resemble brain-derived material.[6–9] Fibril formation by A53T is clearly accelerated relative to both wild-type (WT) and A30P.[6] A30P does not fibrillize unusually rapidly, but, relative to WT, apparently more rapidly forms spherical oligomers with dimensions similar to Aβ protofibrils (diameter ca. 4 nm), intermediates in Aβ amyloid fibril formation.[10–13] Two complementary assays, one that measures the loss of α-synuclein from solution[9] and another, the appearance of α-synuclein in a sedimentable fraction,[8] confirm that A53T aggregates more rapidly than A30P and WT; one of these also reports that A30P is lost from solution more rapidly than is WT.[9]

In order to describe the α-synuclein aggregation/fibrillization process in more detail and to test a possible analogy between PD and AD, we analyzed α-synuclein fibrils formed *in vitro* using a combination of methods that have been used to study amyloid fibrils comprising Aβ and other proteins.[14,15] These include electron microscopy (EM) and atomic-force microscopy (AFM) to assess fibril morphology, Fourier-transform infrared spectroscopy (FTIR), and circular dichroism spectroscopy (CD) to elucidate the constituent secondary structure, and binding of the amyloid histological dyes Congo red and thioflavin T (thio T), as well as protease sensitivity, to correlate species formed *in vitro* with material found in diseased tissue. We report that α-synuclein forms antiparallel β-sheet-containing fibrils, with a similar morphology to those comprising other amyloid proteins,[16] that is, rigid, unbranched fibrils (ca. 10 nm wide) that exhibit birefringence when stained with Congo red and have a predominantly antiparallel β-sheet structure. α-Synuclein fibrils were measured to be 8–10 nm in width by EM and ca. 10 nm in height by AFM, and appeared to be constructed by the winding of two 4–5-nm filaments. The fibrils produced

[a]Address for correspondence: Peter Lansbury, Jr., Ph.D., Center for Neurologic Diseases, Brigham and Women's Hospital, 77 Ave. Louis Pasteur, HIM Room 754, Boston, MA 02115. Tel: (617) 525-5260; fax: (617) 525-5252.
e-mail: plansbury@rics.bwh.harvard.edu

FTIR and CD spectra that are characteristic of antiparallel β-sheet structure. Birefringent staining with Congo red was observed and characteristic shifts in the absorption and fluorescence spectra of fibril-bound Congo red and thioflavin T, respectively, were measured. In contrast to the α-synuclein-soluble monomer, fibrillar α-synuclein is protease resistant, a trait commonly associated with the disease-associated form of the prion protein (PrP^{Sc}),[17] but also observed for Aβ amyloid fibrils.[18] Based on these data, α-synuclein should be added to the growing list of amyloidogenic proteins and PD, DLB, and multiple-system atrophy (MSA) to the list of neurodegenerative amyloid diseases. Furthermore, Lewy bodies can be considered to be cytoplasmic amyloid.

The identity of the pathogenic species and its relationship to the α-synuclein fibril has not been elucidated. In an *in vitro* study, the rates of disappearance of monomeric α-synuclein and appearance of fibrillar α-synuclein were compared for WT and the two PD variants.[19] Monomeric α-synuclein was separated from oligomeric forms by centrifugation to pellet sedimentable material followed by size-exclusion chromatography. The appearance of fibrillar α-synuclein was monitored by two dye-binding assays, thioflavin T and Congo red, and by electron microscopy. Additionally, the conversion from random coil to β-sheet conformation was monitored by circular dichroism.

As reported previously,[6] accelerated fibril formation by the A53T mutation was observed. However, the A30P mutation slowed fibril formation relative to WT. Equimolar mixtures of α-synuclein (200 μM total), containing A53T and WT or A30P and WT, fibrillized at a rate intermediate between the individual components. Circular dichroism spectra collected at several time points demonstrated that the conversion of "random coil" structure to β-sheet structure was most extensive for A53T, followed by WT, then A30P at each time analyzed. This trend paralleled the relative rates of fibril formation.

Yet, under these same conditions, the A30P monomer was consumed at a comparable rate or slightly more rapidly than the WT monomer, while A53T was consumed even more rapidly than WT (as determined by size-exclusion chromatography). The difference between these trends, that is, oligomerization and fibrillization, suggested the existence of nonfibrillar α-synuclein oligomers, which may themselves be pathogenic. To look for such species, the void volume eluate (≥600 kDa, assuming globular structure) from size-exclusion chromatography was concentrated, adsorbed onto atomically smooth mica, and subjected to analysis by atomic force microscopy.[11,12,20] Only apparently spherical oligomers were observed in the void volume eluate; no elongated protofibrils or fibrils were present. Several distinct species, with heights between 2 and 6 nm, were detected. These eluates were concentrated and incubated for 72 h at 4°C. Examination by atomic-force microscopy revealed the presence of ringlike structures in these incubations. Analysis of the population of rings in a 1:1 A53T:WT mixture (total α-synuclein concentration was 300 μM) identified the existence of two general classes: circular rings with diameters in the 35–55-nm range, and elliptical rings (widths between 35 and 55 nm; lengths ranged between 65 and 130 nm). Both species were characterized by regular height fluctuations, between ca. 2 and 4 nm, with a periodicity of ca. 23 nm, corresponding to the measured diameter of the spherical oligomers.

We have observed three discrete nonfibrillar α-synuclein oligomers that seem to be related, since they can share a height (ca. 4–5 nm) and apparent diameter (ca. 20

nm). These are (1) "spheres" of several heights, some of which (4–5 nm)[6] resemble early Aβ protofibrils;[12] (2) chains that appear to comprise linearly associated 4–5-nm spheres, analogous to elongated Aβ protofibrils;[16] and (3) rings, apparently comprising circularized chains.[19] The detailed mechanism of formation of these species and of their possible interconversions has not been determined. By analogy to the Aβ situation,[12] the spheres may be a direct precursor of the chain, and the chain, a direct precursor to the fibril. The circularization of chains to rings may prevent fibril formation. Accordingly, fibrils and rings may arise from α-synuclein by a bifurcated pathway that diverges from a common protofibrillar intermediate.

REFERENCES

1. POLYMEROPOULOS, M.H., C. LAVEDAN, E. LEROY, et al. 1997. Mutation in the α-synuclein gene identified in families with Parkinson's disease. Science 276: 2045–2047.
2. KRUGER, R., W. KUHN, T. MULLER, et al. 1998. Ala30Pro mutation in the gene encoding α-synuclein in Parkinson's disease. Nat. Genet. 18: 106–108.
3. SPILLANTINI, M.G., M.L. SCHMNIDT, V.M. LEE, et al. 1997. α-Synuclein in Lewy bodies. Nature 388: 839–840.
4. BABA, M., S. NAKAJO, P.H. TU, et al. 1998. Aggregation of α-synuclein in Lewy bodies of sporadic Parkinson's disease and dementia with Lewy bodies. Am. J. Pathol. 152: 879–884.
5. SPILLANTINI, M.G., R.A. CROWTHER, R. JAKES, et al. 1998. Filamentous alpha-synuclein inclusions link multiple system atrophy with Parkinson's disease and dementia with Lewy bodies. Neurosci. Lett. 251: 205–208.
6. CONWAY, K.A., J.D. HARPER & P.T. LANSBURY. 1998. Accelerated in vitro fibril formation by a mutant α-synuclein linked to early-onset Parkinson disease. Nat. Med. 4: 1318–1320.
7. HASHIMOTO, M., L.J. HSU, A. SISK, et al. 1998. Human recombinant NACP/alpha-synuclein is aggregated and fibrillated in vitro: relevance for lewy body disease. Brain Res. 799: 301–306.
8. GIASSON, B.I., K. URYU, J.Q. TROJANOWSKI & V.M. LEE. 1999. Mutant and wild type human alpha-synucleins assemble into elongated filaments with distinct morphologies in vitro. J. Biol. Chem. 274: 7619–7622.
9. NARHI, L., S.J. WOOD, S. STEAVENSON, et al. 1999. Both familial Parkinson's disease mutations accelerate alpha-synuclein aggregation. J. Biol. Chem. 274: 9843–9846.
10. HARPER, J.D., C.M. LIEBER & P.T. LANSBURY. 1997. Atomic force microscopic imaging of seeded fibril formation and fibril branching by the Alzheimer's disease amyloid-β-protein. Chem. Biol. 4: 951–959.
11. HARPER, J.D., S.S. WONG, C.M. LIEBER & P.T. LANSBURY. 1997. Observation of metastable Aβ amyloid protofibrils by atomic force microscopy. Chem. Biol. 4: 119–125.
12. HARPER, J.D., S.S. WONG, C.M. LIEBER & P.T. LANSBURY. 1999. Assembly of A beta amyloid protofibrils: an in vitro model for a possible early event in Alzheimer's disease. Biochemistry 38: 8972–8980.
13. WALSH, D.M., A. LOMAKIN, G.B. BENEDEK, et al. 1997. Amyloid beta-protein fibrillogenesis. Detection of a protofibrillar intermediate. J. Biol. Chem. 272: 22364–22372.
14. KELLY, J.W., et al. 1994. A chemical approach to elucidate the mechanism of transthyretin and β-protein amyloid fibril formation. Amyloid: Int. J. Exp. Clin. Invest. 1: 186–205.
15. LANSBURY, P.T., JR. 1992. In pursuit of the molecular structure of amyloid plaque: new technology provides unexpected and critical information. Biochemistry 31: 6865–6870.
16. CONWAY, K.A., J.D. HARPER & P.T. LANSBURY. 2000. Fibrils formed in vitro from α-synuclein and two mutant forms linked to Parkinson's disease are typical amyloid. Biochemistry. 39: 2552–2563.

17. KOCISKO, D.A., P.T. LANSBURY & B. CAUGHEY. 1996. Partial unfolding and refolding of the scrapie-associated prion protein (PrPSc). Biochemistry **35:** 13434–13442.
18. NORDSTEDT, C., J. NASLUND, L.O. TJERNBERG, *et al.* 1994. The Alzheimer Aβ peptide develops protease resistance in association with its polymerization into fibrils. J. Biol. Chem. **269:** 30773–30776.
19. CONWAY, K.A., S.J. LEE, J.C. ROCHET, *et al.* 2000. Acceleration of oligomerization, not fibrillization, is a shared property of both α-synuclein mutations linked to early-onset Parkinson's disease: implications for pathogenesis and therapy. Proc. Natl. Acad. Sci. USA **97:** 571–576.
20. WONG, S.S., *et al.* 1998. Carbon nanotube tips, high-resolution probes for imaging biological systems. J. Am. Chem. Soc. **120:** 603–604.

Classification and Description of Frontotemporal Dementias

D. NEARY,[a,c] J.S. SNOWDEN,[a] AND D.M.A. MANN[b]

[a]*Department of Neurology, Manchester Royal Infirmary, M13 9WL, UK*

[b]*Department of Pathological Sciences, University of Manchester M13 9PT, UK*

ABSTRACT: A number of distinct clinical syndromes have been described that are associated with focal degeneration of the frontal and temporal lobes and have a non-Alzheimer pathology. The nosological status of frontotemporal lobar degeneration (FTLD) has been a matter of controversy, in view of the diversity of clinical manifestations and distribution and nature of histopathological change. This paper describes the major clinical syndromes of frontotemporal dementia, progressive aphasia, and semantic dementia; it discusses their underlying pathologies and considers their molecular status. Common histopathological changes are demonstrated across the three clinical syndromes, highlighting the link between these clinical disorders. It has been suggested that these disorders should be regarded as tauopathies on the basis of the tau pathology seen in a number of cases and the mutations in the tau gene in some familial cases. However, in a series of 47 consecutive autopsy series of FTLD, only 36% had tau pathology and 10% mutations in the tau gene, suggesting that FTLD does not constitute a unitary etiological disorder and that its characterization as a tauopathy may be potentially misleading.

INTRODUCTION

Focal degeneration of the frontotemporal lobes is a relatively common cause of dementia accounting for about 20% of cases of dementia with presenile onset. It gives rise to a variety of clinical syndromes, depending upon the distribution of pathological change within the anterior cerebral hemispheres. The most common syndrome is the behavioral disorder of frontotemporal dementia,[1,2] in which there is bilateral atrophy of the frontal and anterior temporal lobes. Other distinctive syndromes are progressive nonfluent aphasia,[3] in which there is asymmetric involvement of the left anterior hemisphere and semantic dementia[4,5] occurring in association with circumscribed atrophy of the temporal lobes. These prototypical syndromes may be complicated by the development of the amyotrophic form of motor neuron disease.[6,7] The underlying pathology is distinct from that of Alzheimer's disease. There are three main histological types: microvacuolar type, Pick type or motor-neuron disease type.[8] The major prototypical clinical syndromes and their pa-

[c]Address for correspondence: D. Neary, M.D., Professor of Neurology, Department of Neurology, Manchester Royal Infirmary, Manchester M13 9WL, UK. Tel.: 44-(0)161-276-4149; fax: 44-(0)161-276-4681.

e-mail: tross@central.cmht.nwest.nhs.uk

thologies are described, and the nosological status of these focal degenerations of the frontotemporal lobes are considered.

FRONTOTEMPORAL DEMENTIA

Frontotemporal dementia (FTD) typically presents between 45 and 65 years of age, although it may occur more rarely in young adults and the elderly.[9] It affects men and women equally, and a positive family history is found in nearly half of the cases. The clinical presentation is one of profound alteration in social conduct and personality. Patients rapidly become incapable of managing their own affairs and lose their jobs through irresponsibility and impaired judgment. Patients show a dearth of purposive, constructive activity, and they neglect personal hygiene and social and occupational responsibilities. Patients exhibit a blunted or fatuous affect, a lack of sympathy for and empathy with others, and a total lack of concern and insight into their altered mental state. Behavioral changes include mental rigidity, inflexibility, and stereotyped, repetitive behaviors. The latter may range from simple repetitive actions such as grunting, hand rubbing, or foot tapping to complex rituals surrounding activities of daily living. Wandering and pacing are common, often involving a fixed route. Altered eating habits are a salient feature. These may consist of gluttony, food cramming, and a changed preference for sweet foods. Oral exploration of nonedible objects may occur, although typically only in the late stages. Utilization behavior may also be present.

The form of the character change is not uniform across patients. Some patients are disinhibited, overactive and restless, and may clown, pun, sing, and dance. Others are apathetic and inert, lacking in drive and initiative, and showing little response to stimuli. In others, stereotypic, ritualistic behaviors are the dominant clinical feature. Such patients may develop elaborate rituals for dressing or toileting, will adhere to a rigid daily routine, and may be unwilling, for example, to walk on cracks in the pavement.

Speech in FTD is economical, particularly in apathetic patients, although generally linguistically correct. Characteristic features that help to distinguish FTD from Alzheimer's disease include concreteness of thought, echolalia, perseverative responses, and stereotyped use of words and phrases. Mutism invariably ensues later in the disease. Spatial skills remain well preserved, another important feature in distinguishing FTD from Alzheimer's disease. Patients can locate and manipulate objects and can negotiate familiar environments even in late-stage disease. Formal neuropsychological assessment reveals the most profound abnormalities on tasks sensitive to frontal lobe dysfunction, which make demands on abstraction, planning, and self-regulation of behavior. Such tasks elicit a marked concreteness of thought, perseveration, an inability to shift mental set, and strategic, organizational and sequencing difficulties. Performance may, however, be impoverished across a wide spectrum of tests as a secondary result of patients' inattentiveness, impersistence, cursory mode of responding, and unconcern. Memory failures result from frontal executive deficits of poor organizational and retrieval strategies rather than a primary amnesia.

Neurological signs are minimal and in the early stages are confined to primitive reflexes. Akinesia and rigidity emerge typically late in the disease, although they may be relatively early features in patients with a stereotypic presentation of the disorder. The electroencephalogram is normal. Structural imaging reveals cerebral atrophy, and preferential involvement of the frontal and anterior temporal lobes is typically demonstrable on magnetic resonance imaging. SPECT shows selective abnormalities in the frontal and temporal lobes. Although abnormalities are bilateral, there may some asymmetry with more affection of the left or right frontal lobe.

PROGRESSIVE NONFLUENT APHASIA

The demographic features of progressive aphasia (PA) are similar to those of FTD.[9] In this form of lobar degeneration, a progressive decline in language expression occurs in the relative absence of other cognitive deficits. Speech is nonfluent, effortful, and may have a stuttering quality. Word retrieval difficulties are prominent, and there are sound-based (phonemic paraphasic) errors. The ability to repeat, to produce overlearned series such as the days of the week, to read aloud, write and spell, are also affected, and written output has a telegrammatic quality mirroring the spoken output. Spoken and written comprehension is relatively preserved, at least at the single-word level, and patients may retain insight into their language disorder. This, together with the fact that non-language cognitive skills, including visual perception, spatial abilities, and memory function are strikingly preserved, means that patients may continue in productive employment for many years after onset of symptoms. With progression of disease, patients become mute and the development of gestural dyspraxia renders communication virtually impossible. There is a gradual deterioration in comprehension skills over the course of the illness.

Social skills are typically extremely well preserved in the early stages, although behavioral changes akin to FTD may emerge late in the disease. Neurological signs are usually absent, although progressive asymmetric akinesia and rigidity may emerge. Electroencephalography is normal. Structural brain imaging reveals atrophy of the left cerebral hemisphere. Left perisylvian hypometabolism is seen on functional imaging.

SEMANTIC DEMENTIA

Demographic features of semantic dementia are similar to those for FTD.[9] The disorder is characterized by a loss of understanding of the meaning of sensory stimuli, despite preserved perception of those stimuli. Typically patients present with anomia and lack of comprehension of both spoken and written words. Speech is fluent, effortless, grammatically correct and without phonological errors, but empty of content and there are semantic paraphasias (e.g., "dog" for "camel"). Repetition, reading aloud, and writing to dictation of regularly spelled words are essentially intact, reflecting preservation of phonological and articulatory skills. The pattern of language disturbances closely resembles the transcortical sensory aphasia of focal lesions. Failure to recognize the significance of objects and the identity of faces occurs despite a preserved ability to copy accurately and match objects and faces. In contrast to Alzheimer's disease, visuospatial skills are invariably normal. Moreover, day to day memorizing is well preserved, so that patients maintain a degree of functional independence that would be impossible in AD. Behavioral alterations occur, which have a compulsive and stereotypic quality: patients clockwatch, adhere to a rigid behavioral routine, and become preoccupied by a limited range of activities.

With progression of the disease, a systematic deterioration occurs in the patients' understanding of words. Patients' conversational repertoire becomes increasingly contracted and stereotyped until only a few verbal stereotypies remain. Patients eventually become mute. At no time is speech output effortful or nonfluent. Patients also have increasing difficulty recognizing objects, nonverbal sounds and other sensory stimuli, so that they become severely functionally incapacitated. Behavior is repetitive and stereotyped.

Neurological signs are minimal as for FTD. The electroencephalogram is normal throughout the disease. Prominent temporal lobe atrophy is detected by MR imaging, with relative preservation of hippocampi, and functional imaging shows temporal lobe dysfunction. The relative prominence of the semantic disorder for verbal and visual material reflects the relative involvement of left and right temporal lobes demonstrated on neuroimaging.

LOBAR DEGENERATION AND MOTOR NEURON DISEASE

The clinical syndromes of frontotemporal lobar degeneration may occasionally be complicated by the amyotrophic form of motor neuron disease. Typically, the neurological symptoms and signs commence after the development of the dementia and lead to death within three years from respiratory complications. Electrophysiological studies demonstrate widespread denervation of muscles. The association with motor neuron disease (MND) reinforces the link between the distinct clinical syndromes of FTLD.

NEUROPATHOLOGY OF FTLD

In FTD there is typically bilateral and relatively symmetrical atrophy of the frontal and anterior temporal lobes and degeneration of the striatum.[9,10] In overactive, disinhibited patients, the orbitomedial frontal lobes are preferentially affected with relative sparing of the dorsolateral frontal convexity. Inert, apathetic patients, in contrast, have severe atrophy extending into the dorsolateral frontal cortex. In the minority of patients in whom markedly stereotyped behavior predominates, the brunt of the pathology is borne by the striatum with usually severe limbic involvement, but variable cortical and nigral involvement.

In PA, atrophy is markedly asymmetrical, being slight on the right but gross on the left side, particularly affecting frontotemporal, frontoparietal, and lateral parietooccipital regions. The left anterior temporal cortex shows "knife-edge" atrophy. The pattern of atrophy involves the hippocampus, amygdala, the caudate, putamen, globus pallidus, and thalamus on the left side alone. In semantic dementia, the temporal lobes are severely atrophied, in particular, the middle and inferior temporal gyri with preservation of the superior temporal gyrus, parietal and occipital cortices. The frontal lobes are moderately atrophied as are the corpus striatum, globus pallidum, and thalamus. Although bilateral, the temporal atrophy may be asymmetric, the left- and right-hemisphere predominance reflecting the prominence, respectively, of verbal and visual semantic disorder. In patients with MND, cortical atrophy is less marked than in those without MND, presumably reflecting the shorter duration of illness. In FTD/MND, atrophy is mostly frontal chiefly involving the orbitomedial rather than dorsolateral regions. The striatum is less affected than in FTD alone.

Three characteristic histological patterns are seen. The most common histological change is loss of large cortical nerve cells (chiefly from layers III and V), and a spongiform degeneration or microvacuolation of the superficial neuropil (layer II); gliosis is minimal and restricted to subpial regions; layers II and V show no gliosis. No distinctive changes (swellings or inclusions) within remaining nerve cells are seen. The limbic system and the striatum are affected but to a much lesser extent.

The second and less common histological process (Pick type) is characterized by a loss of large cortical nerve cells with widespread and abundant gliosis, but minimal or no spongiform change or microvacuolation. Swollen neurons or inclusions that are both tau and ubiquitin positive are present in some cases, and the limbic system and striatum are more seriously damaged. The two differing histologies nevertheless share a similar distribution within the frontal and temporal cortex. In all cases, the pathological hallmarks of Alzheimer's disease and Lewy body disease are absent.

In patients with lobar degeneration and MND, the histology is typically although not invariably of the microvacuolar type, with loss of large cortical nerve cells, microvacuolation, and mild gliosis. Limbic involvement is slight, though nigral damage is severe with heavy loss of pigmented nerve cells and intense reactive fibrous astrocytosis. Ubiquitinated, but not tau-immunoreactive, inclusions are present within the frontal cortex and hippocampus (dentate gyrus). In the brain stem, the hypoglossus nucleus shows atrophy with loss of neurons. Large Betz cells of the precentral gyrus are largely preserved in number, and there is no obvious demyelination within the corticospinal tracts. Within the anterior horn cells a gross loss of neurons is found at all levels, and many of the surviving anterior horn cells contain large pale ubiquitinated inclusions within the cytoplasm. No Lewy or Pick-type inclusions are typically observed in any cortical or subcortical neurons.

The microvacuolar spongiform type of histological change is most commonly seen, particularly in patients with PA and semantic dementia.

MOLECULAR CLASSIFICATION OF FTLD

Mutations in the tau gene on chromosome 17 have been identified in some familial cases of FTD.[11] In our series of 47 cases of FTLD,[12] encompassing 27 cases of FTD, 7 of PA, 3 of semantic dementia, 9 of FTD + MND, and 1 PA + MND, splice-site mutations were detected in 6 familial FTD cases only, all of whom had the microvacuolar form of histology. Tau pathology in the brain was evidenced by the presence of insoluble tau in the form of neurofibrillary tangles (6 cases with splice-site mutations) or Pick bodies (11 cases: 9 with FTD, 1 with PA, and 1 with PA + MND).

All remaining patients (64% of cases), including all 9 cases of FTD + MND and 3 cases of semantic dementia were completely without tau pathological changes. These findings suggest that mutations in tau represent only a minority of cases and that not all cases of FTLD are tauopathies.

CONCLUSION

FTLD encompasses a clinically heterogeneous group of syndromes, determined by the distribution of pathological change within the brain. The syndromes share common histologies, reinforcing their etiological link. However, cases of FTLD do not have a common molecular basis. Although tau pathology is seen in a minority of cases and splice-site and missense mutations in the tau gene are present in some familial cases, a majority of cases show a total absence of tau pathology. These include cases in which FTD is combined with MND. The data illustrate the need for caution in assuming a single molecular substrate for these conditions and highlight the importance of defining patients on clinical, anatomical, histological, as well as molecular biological, grounds in order to help unravel the nosology of these disorders.

REFERENCES

1. GUSTAFSON, L. 1987. Frontal lobe degeneration of non-Alzheimer type. II. Clinical picture and differential diagnosis. Arch. Gerontol. Geriatrica **6**: 209–223.
2. NEARY, D., J.S. SNOWDEN, B. NORTHEN, *et al.* 1988. Dementia of frontal lobe type. J. Neurol. Neurosurg. Psychiatry **51**: 353–361.
3. MESULAM, M.-M. 1982. Slowly progressive aphasia without generalized dementia. Ann. Neurol. **11**: 592–598.
4. SNOWDEN, J.S., P.J. GOULDING & D. NEARY. 1989. Semantic dementia: a form of circumscribed cerebral atrophy. Behav. Neurol. **2**: 167–182.
5. HODGES, J.R., K. PATTERSON, S. OXBURY, *et al.* 1992. Semantic dementia. Progressive fluent aphasia with temporal lobe atrophy. Brain **115**: 1783–1806.
6. NEARY, D., J.S. SNOWDEN, D.M.A. MANN, *et al.* 1990. Frontal lobe dementia and motor neuron disease. J. Neurol. Neurosurg. Psychiatry **53**: 23–32.
7. CASELLI, R.J., A.J. WINDEBANK, R.C. PETERSEN, *et al.* 1993. Rapidly progressive aphasic dementia and motor neuron disease. Ann. Neurol. **33**: 200–207.
8. THE LUND AND MANCHESTER GROUPS. 1994. Consensus statement. Clinical and neuropathological criteria for fronto-temporal dementia. J. Neurol. Neurosurg. Psychiatry **4**: 416–418.
9. SNOWDEN, J.S., D. NEARY & D.M.A. MANN. 1996. Frontotemporal lobar degeneration: frontotemporal dementia, progressive aphasia and semantic dementia. Churchill Livingstone. London.
10. MANN, D.M.A., P. SOUTH, J.S. SNOWDEN, *et al.* 1993. Dementia of frontal lobe type: neuropathology and immunohistochemistry. J. Neurol. Neurosurg. Psychiatry **56**: 605–614.
11. HUTTON, M., C.L. LENDON, P. RIZZU, *et al.* 1998. Coding and 5' splice mutations in tau associated with inherited dementia (FTDP-17). Nature **393**: 702–705.
12. MANN, D.M.A, A.M. MCDONAGH, J.S. SNOWDEN, *et al.* 2000. Molecular classification of the dementias. Lancet **355**: 626.

Progress in Hereditary Tauopathies: A Mutation in the *Tau* Gene (G389R) Causes a Pick Disease-like Syndrome

BERNARDINO GHETTI,[a,e] JILL R. MURRELL,[a] PAOLO ZOLO,[b] MARIA GRAZIA SPILLANTINI,[c] AND MICHEL GOEDERT[d]

[a]*Indiana University, Indianapolis, Indiana, USA*
[b]*San Donato Medical Center, Arezzo, Italy*
[c]*University of Cambridge, Cambridge, United Kingdom*
[d]*Medical Research Council, Cambridge, United Kingdom*

ABSTRACT: We describe the clinical and pathologic phenotypes of the G389R mutation in exon 13 of the *Tau* gene. Progressive aphasia and memory disturbance are the initial signs and begin in the fourth or fifth decade of life, followed by apathy, indifference, hyperphagia, rigidity, pyramidal signs and dementia. Death occurs after two to five years. Magnetic resonance imaging and neuropathologic studies show frontal and temporal atrophy. Pick body-like and axonal filamentous inclusions found in the neocortex and subcortical white matter, respectively, are tau immunoreactive. Immunoblot analysis of sarkosyl-insoluble tau shows two major bands of 60 and 64 kDa that, upon dephosphorylation, resolve into four bands of three- and four-repeat isoforms. Isolated tau filaments are often straight and occasionally twisted. Recombinant mutant tau protein shows a reduced ability to promote microtubule assembly, suggesting that this may be the primary effect of the mutation. The present findings indicate that the G389R mutation in *Tau* can cause a dementia similar to that in Pick's disease.

INTRODUCTION

Recent work has shown that mutations in *Tau* cause familial frontotemporal dementia and parkinsonism linked to chromosome 17 (FTDP-17).[1–16] Known *Tau* mutations are either intronic, located close to the splice-donor site of the intron following exon 10, or missense, deletion and silent mutations in the coding region. Four intronic mutations have been described in FTDP-17 at positions +3, +13, +14, and +16 of the intron following exon 10 of *Tau,* with the first nucleotide of the splice-donor site taken as +1.[2,3] The S305N mutation in exon 10 is also located close to this splice-donor site.[7] All five mutations destabilize a stem-loop structure located at the exon 10-intron boundary, leading to inclusion of exon 10 in the final tau transcript and resulting in the overproduction of tau isoforms with four repeats.[2,3,9,12,17–20] Where analyzed, these mutations lead to a tau pathology consisting of wide twisted

[e]Address for correspondence: Bernardino Ghetti, M.D., Department of Pathology and Laboratory Medicine, Division of Neuropathology, Indiana University School of Medicine, 635 Barnhill Drive, MS A142, Indianapolis, IN 46202. Tel.: (317) 274-7818; fax: (317) 274-4882.
e-mail: bghetti@iupui.edu

ribbons made of four-repeat tau isoforms that are present in neurons and glia.[9,15,21,22] Coding region mutations are missense, deletion or silent. Experimental studies have shown that most of these mutations reduce the ability of tau to interact with microtubules,[16,23,24] whereas others influence splicing in of exon 10.[5,12,15,18,19] Moreover, several missense mutations also stimulate heparin-induced assembly of tau into filaments.[25,26] Coding region mutations are concentrated in the microtubule-binding repeat region, where they are located in exons 9 (G272V), 10 (N279K, L284L, ΔK280, P301L, P301S, S305N), and 12 (V337M). The mutations in exon 10 that reduce the ability of tau to interact with microtubules lead to a pathology made of narrow twisted ribbons that consist predominantly of four-repeat tau isoforms and are found in neurons and glial cells.[23,27,28] By contrast, the missense mutations located outside exon 10 that have been examined lead to a neuronal tau pathology made of Alzheimer-type paired helical and straight filaments that consist of all six tau isoforms.[16,29]

To date, only one mutation (R406W) has been described in exon 13 which is located outside the microtubule-binding repeats.[2,16] We are studying a familial form of frontotemporal dementia in an Italian family with a missense mutation in exon 13 of *Tau*.[30] It changes glycine residue 389 to arginine (G389R). Neuropathologically, this tauopathy is characterized by large numbers of Pick body-like inclusions and an extensive filamentous tau pathology in axons. Tau filaments are straight or twisted and contain three- and four-repeat tau isoforms. The straight filaments closely resemble the straight filaments found in Alzheimer's disease and in tauopathies with the V337M and R406W mutations. By contrast, the twisted filaments differ from the paired helical filaments of Alzheimer's disease.

RESULTS

Family History and Clinical Studies

Three members of this Italian family are known to have suffered from dementia; they are the proband, his paternal uncle, and his paternal grandfather. Their disease was characterized by personality changes, deterioration of social skills, apathy, aphasia, hyperactivity, memory disturbance, apraxia and other features of dementia that were accompanied by extrapyramidal and pyramidal signs. The presenting symptoms were consistent with damage to the prefrontal and temporal cortices.

The proband showed initial signs of cognitive dysfunction at 38 years of age. The initial complaints were memory disturbance related to his professional activities and language disturbance manifesting as anomia. Over the ensuing months, the language difficulties became more severe and apathy, indifference, and inertia became apparent.

Early in the course of the disease, the patient's score on the Mini-Mental State Examination (MMSE) was significantly lower than the normal range (10/30). Language abilities were evaluated with the Aachener Aphasie Test (AAT) and the patient's deficits were classified as Wernicke aphasia with prevalent disturbances in comprehension and naming. Repetition was relatively well preserved. There was a severe deficit of verbal fluency in the analysis of semantic categories with semantic intrusions and perseverations. Short-term memory was tested in order to assess verbal and visual-spatial memory. The Wechsler Memory Scale (WMS) gave a score of 62/100, and the Buschke-Fuld test for verbal learning showed a complete lack of performance. Visual-spatial learning tested by the Rey complex figure showed the following scores: 28/36 for simple copying, 12/36 for memory reproduction, and 42/100 for recall. Perception tested with Benton's visual discrimination test showed a borderline performance with a score of 26/32.

Serial magnetic resonance image (MRI) studies showed: (i) a moderate atrophy localized to the left frontal and temporal operculi and the insular cortex, (ii) a moderate bilateral atrophy of hippocampal formation and a dilatation *ex vacuo* of the temporal horn of the left ventricle, (iii) a moderate atrophy of the anterior third of the left parahippocampal gyrus and the inferior medial and superior temporal gyri, (iv) moderate dilatation of the third ventricle and lateral ventricles, and (v) a hypodensity of the left insular subcortical white matter.

Eight months after the initial evaluation, the patient's MMSE score was 7/30, and he showed lower than normal scores on the Wechsler Adult Intelligence Scale (WAIS). One year after the initial evaluation, the patient became completely aphasic and his behavior deteriorated dramatically. A neuropsychological evaluation was repeated at which no verbal production could be elicited. The activities of daily living were reduced to a few routines, such as self-dressing and sphincteric control. The patient showed perseverations, hyperphagia, and nonfinalized hyperactivity.

A MRI performed three years after onset showed a severe bilateral symmetric atrophy of the temporal and frontal lobes and of the hippocampal formation, with dilatation of the Sylvian and perihippocampal fissures, as well as a knife-edge appearance of the cerebral gyri in several regions and an increased depth of cerebral sulci. A dilatation *ex vacuo* of the lateral ventricles and the third ventricle was present, as was a marked atrophy of the corpus callosum. The MRI also showed a hyperintensity of the frontal insular and temporal subcortical white matter, the posterior arms of the internal capsules, and the corticospinal tracts down to the brain stem with atrophy of the pyramids (Wallerian degeneration). At this time examination showed marked rigidity, hyperreflexia of all four limbs, clonus of the wrists, persistent contracture of the masseters with bruxism, postural and kinetic tremor of upper limbs, bilateral grasping following palmar stimulation and incontinence.

By the fourth year, the rigidity had worsened and the patient presented with automatic movements of the limbs and bruxism. On subsequent examination, he showed spastic hypertonus with clonus of wrists, patella, and ankles. Tendon reflexes were hyperactive with clonus, and there was a Babinski sign bilaterally. Later that year, the patient showed accentuation of the spasticity, opisthotonus, dysphagia, and continuous bruxism. By the fifth year, he was tetraplegic with hypothonus on the right and spastic hypothonus on the left. The patient died in the fifth year of symptoms.

Genetic Analysis

Sequencing of the proband's genomic DNA showed wild-type sequence in all exons of *Tau*, with the exception of exon 13, where a G to C transversion was present at codon 389. It changes glycine residue 389 to arginine (G389R). This change was not seen in DNA of 50 individuals from the Indiana University DNA Bank and in DNA of 30 individuals from the region of Italy that the proband originated from. The nucleotide change creates *NciI* and *MspI* restriction sites. When the amplified exon 13 product from the proband was digested with *NciI*, four bands of 338, 236, 102, and 89 base pairs (bp) were observed. Only two bands of 338 and 89 bp were seen in controls. When *MspI* was used for digestion, five bands of 179, 159, 102, 89, and 77 bp were observed in the proband's DNA. Three bands of 179, 159, and 89 bp were seen in controls.

Neuropathology

The proband's brain showed: (i) a severe atrophy of the frontal and temporal lobes with a knife-edge atrophy of the convolutions, (ii) atrophy of the white matter of the centrum semiovale and corpus callosum, (iii) atrophy of the subcortical nuclei, particularly the caudate nucleus, (iv) atrophy of the hippocampus and amygdala, (v) a moderate atrophy of the pons. The lateral and third ventricles were severely dilated. In the midbrain, the substantia nigra showed loss of pigmentation, and the medulla was unremarkable.

Neuronal loss was severe in the frontal, cingulate, temporal, and insular cortices, with relative sparing of parietal and occipital cortices, caudate nucleus, putamen, globus pallidus, and substantia nigra. Spongiosis was present in the second cortical layer and in the lower layers of the temporal cortex. In the cerebellum, a moderate loss of Purkinje cells was observed, while the dentate nucleus was relatively spared. Gliosis was present in grey matter areas in which neuronal loss and spongiosis were most pronounced. In the neocortex, it was most marked in the first, second, fifth, and sixth layers. In the white matter, gliosis was diffuse. It was particularly severe in the frontal and temporal lobes.

By Bodian silver stain, the most prominent changes were Pick body-like inclusions in neurons of the neocortex. They were particularly prominent in the second, fifth, and sixth layers of the frontal, cingulate, temporal, and insular cortices, while they were rare in the occipital cortex. Some neurons of the cortex showed discrete tangle-like, silver-positive deposits. Pick body-like inclusions were also abundant in the fascia dentata. Argentophilia of the cytoplasm of glial cells was only rarely noticed in neocortex and subcortical white matter. Argentophilic neuronal inclusions were infrequent in caudate nucleus, putamen, and thalamus. In the amygdala, numerous nerve cells had intracytoplasmic deposits. In the cerebellum, some Purkinje cells showed axonal torpedoes. No argentophilia was seen in neurons of the substantia nigra, while in the pons, argentophilic inclusions were seen in the raphe nuclei and occasionally in the pontine grey nuclei.

In subcortical white matter of the centrum semiovale, the internal, external, and extreme capsules, as well as within grey matter of subcortical nuclei, argentophilic elongated structures ranging between 4 and 40 μm were observed. They appeared either as long threads or focal axonal swellings, or as dystrophic axons. With the Heidenhain-Woelcke method for myelin, extensive loss of stain was seen. The most severe pallor, resulting from an almost complete loss of myelin, was observed in white matter of the temporal lobe, whereas the pallor observed in the frontal lobe, corpus callosum, and in the internal, external, and extreme capsules was also severe. No loss of myelin was detected in the occipital lobe. In the pons, loss of myelin was severe at the level of the basis pontis and appeared to involve mostly the descending fibers of the corticospinal and corticobulbar tracts, while sparing the transverse bundles of pontocerebellar fibers.

Immunohistochemical studies showed no immunolabeling using a monoclonal antibody against Aβ (10D5) or a polyclonal antibody against α-synuclein. In contrast, strong cytoplasmic immunopositivity was seen in nerve cells using anti-tau antibodies. The latter also stained axonal inclusions in grey matter structures and in the white matter. When comparing adjacent sections that were either immunolabeled with anti-tau antibodies or stained with the Bodian silver stain, immunopositive neurons were more numerous than those showing silver deposits.

To study the tau pathology, phosphorylation-dependent (p), phosphorylation-independent (pi), and dephosphorylation-dependent (dd) anti-tau monoclonal antibodies were used. From the first group (p), we used AT270 (Innogenetics) (1:400), AT8 (Innogenetics) (1:200), AT100 (Innogenetics) (1:400), AT180 (Innogenetics) (1:400), 12E8 (Athena Neurosciences) (1:5,000), PHF-1 (donated by P. Davies) (1:400), and AP422 (1:3,000). These antibodies recognize phosphorylated (p) Thr181 [AT270], pSer202/pThr205 [AT8], pThr212/pSer214 [AT100], pThr231 [AT180], pSer262, and/or pSer356 [12E8], pSer396/pSer404 [PHF1], and pSer422 [AP422]. From the second group (pi), we used Alz50 (donated by P. Davies) (1:250), E10 (donated by A. Delacourte) (1:500), BR134 (1:500), BR304 (1:500), and BR189 (1:500). Alz50 preferentially recognizes a conformation of assembled tau protein. E10 is largely specific for tau isoforms with four repeats. BR134 was raised against amino acids 428–441 of human tau. BR304 and BR189 were raised against amino acids 45–73 and 76–87 of human tau; they are specific for the amino-terminal 29- and 58-amino acids inserts of tau, respectively. From the third group (dd), we used Tau-1 (donated by P. Davies) (1:100), which recognizes an epitope including residues 189–207 of tau.

Using antibody AT8, tau immunopositivity was strong in many regions of the grey and white matter. In the cerebral cortex, especially in the frontal, insular, and temporal regions, the majority of neurons in layer two and many neurons in layers five and six showed strong tau immunoreactivity. In layer two, neurons showed either a diffuse cytoplasmic immunopositivity or the presence of round, well-circumscribed, densely immunolabeled inclusions, resembling Pick bodies. In layers five and six, there were numerous neurons with Pick body-like inclusions and others with diffuse cytoplasmic immunopositivity, which occasionally extended into the main dendritic process. Immunopositive neurons with Pick body-like inclusions were sometimes seen in parietal and occipital cortices. Occasionally, tangle-like inclusions were observed. Pick body-like inclusions were also present in the fascia dentata of the hippocampus. Tau immunopositive neurons were numerous in the amygdala, while they were only occasionally seen in the caudate nucleus, putamen and globus pallidus. No Pick body-like inclusions were seen in these brain regions. Anti-tau immunopositive neuronal perikarya were also present in brain stem, particularly the pons. A small number of neurons in the raphe and pontine nuclei were diffusely tau-positive. Tau immunopositivity of glial cell perikarya was only rarely seen.

Besides perikaryal accumulations of hyperphosphorylated tau, a most striking change was the presence in white matter of fine, elongated, thread-like structures that were reactive with anti-tau antibodies. They were of uneven thickness and sometimes had a beaded appearance. They were strongly labeled with antibody AT8 and were most numerous in the lowest cortical layers, as well as in the adjacent white matter, where they ran tangentially to the cortex. They were abundant in white matter of the centrum semiovale and particularly numerous in white matter of the temporal lobe. They were also present within the internal, external, and extreme capsules. Rarely, these structures were found in white matter of the cerebellar folia and the pons. They were also present in grey matter structures, including cortex, putamen, globus pallidus, and thalamus.

Anti-tau antibodies AT270, AT100, AT180, 12E8, PHF1, AP422, Alz50, BR134, BR304, BR189, and Tau-1 all recognized neurons in a pre-tangle state, as well as Pick body-like inclusions, tangles, and axonal inclusions. AT270, AT100, AT180, 12E8, PHF1, AP422, BR134, and BR304 showed staining similar to AT8, whereas BR189 stained some neurons in a pre-tangle state and Pick body-like inclusions, but only few axonal inclusions. To determine the cellular origin of the tau-positive inclusions, white matter was studied by double-labeling immunohistochemistry using AT8 and SMI 32, an antibody against the high molecular weight neurofilament protein. In some instances, elongated processes were labeled by both AT8 and SMI 32. In most of these, a thin segment labeled with SMI 32 was seen in continuation with a widening segment labeled with AT8.

Tau Extraction, Dephosphorylation, and Immunoblotting

We extracted sarkosyl-insoluble tau from frontal and occipital cortices of the proband. By immunoblotting with anti-tau serum BR134, it resolved into two major bands of 60 and 64 kDa apparent molecular mass and two minor bands of 68 and 72 kDa. Antiserum E10 labeled the 64 kDa band. Antiserum BR304 stained the 64 kDa band, whereas antiserum BR189 failed to label the sarkosyl-insoluble tau bands. When compared with sarkosyl-insoluble tau extracted from Alzheimer's disease brain, the 68 and 72 kDa bands were much weaker. After alkaline phosphatase treatment, sarkosyl-insoluble tau from the proband resolved into four bands that probably corresponded to the three-repeat tau isoforms of 352 and 381 amino acids and the four-repeat tau isoforms of 383 and 412 amino acids. The 410 and 441 amino acid isoforms of human brain tau were not seen. Following alkaline phosphatase treatment, the shortest tau band failed to align with the 352 amino acid recombinant tau isoform, probably because it co-ran with alkaline phosphatase. A similar phenomenon has previously been observed for sarkosyl-insoluble tau extracted from Alzheimer's disease brain.[31] Soluble, dephosphorylated tau extracted from the frontal cortex of the patient resolved into six bands, with a pattern that was indistinguishable from that of soluble tau extracted from the frontal cortex of controls.

Electron Microscopy of Dispersed Filaments

Electron microscopy of preparations of extracted, sarkosyl-insoluble filaments[32] showed filaments with two morphologies. The major species was a straight filament with a twisted stranded sub-structure very similar in appearance to straight filaments in Alzheimer's disease[32] or in the V337M and R406W tauopathies.[16,24] The minor species was an open-looking, low-contrast twisted filament with a crossover spacing of about 120 nm and a projected width varying between about 6 and 23 nm. In the wider parts, the image showed a strong central white stain-excluding axial line flanked by two somewhat weaker stain-excluding lines. Both kinds of filament were strongly labeled by antibodies directed against nonphosphorylated and phosphorylated epitopes of tau. No examples of standard Alzheimer-type paired helical filaments were observed.

DISCUSSION

The G389R mutation in *Tau* causes a syndrome of frontotemporal dementia, beginning in the fourth decade of life and characterized by a rapidly progressing decline of cognitive and behavioral abilities, and severe frontal and temporal atrophy. Histologically, this syndrome is characterized by large numbers of filamentous Pick body-like and axonal inclusions that are made of hyperphosphorylated tau protein.

Shortly after the onset of symptoms, neuroradiological studies revealed atrophy of the frontal and temporal regions. The MRI performed two months after the initial clinical evaluation revealed atrophy of the frontal and temporal structures that was more prominent on the left side, being particularly evident at the level of the superior temporal and parahippocampal gyri. Focal atrophy with predominance of the left temporal lobe has been known ever since the first descriptions of Pick's disease.[33,34] Asymmetry of the atrophy is observed in approximately 60% of these patients, with the atrophy being usually more conspicuous on the left.[35] The clinical, neuropsychological, and imaging investigations of the proband are consistent with a diagnosis of Pick's disease.

The gross neuropathologic findings of the proband's brain showed severe frontal and temporal lobar atrophy, consistent with the brain imaging data and with a clinical diagnosis of Pick's disease. The histopathological findings would also have fulfilled the criteria for this diagnosis, because the Bodian stain revealed a large number of argentophilic intracytoplasmic inclusions that were indistinguishable from Pick bodies. The clinicopathologic concept of Pick's disease is being re-evaluated following the discovery of *Tau* mutations.[1–3] Familial diseases that had previously been identified as hereditary Pick's disease have now been subsumed under the heading of FTDP-17.[2,36–39] So far, more than 15 different mutations have been found in exons 9, 10, 12, and 13 of *Tau*, as well as in the intron following exon 10.[1–16] Neuropathologically, Pick body-like inclusions have been seen in some families with FTDP-17,[9,10,13,14] especially in Dutch family 2 with the G272V in exon 9 of *Tau*.[2,35] The concept of "Pick body"[40] has evolved recently, largely due to the availability of phosphorylation-dependent anti-tau antibodies, such as AT270, AT8, AT180, 12E8, PHF-1, and AT100. These antibodies stain both Pick bodies and the neurofibrillary pathology of Alzheimer's disease. The only exception is antibody 12E8, which stains neurofibrillary lesions but not Pick bodies.[41,42] In the present case, the intracytoplamic inclusions were indistinguishable from Pick bodies when using the Bodian stain and many anti-tau antibodies. However, unlike Pick bodies, they were immunoreactive with 12E8. Previously, the Pick body-like inclusions in Dutch family 2 were found to be 12E8-negative,[39] like the Pick bodies of Pick's disease.[41,42]

Besides Pick body-like inclusions, a second major histological feature of the proband's brain was the presence in white matter of a large number of inclusions of variable length, irregular shape and variable width. These inclusions were argyrophilic and strongly immunoreactive with phosphorylation-dependent anti-tau antibodies. Antibody BR189, which recognizes tau isoforms with the 58 amino acid amino-terminal insert,[31] only labeled a small number of the white matter inclusions. Using double immunolabeling, these inclusions were also labeled with anti-neurofilament antibody SMI 32. By electron microscopy, they were surrounded by a myelin sheath, supporting their axonal nature. Interestingly, in recent years, tau-positive neuropil threads of axonal origin have been recognized as an essential characteristic of Pick's disease.[41,43] We speculate that the axonal inclusions belonged to axons derived from neuronal perikarya containing Pick body-like inclusions. In the proband, Pick body-like inclusions were mostly present in the second, fifth, and sixth cortical layers. The neurons of the second layer are small pyramidal cells from which cortico-cortical fibers originate; these fibers may have contained the axonal inclusions found subcortically in the vicinity of the lowest cortical layers. The neurons of the fifth and sixth cortical layers provide corticospinal fibers, as well as cortico-cortical, callosal, and corticothalamic fibers. These fibers may have contained the axonal inclusions found in deeper white matter and in the corpus callosum.

Immunoblotting of sarkosyl-insoluble tau extracted from cerebral cortex of the proband showed two strong bands of 60 and 64 kDa and two weak bands of 68 and 72 kDa. This pattern is reminiscent of that found in Pick's disease[44] and differs from that of Alzheimer's disease by the low levels of the 68 and 72 kDa bands. Following dephosphorylation, the sarkosyl-insoluble tau resolved into four bands corresponding to the 352 and 381 amino acid tau isoforms with three repeats, and the 383 and 412 amino acid isoforms with four repeats. The 410 and 441 amino acid isoforms of tau were not seen. This pattern differs from that of Pick's disease, where only three-repeat tau isoforms are present.[45] By contrast, in Alzheimer's disease, all six brain tau isoforms are found in sarkosyl-insoluble tau.[31] It is unclear whether the absence of the 410 and 441 amino acid tau isoforms merely reflected the normally low levels of these isoforms, or whether they were truly excluded from pathological tau.

Tau filaments isolated from cerebral cortex of the proband showed two distinct morphologies. The major species was a straight filament and the minor species a twisted filament. Similar filaments were seen in tissue sections by immunoelectron microscopy, although it was not possible to define their exact morphologies. The straight filament had the same morphology as the straight filament of Alzheimer's disease.[32] However, in the latter disease, straight filaments account for only about 10% of isolated filaments, with paired helical filaments constituting the major species. Alzheimer-type paired helical filaments were not present in sarkosyl-insoluble tau prepared from the proband's cerebral cortex. Instead, small numbers of open-looking twisted filaments with a width of 6–23 nm and crossover spacing of 120 nm were present. Isolated filaments with this morphology have thus far not been described in either sporadic tauopathies or in familial cases with mutations in the *Tau* gene.[28] Electron microscopy on tissue sections from Pick's disease brain has shown a large number of straight filaments and a smaller number of twisted filaments,[43,46–48] further underlining the similarities between Pick's disease and the pathology resulting from the G389R mutation in *Tau*.

Comparison with the characteristics of other cases of FTDP-17 shows that the G389R mutation leads to a unique neuropathological phenotype. Mutations in exon

10 and in the intron following exon 10 produce a neuronal and glial tau pathology consisting of twisted ribbons that are made predominantly of tau isoforms with four repeats.[22,39] By contrast, mutations located in exons 9, 12, and 13 lead to a largely neuronal tau pathology. Where analyzed, the tau filaments are paired helical and straight filaments that are made of all six brain tau isoforms. This has been shown for the V337M mutation in exon 12 and the R406W mutation in exon 13.[16,29]

Biochemically, most coding region mutations lead to a reduced ability of tau to promote microtubule assembly.[6,13,23] The same was found for the G389R mutation, suggesting that a reduced ability of mutant tau to interact with microtubules may be the primary effect of this mutation. Consistent with its location in exon 13, the G389R mutation produced a largely neuronal tau pathology. However, unlike the V337M and R406W mutations,[16,29] the tau filament morphologies and the pattern of sarkosyl-insoluble tau bands differed from those found in Alzheimer's disease and resembled most closely the characteristics of Pick's disease. These findings indicate that depending on the positions of *Tau* missense mutations in exons 12 and 13, and perhaps the nature of these mutations, a filamentous tau pathology ensues that resembles either that of Alzheimer's disease or that of Pick's disease. The mechanisms underlying this exquisite specificity remain to be established. Meanwhile, the present findings indicate that the G389R mutation in *Tau* in the proband causes a dementing disease that is similar to Pick's disease in its clinical, neuroradiological, neuropathological, and biochemical characteristics.

ACKNOWLEDGMENTS

This work was supported by PHS grants AG10133, NS14426 (B.G.), and NS37431 (J.R.M.); U.K. Parkinson's Disease Society (M.G.S.); U.K. Medical Research Council (M.G.).

REFERENCES

1. POORKAJ, P., T.D. BIRD, E. WIJSMAN, *et al.* 1998. Tau is a candidate gene for chromosome 17 frontotemporal dementia. Ann. Neurol. **43:** 815–825.
2. HUTTON, M., C.L. LENDON, P. RIZZU, *et al.* 1998. Association of missense and 5'-splice-site mutations in *tau* with inherited dementia FTDP-17. Nature **393:** 702–705.
3. SPILLANTINI, M.G., J. MURRELL, M. GOEDERT, M.R. FARLOW, A. KLUG & B. GHETTI. 1998. Mutation in the tau gene in familial system tauopathy with presenile dementia. Proc. Natl. Acad. Sci. USA **95:** 7737–7741.
4. DUMANCHIN, C., A. CAMUZAT, D. CAMPION, *et al.* 1998. Segregation of a missense mutation in the microtubule-associated protein tau gene with familial frontotemporal dementia and parkinsonism. Hum. Mol. Genet. **7:** 1825–1829.
5. CLARK, L.N., P. POORKAJ, Z. WSZOLEK, *et al.* 1998. Pathogenic implications of mutations in the tau gene in pallido-ponto-nigral degeneration and related neurodegenerative disorders linked to chromosome 17. Proc. Natl. Acad. Sci. USA **98:** 13103–13107.
6. RIZZU, P., J.C. VAN SWIETEN, M. JOOSSE, *et al.* 1999. High prevalence of mutations in the microtubule-associated protein tau in a population study of frontotemporal dementia in the Netherlands. Am. J. Hum. Genet. **64:** 414–421.
7. IIJIMA, M., T. TABIRA, P. POORKAJ, *et al.* 1999. A distinct familial presenile dementia with a novel missense mutation in the tau gene. Neuroreport **10:** 497–501.

8. MORRIS, H.R., J. PEREZ-TUR, J.C. JANSSEN, *et al.* 1999. Mutation in the tau exon 10 splice site region in familial frontotemporal dementia. Ann. Neurol. **45:** 270–271.
9. GOEDERT, M., M.G. SPILLANTINI, R.A. CROWTHER, *et al.* 1999. Tau gene mutation in familial progressive subcortical gliosis. Nature Med. **5:** 454–457.
10. MIRRA, S.S., J.R. MURRELL, M. GEARING, *et al.* 1999. Tau pathology in a family with dementia and a P301L mutation in tau. J. Neuropathol. Exp. Neurol. **58:** 335–345.
11. BIRD, T.D., D. NOCHLIN, P. POORKAJ, *et al.* 1999. A clinical pathological comparison of three families with frontotemporal dementia and identical mutations in the tau gene (P301L). Brain **122:** 741–756.
12. D'SOUZA, I., P. POORKAJ, M. HONG, *et al.* 1999. Missense and silent tau gene mutations cause frontotemporal dementia with parkinsonism-chromosome 17 type, by affecting multiple alternative RNA splicing regulatory elements. Proc. Natl. Acad. Sci. USA **96:** 5598–5603.
13. BUGIANI, O., J.R. MURRELL, G. GIACCONE, *et al.* 1999. Frontotemporal dementia and corticobasal degeneration in a family with a P301S mutation in tau. J. Neuropathol. Exp. Neurol. **58:** 667–677.
14. NASREDDINE, Z.S., M. LOGINOV, L.N. CLARK, *et al.* 1999. From genotype to phenotype: a clinical, pathological, and biochemical investigation of frontotemporal dementia and parkinsonism (FTDP-17) caused by the P301L tau mutation. Ann. Neurol. **45:** 704–715.
15. DELISLE, M.B., J.R. MURRELL, R. RICHARDSON, *et al.* 1999. A mutation at codon 279 (N279K) in exon 10 of the *Tau* gene causes a tauopathy with dementia and supranuclear palsy. Acta Neuropathol. **98:** 62–77.
16. VAN SWIETEN, J.C., M. STEVENS, S.M. ROSSO, *et al.* 1999. Phenotypic variation in hereditary frontotemporal dementia with tau mutations. Ann. Neurol. **46:** 617–626.
17. HONG, M., V. ZHUKAREVA, V. VOGELSBERG-RAGAGLIA, *et al.* 1998. Mutation-specific functional impairments in distinct tau isoforms of hereditary FTDP-17. Science **282:** 1914–1917.
18. HASEGAWA, M., M.J. SMITH, M. IIJIMA, T. TABIRA & M. GOEDERT. 1999. FTDP-17 mutations N279K and S305N in tau produce increased splicing of exon 10. FEBS Lett. **443:** 93–96.
19. GROVER, A., H. HOULDEN, M. BAKER, *et al.* 1999. 5'-Splice site mutations in tau associated with the inherited dementia FTDP-17 affect a stem-loop structure that regulates alternative splicing of exon 10. J. Biol. Chem. **274:** 15134–15143.
20. VARANI, L., M. HASEGAWA, M.G. SPILLANTINI, *et al.* 1999. Structure of tau exon 10 splicing regulatory element RNA and destabilization by mutations of frontotemporal dementia and parkinsonism linked to chromosome 17. Proc. Natl. Acad. Sci. USA **96:** 8229–8234.
21. REED, L.A., M.L. SCHMIDT, Z.K. WSZOLEK, *et al.* 1998. The neuropathology of a chromosome 17-linked autosomal dominant parkinsonism and dementia ("pallido-ponto-nigral degeneration"). J. Neuropathol. Exp. Neurol. **57:** 588–601.
22. SPILLANTINI, M.G., M. GOEDERT, R.A. CROWTHER, J.R. MURRELL, M.R. FARLOW & B. GHETTI. 1997. Familial multiple system tauopathy with presenile dementia: a disease with abundant neuronal and glial tau filaments. Proc. Natl. Acad. Sci. USA **94:** 4113–4118.
23. HASEGAWA, M., M.J. SMITH & M. GOEDERT. 1998. Tau proteins with FTDP-17 mutations have a reduced ability to promote microtubule assembly. FEBS Lett. **437:** 207–210.
24. DAYANANDAN, R., M. VAN SLEGTENHORST, T.G.A. MACK, *et al.* 1999. Mutations in tau reduce its microtubule binding properties in intact cells and affect its phosphorylation. FEBS Lett. **446:** 228–232.
25. NACHARAJU, P., J. LEWIS, C. EASSON, *et al.* 1999. Accelerated filament formation from tau protein with specific FTDP-17 missense mutations. FEBS Lett. **447:** 195–199.
26. GOEDERT, M., R. JAKES & R.A. CROWTHER. 1999. Effects of frontotemporal dementia FTDP-17 mutations on heparin-induced assembly of tau filaments. FEBS Lett. **450:** 306–311.
27. SPILLANTINI, M.G., T. BIRD & B. GHETTI. 1998. Frontotemporal dementia and parkinsonism linked to chromosome 17: a new group of tauopathies. Brain Pathol. **8:** 387–402.

28. GOEDERT, M., R.A. CROWTHER & M.G. SPILLANTINI. 1998. Tau mutations cause fronto-temporal dementias. Neuron 21: 955–958.
29. SPILLANTINI, M.G., R.A. CROWTHER & M. GOEDERT. 1996. Comparison of the neurofibrillary pathology in Alzheimer's disease and familial presenile dementia with tangles. Acta Neuropathol. 92: 42–48.
30. MURRELL, J.R., M.G. SPILLANTINI, P. ZOLO, et al. 1999. Tau gene mutation G389R causes a tauopathy with abundant Pick body-like inclusions and axonal deposits. J. Neuropathol. Exp. Neurol. 58: 1207–1226.
31. GOEDERT, M., M.G. SPILLANTINI, N.J. CAIRNS & R.A. CROWTHER. 1992. Tau proteins of Alzheimer paired helical filaments: abnormal phosphorylation of all six brain isoforms. Neuron 8: 159–168.
32. CROWTHER, R.A. 1992. Straight and paired helical filaments in Alzheimer disease have a common structural unit. Proc. Natl. Acad. Sci. USA 88: 2288–2292.
33. PICK, A. 1892. Über die Beziehungen der senilen Hirnatrophie zur Aphasie. Prager Med. Wochenschr. 16: 765–767.
34. PICK, A. 1904. Zur Symptomatologie der linksseitigen Schläfenlappenatrophie. Monatsschr. Psychiat. Neurol. 16: 378–388.
35. BINETTI, G., J.H. GROWDON & J.-P.G. VONSATTEL. 1998. Pick's disease. In The Dementias. J.H. Growdon & M.N. Rossor, Eds.: 7–44. Butterworth Heinemann. Boston, MA.
36. SCHENK, V.W.D. 1959. Re-examination of a family with Pick's disease. Ann. Hum. Genet. 23: 325–333.
37. GROEN, J.J. & L.J. ENDTZ. 1982. Hereditary Pick's disease. Second re-examination of a large family and discussion of other hereditary cases, with particular reference to electroencephalography and computerized tomography. Brain 105: 443–459.
38. HEUTINK, P., M. STEVENS, P. RIZZU, et al. 1997. Hereditary fronto-temporal dementia is linked to chromosome 17q21-22: a genetic and clinico-pathological study of three Dutch families. Ann. Neurol. 41: 150–159.
39. SPILLANTINI, M.G., R.A. CROWTHER, W. KAMPHORST, P. HEUTINK & J.C. VAN SWIETEN. 1998. Tau pathology in two Dutch families with mutations in the microtubule-binding region of tau. Am. J. Pathol. 153: 1359–1363.
40. ALZHEIMER, A. 1911. Über eigenartige Krankheitsfälle des späteren Alters. Z. Neurol. Psychiat. 4: 356–385.
41. PROBST, A., M. TOLNAY, D. LANGUI, M. GOEDERT & M.G. SPILLANTINI. 1996. Pick's disease: hyperphosphorylated tau protein segregates to the somatoaxonal compartment. Acta Neuropathol. 92: 588–596.
42. DELACOURTE, A., N. SERGEANT, A. WATTEZ, D. GAUVREAU & Y. ROBITAILLE. 1998. Vulnerable neuronal subsets in Alzheimer's and Pick's disease are distinguished by their tau isoform distribution and phosphorylation. Ann. Neurol. 43: 193–204.
43. MURAYAMA, S., H. MORI, Y. IHARA & M. TOMONAGA. 1990. Immunocytochemical and ultrastructural studies of Pick's disease. Ann. Neurol. 27: 394–404.
44. DELACOURTE, A., Y. ROBITAILLE, N. SERGEANT, et al. 1996. Specific pathological tau protein variants characterize Pick's disease. J. Neuropathol. Exp. Neurol. 55: 159–168.
45. SERGEANT, N., J.P. DAVID, D. LEFRANC, P. VERMERSCH, A. WATTEZ & A. DELACOURTE. 1997. Different distribution of phosphorylated tau protein isoforms in Alzheimer's and Pick's disease. FEBS Lett. 412: 578–582.
46. SHIBAYAMA, H., J. KITOH, Y. MARUI, et al. 1983. An unusual case of Pick's disease. Acta Neuropathol. 59: 79–87.
47. MUNOZ-GARCIA, D. & S.K. LUDWIN. 1984. Classic and generalized variants of Pick's disease: a clinico-pathological, ultrastructural and immunocytochemical comparative study. Ann. Neurol. 16: 467–480.
48. KATO, S. & H. NAKAMURA. 1990. Presence of two different fibril subtypes in the Pick body: an immunoelectron microscopic study. Acta Neuropathol. 81: 125–129.

Molecular Genetics of Chromosome 17 Tauopathies

MICHAEL HUTTON[a]

Mayo Clinic Jacksonville, Jacksonville, Florida, USA

ABSTRACT: The identification of mutations in the gene encoding the micro-tubule associated protein tau in frontotemporal dementia and parkinsonism linked to chromosome 17 (FTDP-17) demonstrated that tau dysfunction can lead to neurodegeneration. At least 11 missense mutations and 1 deletion mutation (ΔK280) have been identified in exons 9–13 that encode the microtubule binding domains of tau. In addition, five mutations have been found close to the 5′ splice site of exon 10. The different FTDP-17 mutations have multiple effects on the biology and function of tau. These varied pathogenic mechanisms likely explain the wide range of clinical and neuropathological features observed in different families with FTDP-17. In addition to the highly penetrant mutations that are found in large families with FTDP-17, a common extended haplotype in the *tau* gene also appears to be a risk factor in the development of the apparently sporadic tauopathy, progressive supranuclear palsy (PSP). The mechanism by which this common variability in the *tau* gene influences the development of PSP is unclear; however, it further suggests a central role for tau in the pathogenesis of several neurodegenerative conditions including Alzheimer's disease (AD).

INTRODUCTION

Abnormal intraneuronal inclusions that consist of the microtubule-associated protein tau are a feature of multiple neurodegenerative diseases including Alzheimer's disease (AD), Pick's disease (PiD), progressive supranuclear palsy (PSP), and corticobasal degeneration (CBD).[1] As a result, these diseases have come to be known as tauopathies. The deposited tau protein is insoluble, hyperphosphorylated, and composed of filaments of varying morphology.[2]

In the normal brain, tau binds to microtubules (MT) and is thought to regulate the assembly, dynamic behavior, and spatial organization of MTs in neurons and probably glial cells.[3–4] In addition, recent studies have demonstrated that tau regulates the axonal transport of organelles including mitochondria.[5] Tau is a soluble protein in the normal brain that exists as six major isoforms generated by alternative splicing (exons 2, 3, and 10). The interaction between tau and tubulin is mediated by four imperfect repeat domains (31–32 residues) encoded by exons 9–12.[6] Alternative splicing of exon 10 gives rise to isoforms with 3 (exon 10–) or 4 (exon 10+) binding domains (3R and 4R tau)[7] (FIG. 1). In adult human brain the ratio of 3R and 4R isoforms is approximately 1:1; in fetal brain, however, only 3R tau is present, demon-

[a]Address for correspondence: Michael Hutton, Mayo Clinic Jacksonville, 4500 San Pablo Road, Jacksonville, FL 32224. Tel.: (904) 953-0159; fax: (904) 953-7370.
e-mail: hutton.michael@mayo.edu

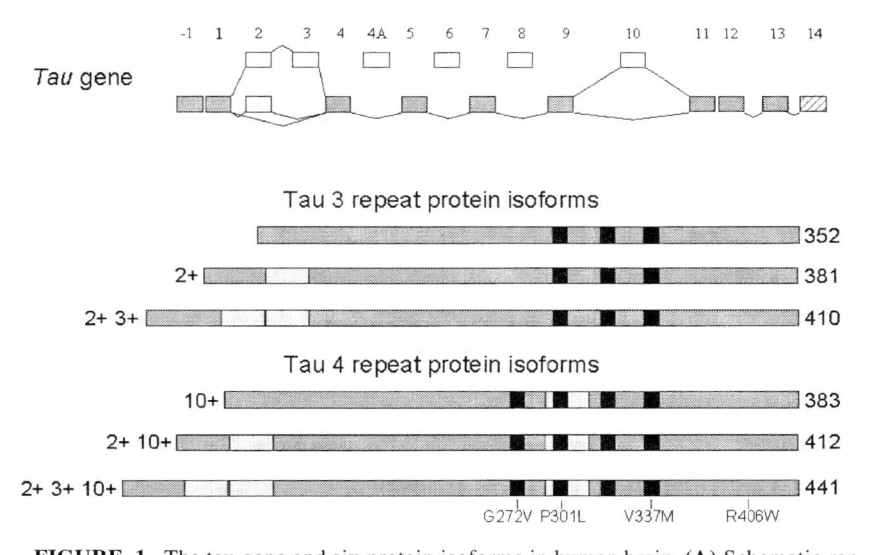

FIGURE 1. The tau gene and six protein isoforms in human brain. **(A)** Schematic representation of the *tau* gene. Alternatively spliced exons 2, 3, and 10 are shown above the constitutive exons. Exons 4A, 6, and 8 are generally not spliced into human *tau* mRNA, and most transcripts retain the intron between exons 13 and 14. **(B)** The six tau isoforms with alternatively spliced exons 2, 3, and 10 indicated by *shaded boxes*. Exons 9–12 encode microtubule binding repeats (*filled boxes*). Alternative splicing of exon 10 gives rise to tau isoforms with 4 (exon 10+) or 3 (exon 10–) binding repeats. Position of FTDP-17 missense mutations in C-terminal region is indicated.

strating developmental regulation of exon 10 splicing. Different brain regions also differ in the relative levels of 3R and 4R isoforms with granule cells in the hippocampal formation reported to have only 3R tau.[7]

IDENTIFICATION OF TAU MUTATIONS IN FTDP-17

FTDP-17[8] is inherited as an autosomal dominant condition characterized by behavioral, cognitive, and motor disturbance; age of onset is usually 45–65 years. At autopsy, patients with FTDP-17 display frontotemporal atrophy with neuronal loss, gray and white matter gliosis, and superficial cortical spongiform change. In addition, intraneuronal tau inclusions are present, with glial inclusions observed in some families.[2,8–13] The morphology and isoform composition of the tau filaments that compose the inclusions is also variable.[2,8–13]

The identification in June 1998 of missense mutations[14–15] and splice site mutations[15–16] in *tau* associated with FTDP-17 established the link between tau dysfunction and neurodegeneration.[14–16] These and subsequent reports have to date identified 11 missense mutations, a deletion of lysine 280 (ΔK280) and five mutations that affect the exon 10 5′ splice site[12–19] in over 50 FTDP-17 families (FIG. 2). All the mutations occur in exons 9–13, which encode the C-terminal part of tau, including the microtubule binding repeats (exons 9–12).

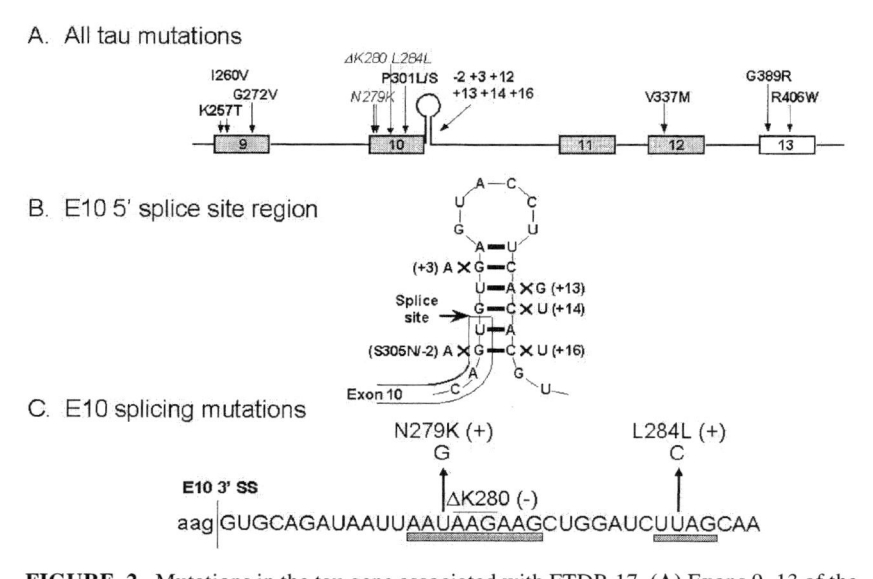

FIGURE 2. Mutations in the tau gene associated with FTDP-17. **(A)** Exons 9–13 of the *tau* gene are shown with mutations indicated. To date all pathogenic mutations have been found in exons 9–13. Eleven missense mutations, a deletion mutation (ΔK280) and five mutations in the 5′ splice site of exon 10 have been identified. Internal exon 10 mutations in italics alter alternative splicing and are shown in detail in panel **C**. **(B)** Mutations in the 5′ splice site of exon 10 [−2(S305N) to +16] are predicted to disrupt a stem-loop that regulates alternative splicing of exon 10. Disruption of the stem-loop is predicted to increase recognition of exon 10 by the U1 snRNP. **(C)** Splicing mutations *within* exon 10 (N279K, ΔK280, and L284L). The N279K and ΔK280 mutations alter a polypurine positive *cis*-element. The N279K mutation strengthens this element resulting in increased exon 10+ RNA whereas the ΔK280 mutation abolishes the polypurine tract and reduces exon 10 splicing. The L284L mutation eliminates a proposed negative regulatory element and thus causes increased incorporation of exon 10 into *tau* mRNA. (+) and (−) symbols beside each mutation indicates its effect on exon 10 splicing.

The identification of mutations in *tau* has largely explained the variability in tau pathology observed in FTDP-17 (TABLE 1).[19] Families with missense mutations (G272V, V337M, R406W) outside exon 10, which affect 3R and 4R tau, have inclusions composed of all six isoforms with filaments that are similar to the paired helical filaments (PHFs) and straight filaments observed in AD.[2,10,11,20] These mutations are usually associated with tau pathology that is predominantly neuronal in distribution.[2,10,11,20] In contrast, families with missense (P301L, N279K) or splice site mutations that affect exon 10, and thus 4R isoforms, have tau inclusions consisting predominantly of 4R tau.[2,10,12,13,17,20] The filaments in these cases are variable, but have a different morphology (often including longer periodicity) than the PHFs that comprise the neurofibrillary tangles observed in AD. These mutations are associated with prominent tau pathology in both neurons and glia.

TABLE 1. Correlation between FTDP-17 mutations and Tau pathology

Mutation type	Mutations	Soluble Tau	Tau Inclusions	Tau Filaments
Missense NOT exon 10	G272V V337M G389R R406W	normal ratio of 4 to 3 repeat	all six isoforms	AD-like PHF
Missense in exon 10	P301L P301S	reduced 4 repeat in affected brain regions**	4 repeat predominates	variable, long periodicity
Exon 10 splice mutations	+3, +13, +14, +16*** N279K*	increased 4 repeat	4 repeat predominates	long periodicity

NOTE: Only mutations with studied Tau neuropathology are presented. Data taken from Refs. 2, 9–13, 16, and 20, and from unpublished data (G389R and E10+13Mutations).
*The N279K missense mutation alters E10 alternative splicing and is thus included with the splice mutations.[20]
**P301L mutation causes the selective incorporation of 4R Tau into inclusions reducing the soluble 4R to 3R ratio, however, this effect is limited to brain regions affected in FTDP-17; unaffected regions have a normal ration in soluble tau.[20]
***Exon10 5' splice site intronic mutations numbered from 3' end of exon 10.

POTENTIAL PATHOGENIC MECHANISMS OF TAU MUTATIONS IN FTDP-17

The Majority of Missense Mutations Disrupt Tau–Microtubule Interactions

The missense mutations identified to date affect the C-terminal region of tau that contains the microtubule binding domains. Consistent with this observation, in vitro studies[18,20–22] have demonstrated that the majority of FTDP-17 missense mutations disrupt tau-microtubule binding. Recombinant 4R tau binding to taxol stabilized microtubule dimers is reduced by the missense mutations (G272V, P301L, P301S, V337M, R406W) and by the ΔK280 deletion mutation. In each case the mutation affects both the affinity of tau (Kd) for microtubules and the binding capacity (βmax).[20] The majority of missense mutations also reduce the ability of tau to polymerize tubulin. The mutations increased the lag time, reduced the rate of polymerization and reduced the total polymerized tubulin formed.[18,20,21] The missense tau mutations P301L, V337M, and R406W were also shown to reduce the ability of transfected CHO cells to form microtubule-filled processes after cytochalasin B treatment.[22] These results are consistent with the majority of missense mutations causing a partial loss of tau-microtubule binding. In contrast, two missense mutations in exon 10 (N279K and S305N) do not affect tau-microtubule binding in similar assays.[20,23] However these mutations are thought to alter the alternative splicing of exon 10 (see below) and thus involve an alternative pathogenic mechanism.

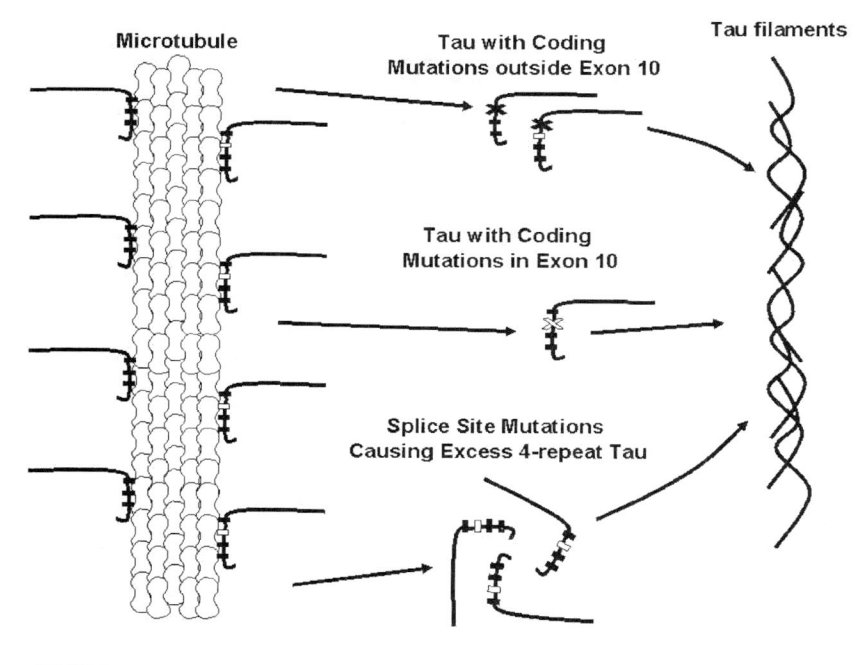

FIGURE 3. Proposed pathogenic mechanism of missense and splicing mutations. The majority of missense mutations inside and outside exon 10 reduce tau binding to microtubules and directly accelerate tau aggregation. Mutations in exon 10 only affect 4R tau while those outside exon 10 affect all isoforms. Splicing mutations (except ΔK280) increase the level of 4R tau which results in neurodegeneration, possibly through an increase in unbound 4R tau or through a direct acceleration in aggregation.

Missense Mutations Alter Tau Polymerization into Filaments

Aggregation studies in which recombinant wild-type and mutant tau is incubated in the presence of either heparin or archidonic acid have indicated that at least some of the FTDP-17 missense mutations are able to accelerate tau filament formation.[24,25] This is consistent with observations that the microtubule binding domains are required for tau self-interaction and the formation of aggregates.[26,27] In the two studies published to date, the P301L and P301S mutations were associated with the greatest increase in filament formation compared to wild-type tau.[24,25] The proportion of FTDP-17 missense mutations that have a significant impact on tau aggregation is unclear; however, the polymerization studies suggest that these mutations potentially have a double pathogenic mechanism that initially involves reduction of microtubule binding and a corresponding increase in unbound tau. Second, the mutations directly increase the tendency of the unbound tau to polymerize into insoluble filaments (FIG. 3). A recent report has further suggested that a third potential pathogenic effect of the missense mutations may be to decrease tau degradration by calpain, further increasing the level of tau available for aggregation.[28]

Mutations that Alter Alternative Splicing of Tau Exon 10
(Missense and 5' Splice Site)

Both intronic and exonic mutations have been described that alter the alternative splicing of exon 10. The largest group of splicing mutations occurs in the intron downstream of exon 10 (at positions +3, +13, +14, and +16 relative to the splice site) and affect recognition of the 5' splice site (FIG. 2).[15,16] Studies of the mechanism of the intronic mutations utilized RT-PCR analysis of FTDP-17 brains and exon trapping to demonstrate that they cause increased recognition of exon 10 and thus increase the ratio of exon 10+ to 10− *tau* mRNA.[15] Analysis of soluble tau from the brains of splice site mutation cases also revealed a preponderance of four repeat tau.[16,20] Examination of the intronic sequence downstream of exon 10 revealed that each mutation is predicted to disrupt a potential stem-loop structure that is thought to be involved in regulating exon 10 alternative splicing by competing with the U1 snRNP for binding to the 5' splice site.[15,16] Stem-loop structures have been implicated in regulating the selection of alternative 5' splice sites[29] and distant branch points[30] and also in tissue-specific splicing of β-tropomyosin exons.[31] However, this is the first time that splicing mutations in a stem-loop have been implicated in human disease.[32]

Analysis of the secondary structure of *in vitro* transcribed RNA demonstrated that a stable stem-loop can form at this position and is disrupted by the intronic mutations.[32,33] In addition, detailed exon trapping analysis using artificial exon 10 constructs with stem-loops of varying stability have produced results that are consistent with alternative splicing being regulated by the predicted stem-loop.[32,33] In contrast, splicing assays in which the effects of stem-loop mutations are rescued by altering the complementary residue on the opposite side of the stem-loop such that base pairing is restored have given variable results.[23,32] This has led to controversy over the significance of the stem-loop.[23,32] An alternative hypothesis is that the intronic mutations disrupt a novel type of negative regulatory element that acts as a recognition sequence for a *trans*-acting splice factor.[23] However, whichever mechanism is involved, it is clear that mutations in the intronic mutations close to the 5' splice site of exon 10 increase the proportion of exon 10+ RNA and 4R tau.

Four other mutations *within* exon 10 have also been demonstrated to alter alternative splicing.[23] Two mutations N279K and ΔK280 have opposite effects on a polypurine element that is a splice enhancer element within exon 10. The N279K mutation[12] strengthens this element (AAUAAGAAG to AAGAAGAAG), which results in an increase in exon 10+ RNA.[20,23] In contrast, the ΔK280 mutation[19] eliminates the polypurine tract (AAUAAGAAG to AAUAAG) resulting in reduced exon 10 splicing; this effect has only been observed using *in vitro* exon trapping assays because brain tissue from a ΔK280 individual is not available.[23] The ΔK280 mutation is interesting because in addition to eliminating exon 10 splicing *in vitro* it also disrupts tau-microtubule binding.[18,23] It is unclear whether the effect of the ΔK280 mutation on splicing or on tau–microtubule interactions is most significant to pathogenesis. Indeed, it is possible that the negative effect of ΔK280 on exon 10 splicing is coincident and even protective in that it reduces the level of the pathogenic ΔK280 mutant 4R tau in the affected brain.

A third mutation in exon 10 that alters alternative splicing is a silent change in codon L284.[2,3] This mutation eliminates a potential negative *cis*-acting splice element (UUAG to UCAG) that lies adjacent to the polypurine positive element altered by N279K and ΔK280.[23] The elimination of this negative splice element causes an increase in exon 10 incorporation and thus an increase in the level of 4R tau (similar to the 5′ splice site and N279K mutations).[23] The fourth internal exon 10 splicing mutation, S305N, alters the −2 residue relative to the 5′ splice site.[23] This residue is predicted to be part of the stem-loop that is disrupted by the 5′ splice site intronic mutations (+3, +13, +14, and +16).[15,16,32] In addition, the S305N(-2) mutation is predicted to directly increase U1 snRNP binding to the 5′ splice site.[23] The combined effect of this mutation is thus to increase the splicing-in of exon 10 and the level of 4R tau.

The identification of mutations that disrupt alternative splicing of exon 10 has revealed three different *cis*-acting splice regulatory elements:[15,16,23,32] (1) a polypurine tract splice enhancer in exon 10; (2) a negative element (possibly UUAG) adjacent to the polypurine tract; and (3) a negative element in the 5′ splice site, which is probably the proposed stem-loop structure. Preliminary data would also suggest that further intronic and exonic *cis*-elements are also present (author's unpublished results). This indicates that regulation of exon 10 alternative splicing is a complex process involving interaction between multiple *cis*- and presumably *trans*-acting factors. This likely explains why there are different ratios of 4R to 3R tau in different brain regions and why during fetal development only 3R tau is produced in the brain; 4R isoforms appear some time after birth.[7]

TAU POLYMORPHISMS IN PSP

In addition to the identification of highly penetrant *tau* mutations in FTDP-17 families, variability in the *tau* gene has also been shown to be a risk factor for another tauopathy, PSP.[34,35] PSP is a rare parkinsonian movement disorder that is associated with early postural instability and supranuclear vertical gaze palsy.[36] The brains of patients display neurofibrillary tangles that are primarily subcortical in distribution. The tau deposited in the tangles is predominantly the 4R isoforms. PSP appears to be a "sporadic" disorder with few familial cases.[36] However, in 1997 an initial study[34] of *tau* variability in PSP demonstrated that one allele (A0) of a dinucleotide polymorphism, between exon 9 and exon 10, was associated with the development of PSP. This association was due to an excess of A0/A0 homozygotes among the PSP cases. Subsequent studies[35] have further shown that this polymorphism is inherited as part of two extended haplotypes (H1 and H2) that extend over the entire *tau* gene (>100 kb). No recombination has been observed between the H1 and H2 haplotypes (FIG. 4).[35] Inheritance of two copies of the common haplotype (H1) in the *tau* gene is strongly associated with the development of PSP (87.5% in PSP cases, 62.8% in controls; $\chi^2 = 13.85$, $p < 0.001$).[35] It is currently unclear, however, which specific polymorphism or combination of polymorphisms within the *tau* H1 haplotype produces the increased risk for the development of PSP.[35] One possibility is that exon 10 splicing is altered in PSP, consistent with the selective deposition of 4R tau; however, no polymorphisms have yet been identified that are likely to alter alternative splicing. Whichever mechanism is involved, these data clearly provide further genetic evidence for a central role for tau in the pathogenesis of PSP.

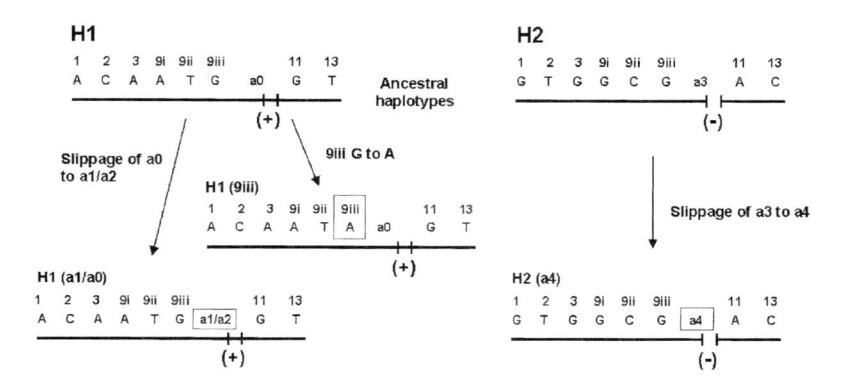

FIGURE 4. Human *tau* haplotypes and association with PSP. Schematic representation of human *tau* gene haplotypes. Ancestral haplotypes H1 and H2 are defined by a series of polymorphisms throughout the tau gene (>100 kb) that are in complete linkage disequilibrium with each other. H1 and H2 have been modified by subsequent mutational events (examples are shown); however, no recombination is observed between H1 and H2 haplotypes (H1–H1 and H2–H2 recombination may occur). +/− symbols indicate a deletion/insertion polymorphism upstream of exon 10. a0–a4 are alleles of the dinucleotide polymorphism between exons 9 and 10. Inheritance of the H1/H1 genotype is a significant genetic risk factor for the development of PSP; however, the critical polymorphism(s) that influence pathogenesis have not yet been identified.

SUMMARY AND CONCLUSIONS

A mixture of missense and splice site mutations in *tau* is the genetic cause of the group of tauopathies known collectively as FTDP-17. This is significant first because this locus is a major cause of autosomal dominant neurodegenerative dementia with 16 mutations in more than 50 families identified to date. In addition, these data have provided clear evidence that tau dysfunction can result in neurodegeneration. In turn, this suggests that tau plays a central, if not primary, role in the pathogenesis of other tauopathies including AD, PiD, PSP, and CBD. Indeed, variability in the *tau* gene has also been shown to be a risk factor for the development of PSP.[34,35]

The identified FTDP-17 mutations have multiple effects on tau biology. The exon 10 splicing mutations (N279K, L284L, and E10 5′ splice site −2 to +16) increase the proportion of exon 10+ mRNA and thus the ratio of 4R to 3R isoforms.[15,16,20,23,32] Increasing the ratio of 4R to 3R tau, by as little as twofold,[15] results in FTDP-17; however, the mechanism by which this shift in ratio leads to neurodegeneration remains unclear. One possibility is that saturation of specific 4R tau binding sites on microtubules causes an increase in unbound tau available for aggregation into filaments (FIG. 3). It is also possible that an increase in 4R tau directly accelerates at least part of the aggregation process *in vivo* (FIG. 3), although it is not clear how this hypothesis fits with current nucleated assembly models of tau aggregation.[37] In contrast, the ΔK280 mutation reduces the proportion of exon 10+ transcripts in exon trapping assays.[23] However, the pathogenic significance of this reduction in exon 10 splicing by ΔK280 remains unclear because pathological findings are not available, and, in addition, this mutation also produces a dramatic reduction in tau-microtubule binding.[18]

In contrast, the majority of missense mutations disrupt the interaction between tau and microtubules.[18,20–22] The disruption of this interaction is expected to increase the level of unbound tau in neurons that is available for aggregation. In addition, at least some missense mutations also appear to directly increase the tendency of tau to self-interact and form filaments.[24,25] The overall effect of the majority of FTDP-17 missense mutations is thus predicted to be an increase in the rate of tau aggregation and eventually the formation of the insoluble tau inclusions that are a feature of FTDP-17.

ACKNOWLEDGMENTS

This work was supported by grants from the NIA, NINDS, the Mayo Foundation, and the Smith-Mayo Scholar Program.

REFERENCES

1. DICKSON, D. 1997. Neurodegenerative diseases with cytoskeletal pathology: a biochemical classification. Ann. Neurol. **42:** 541–543.
2. SPILLANTINI, M.G., T.D. BIRD & B. GHETTI. 1998. Frontotemporal dementia and parkinsonism linked to chromosome 17: a new group of tauopathies. Brain Pathol. **8:** 387–402.
3. DICKSON, D.W., M.B. FEANY, S.H. YEN, L.A. MATTIACE & P. DAVIES. 1996. Cytoskeletal pathology in non-Alzheimer degenerative dementia: new lesions in diffuse Lewy body disease, Pick's disease, and corticobasal degeneration. J. Neural Transm. **47:** 31–46.
4. LOPRESTI, P., S. SZUCHET, S.C. PAPASOZOMENOS, R.P. ZIJNKOWSKI & L.I. BINDER. 1995. Functional implications for the microtubule-associated protein tau: localization in oligodendrocytes. Proc. Natl. Acad. Sci. **92:** 10369–10373.
5. EBNETH, A., R. GODEMANN, K. STAMER, et al. 1998. Overexpression of tau protein inhibits kinesin-dependent trafficking of vesicles, mitochondria, and endoplasmic reticulum: implications for Alzheimer's disease. J. Cell Biol. **143:** 777–794.
6. LEE, G., R.L. NEVE & K.S. KOSIK. 1989. The microtubule binding domain of tau protein. Neuron **2:** 1615–1624.
7. GOEDERT, M., M.G. SPILLANTINI, M.C. POTIER, J. ULRICH & R.A. CROWTHER. 1989a. Cloning and sequencing of the cDNA encoding an isoform of microtubule-associated protein *tau* containing four tandem repeats: differential expression of tau protein mRNAs in human brain. EMBO J. **8:** 393–399.
8. FOSTER, N.L., K. WILHELMSEN, A.A. SIMA, M.Z. JONES, C.J. D'AMATO & S. GILMAN. 1997. Frontotemporal dementia and parkinsonism linked to chromosome 17: a consensus statement. Ann. Neurol. **41:** 706–715.
9. SPILLANTINI, M.G., M. GOEDERT, R.A. CROWTHER, J.R. MURRELL, M.R. FARLOW & B. GHETTI. 1997. Familial multiple system tauopathy with presenile dementia: a disease with abundant neuronal and glial tau filaments. Proc. Natl. Acad. Sci. USA **94:** 4113–4118.
10. SPILLANTINI, M.G., R.A. CROWTHER, W. KAMPHORST, P. HEUTINK & J.C. VAN SWIETEN. 1998. Tau pathology in two Dutch families with mutations in the microtubule-binding region of tau. Am. J. Pathol. **153:** 1359–1363.
11. REED, L.A., T.J. GRABOWSKI, M.L. SCHMIDT, et al. 1997. Autosomal dominant dementia with widespread neurofibrillary tangles. Ann. Neurol. **42:** 564–572.

12. CLARK, L.N., P. POORKAJ, Z. WSZOLEK, et al. 1998. Pathogenic implications of mutations in the tau gene in pallido–ponto-nigral degeneration and related neurodegenerative disorders linked to chromosome 17. Proc. Natl. Acad. Sci. USA **95:** 13103–13107.
13. GOEDERT, M., M.G. SPILLANTINI, R.A. CROWTHER, et al. 1999. Tau gene mutation in familial progressive subcortical gliosis. Nat. Med. **5:** 454–457.
14. POORKAJ, P., T.D. BIRD, E. WIJSMAN, et al. 1998. *Tau* is a candidate gene for chromosome 17 frontotemporal dementia. Ann. Neurol. **43:** 815–825.
15. HUTTON, M., C.L. LENDON, P. RIZZU, et al. 1998. Association of missense and 5′–splice-site mutations in *tau* with the inherited dementia FTDP-17. Nature **393:** 702–705.
16. SPILLANTINI, M.G., J.R. MURRELL, M. GOEDERT, M.R. FARLOW, A. KLUG & B. GHETTI. 1998. Mutation in the *tau* gene in familial multiple system tauopathy with presenile dementia. Proc. Natl. Acad. Sci. USA **95:** 7737–7741.
17. DUMANCHIN, C., A. CAMUZAT, D. CAMPION, et al. 1998. Segregation of a missense mutation in the microtubule-associated protein tau gene with familial frontotemporal dementia and parkinsonism. Hum. Mol. Genet. **7:** 1825–1829.
18. RIZZU, P., J.C. VAN SWIETEN, M. JOOSSE, et al. 1999. High prevalence of mutations in the microtubule-associated protein tau in a population study of frontotemporal dementia in the Netherlands. Am. J. Hum. Genet. **64:** 414–421.
19. HARDY, J., K. DUFF, K.G. HARDY, J. PEREZ-TUR & M. HUTTON. 1998. Genetic dissection of Alzheimer's and related dementias: amyloid and its relationship to tau. Nature Neurosci. **1:** 355–358.
20. HONG, H., V. ZHUKAREVA, W. VOGELSBERG-RAGAGLIA, et al. 1998. Mutation-specific functional impairments in distinct tau isoforms of hereditary FTDP-17. Science **282:** 1914–1917.
21. HASEGAWA, M., M.J. SMITH & M. GOEDERT. 1998. Tau proteins with FTDP-17 mutations have a reduced ability to promote microtubule assembly. FEBS Lett. **437:** 207–210.
22. DAYANANDAN, R., M. VAN SLEGTENHORST, T.G. MACK, et al. 1999. Mutations in tau reduce its microtubule-binding properties in intact living cells. FEBS Lett. **446:** 228–232.
23. D'SOUZA, I., P. POORKAJ, M. HONG, et al. 1999. Missense and silent tau gene mutations cause frontotemporal dementia with parkinsonism-chromosome 17 type, by affecting multiple alternative RNA splicing regulatory elements. Proc. Natl. Acad. Sci. USA **96:** 5598–5603.
24. NACHARAJU, P., J. LEWIS, C. EASSON, et al. 1999. Accelerated filament formation from tau protein with specific FTDP-17 missense mutations. FEBS Lett. **447:** 195–199.
25. GODERT, M., R. JAKES & R.A. CROWTHER. 1999. Effects of frontotemporal dementia FTDP-17 mutations on heparin-induced assembly of tau filaments. FEBS Lett. **450:** 306–311.
26. WILLE, H., G. DREWES, J. BIERNAT, E.M. MANDELKOW & E. MANDELKOW. 1992. Alzheimer-like paired helical filaments and antiparallel dimers formed from microtubule associated protein tau *in vitro*. J. Cell Biol. **118:** 573–584.
27. PEREZ, M., J.M. VALPUESTA, M. MEDINA, E. MONTEJO DE GARCINI & J. AVILA. 1996. Polymerization of τ into filaments in the presence of heparin: the minimal sequence required for τ–τ interaction. J. Neurochem. **67:** 1183–1190.
28. YEN, S., C. EASSON, P. NACHARAJU, M. HUTTON & S.H. YEN. 1999. FTDP-17 tau mutations decrease the susceptibility of tau to calpain digestion. FEBS Lett. **461:** 91–95.
29. DOMENJOUD, L., H. GALLINARO, L. KISTER, S. MEYER & M. JACOB. 1991. Identification of a specific exon sequence that is a major determinant in the selection between a natural and a cryptic 5′ splice site. Mol. Cell. Biol. **11:** 4581–4590.
30. CHEBLI, K., R. GATTONI, P. SCHMITT, G. HILDWEIN & J. STEVENIN. 1989. The 216-nucleotide intron of the E1A pre-mRNA contains a hairpin structure that permits utilization of unusually distant branch acceptors. Mol. Cell. Biol. **9:** 4852–4861.
31. D'ORVAL, B., Y. CARAFA, P. SIRAND-PUGNET, M. GALLEGO, E. BRODY & J. MARIE. 1991. RNA secondary structure repression of a muscle exon in HeLa cell nuclear extracts. Science **252:** 1823–1828.
32. GROVER, A., H. HOULDEN, M. BAKER, et al. 1999. 5′ Splice site mutations in *tau* associated with the inherited dementia FTDP-17 affect a stem-loop structure that regulates alternative splicing of exon 10. J. Biol. Chem. **274:** 15134–15143.

33. VARANI, L., M. HASEGAWA, M.G. SPILLANTINI, *et al.* 1999. Structure of tau exon 10 splicing regulatory element RNA and destabilization by mutations of frontotemporal dementia and parkinsonism linked to chromosome 17. Proc. Natl. Acad. Sci. USA **96:** 8229–8234.
34. CONRAD, C., A. ANDREADIS, J.Q. TROJANOWSKI, *et al.* 1997. Genetic evidence of the involvement of τ in progressive supranuclear palsy. Ann. Neurol. **41:** 277–281.
35. BAKER, M., I. LITVAN, H. HOULDEN, *et al.* 1999. Association of an extended haplotype in the *tau* gene with progressive supranuclear palsy. Hum. Mol. Genet. **8:** 711–715.
36. LITVAN, I. & M. HUTTON. 1998. Clinical and genetic aspects of progressive supranuclear palsy. J. Geriatr. Psychiatry Neurol. **11:** 107–114.
37. FRIEDHOFF, P., M. VON BERGEN, E.M. MANDELKOW, P. DAVIES & E. MANDELKOW. 1998. A nucleated assembly mechanism of Alzheimer paired helical filaments. Proc. Natl. Acad. Sci. USA **95:** 15712–15717.

Tau Gene Mutations in Frontotemporal Dementia and Parkinsonism Linked to Chromosome 17 (FTDP-17)

Their Relevance for Understanding the Neurogenerative Process

MICHEL GOEDERT,[a,d] BERNARDINO GHETTI,[b] AND MARIA GRAZIA SPILLANTINI[c]

[a]*Medical Research Council Laboratory of Molecular Biology, Cambridge, UK*

[b]*Department of Neuropathology, Indiana University School of Medicine, Indianapolis, Indiana, USA*

[c]*Department of Neurology and Brain Repair Centre, University of Cambridge, Cambridge, UK*

ABSTRACT: Tau is a microtubule-associated protein that binds to microtubules and promotes microtubule assembly. Six tau isoforms are produced in adult human brain by alternative mRNA splicing from a single gene. Inclusion of a 31 amino acid repeat encoded by exon 10 of the *tau* gene gives rise to the three isoforms with four microtubule-binding repeats each. The other three tau isoforms have three repeats each. Abundant neurofibrillary lesions made of tau protein constitute a defining neuropathological characteristic of Alzheimer's disease. Filamentous tau protein deposits are also the defining characteristic of other neurodegenerative diseases, many of which are frontotemporal dementias or movement disorders, such as Pick's disease, progressive supranuclear palsy, and corticobasal degeneration. It is well established that the distribution of tau pathology correlates with the presence of symptoms of disease. However, until recently, there was no genetic evidence linking *tau* to neurodegeneration. This has now changed with the discovery of more than 15 mutations in the *tau* gene in frontotemporal dementia and parkinsonism linked to chromosome 17 (FTDP-17). The new work has shown that dysfunction of tau protein causes neurodegeneration.

INTRODUCTION

Arnold Pick provided the first clinical description of frontotemporal dementia in 1892.[1] In 1911, Alois Alzheimer described the neuropathological lesions characteristic of Pick's disease.[2] In the 1960s, these so-called Pick bodies were shown to contain abnormal filaments,[3] which are now known to be made of hyperphosphorylated

---

[d]Address for correspondence: M. Goedert, Medical Research Council Laboratory of Molecular Biology, Cambridge, UK. Tel.: 44-1-223-402036; fax: 44-1-223-402197.
e-mail: mg@mrc-lmb.cam.ac.uk

microtubule-associated protein tau.[4,5] They resemble the neurofibrillary lesions described by Alzheimer in 1907 in the disease subsequently named after him.[6,7]

Frontotemporal dementias occur in familial forms and more commonly as sporadic cases. Neuropathologically, they are characterized by a remarkably circumscribed atrophy of the frontal and temporal lobes of the cerebral cortex, often with additional, subcortical changes. In 1994, an autosomal dominantly inherited familial form of frontotemporal dementia with parkinsonism was linked to chromosome 17q21.2.[8] This was followed by the identification of other familial forms of frontotemporal dementia that are linked to this region, resulting in the denomination frontotemporal dementia and parkinsonism linked to chromosome 17 (FTDP-17) for this class of disease.[9] A major neuropathological characteristic of FTDP-17 is a filamentous pathology made of hyperphosphorylated tau protein.[10] Tau is a microtubule-associated protein that binds to microtubules and promotes microtubule assembly.[7] Tau filaments are space-occupying lesions that may interfere with a host of cellular processes, leading to the degeneration of affected nerve cells and glial cells. Importantly, the *tau* gene maps to the FTDP-17 locus on chromosome 17. Genetic linkage and neuropathology thus made *tau* a strong candidate gene for FTDP-17. The discovery of the *tau* coding region and intronic mutations has shown that the FTDP-17 locus is indeed the *tau* gene.[11–13]

TAU MUTATIONS

In adult human brain, six tau isoforms are produced from a single gene by alternative mRNA splicing (FIG. 1a, A–F).[14–18] They differ from each other by the presence or absence of 29- or 58-amino acid inserts located in the amino-terminal half and a 31 amino acid repeat located in the carboxy-terminal half. Inclusion of the latter, which is encoded by exon 10 of the *tau* gene, gives rise to the three tau isoforms (FIG. 1a, D–F) with four repeats each. The other three isoforms (FIG. 1a, A–C) have three repeats each. In normal cerebral cortex, similar levels of three-repeat and four-repeat tau isoforms are observed. The repeats and some adjoining sequences constitute the microtubule-binding domains of tau.[19,20]

Tau mutations in FTDP-17 are either missense, deletion or silent mutations in the coding region, or intronic mutations located close to the splice-donor site of the intron following the alternatively spliced exon 10 (FIG. 1).[11–13,21–39] Missense mutations are located in the microtubule-binding repeat region or close to it. Mutations in exon 9 (G272V), exons 12 (V337M), and exon 13 (G389R and R406W) affect all six tau isoforms (FIG. 1a). By contrast, mutations in exon 10 (N279K, ΔK280, L284L, P301L, P301S, and S305N) only affect tau isoforms with four microtubule-binding repeats or their expression (FIG. 1a). Most missense mutations reduce the ability of tau to interact with microtubules, as reflected by a marked reduction in the ability of mutant tau to promote microtubule assembly.[23,30,38,40–42] Mutations in exon 10 (ΔK280, P301L, and P301S) produce the largest effects, with intermediate reductions for mutations in exons 9 (G272V) and 12 (V337M), and a smaller reduction for the G389R and R406W mutations in exon 13. Moreover, a number of missense mutations have a direct stimulatory effect on heparin-induced assembly of tau into filaments.[43,44] This effect is particularly marked for the P301L and P301S mutations, with smaller effects for the G272V and V337M mutations. A study using synthetic

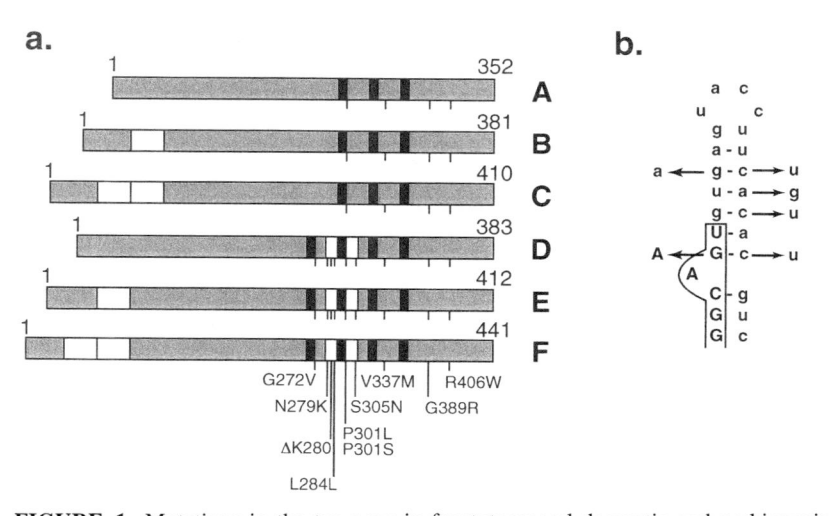

FIGURE 1. Mutations in the tau gene in frontotemporal dementia and parkinsonism linked to chromosome 17 (FTDP-17). (**a**) Schematic diagram of the six tau isoforms (**A–F**) that are expressed in adult human brain. Alternatively spliced exons 2, 3, and 10 are shown in *white; black bars* indicate the microtubule-binding repeats. Eight missense mutations, one deletion mutation, and one silent mutation in the coding region are shown. Amino acid numbering corresponds to the 441 amino acid isoform of human brain tau. (**b**) Stem-loop structure in the pre-mRNA at the boundary between exon 10 and the intron following exon 10. Six mutations that reduce the stability of the stem-loop structure are shown (at positions −1, +3, +12, +13, +14, and +16, with the first nucleotide of the splice-donor site taken as +1). Exon sequences are shown in capital and intron sequences in lower-case letters.

peptides derived from each of the four microtubule-binding repeats of tau has also shown increased heparin-induced filament formation for the P301L mutation in the second repeat.[45]

Intronic mutations are located at positions +3, +12, +13, +14, and +16 of the intron following exon 10, with the first nucleotide of the splice-donor site taken as +1 (FIG. 1b).[12,13,25,26,34,39] Secondary structure predictions have suggested the presence of an RNA stem-loop structure at the exon 10-intron boundary that is disrupted by the intronic mutations.[12,13] In addition, the +3 mutation is predicted to lead to increased binding of U1 snRNA to the 5′ splice site.[13] Exon trapping experiments have shown that intronic mutations increase splicing in of exon 10.[12,26,29,32,39,46,47] Increased production of transcripts encoding exon 10 has also been demonstrated in brain tissue from patients with *tau* intronic mutations.[12,39] This increase is in turn reflected by a change in the ratio of three-repeat to four-repeat tau isoforms, resulting in a net overproduction of four-repeat isoforms.[13,26,34,39,41]

The proposed existence of a stem-loop structure at the boundary between exon 10 and the intron following exon 10 has received support from the determination of the three-dimensional structure of a 25 nucleotide-long RNA (extending from positions −5 to +19) by NMR spectroscopy (FIG. 1b).[46] It has shown that this sequence forms a stable, folded structure. The stem of this exon 10 regulatory element consists of a single G-C base pair that is separated from a double helix of six base pairs by an unpaired adenine. The apical loop consists of six nucleotides that adopt multiple conformations in rapid exchange. The structure differs in several respects from the two proposed representations of the stem-loop.[12,13] Known intronic mutations are located in the upper part of the stem of the *tau* exon 10 regulatory element. All five mutations reduce the thermodynamic stability of the stem-loop structure, but to various extents. The largest drop in melting temperature was observed for the +3 mutation.[46] The +12 and +14 mutations also produced a large reduction in melting temperature, whereas the effects of the +13 and +16 mutations were smaller.[39,46] The aminoglycoside antibiotic neomycin binds to the tau exon 10 regulatory element and markedly increases the thermodynamic stability of both wild-type and mutated elements.[47] The differential reductions in stem-loop stability resulting from the various intronic FTDP-17 mutations were reflected in the magnitude of increased splicing in of exon 10, as revealed by exon trapping.[12,29,39,46,48]

The emerging picture is one of missense mutations that lead to a reduced ability of tau to interact with microtubules and to a stimulatory effect on tau filament assembly, and of intronic mutations whose primary effects are at the RNA level, resulting in an overproduction of tau isoforms with four microtubule-binding repeats. However, two missense mutations in exon 10 (N279K and S305N) deviate from this rule in that they do not lead to a reduction in the ability of tau to promote microtubule assembly.[49] Instead, they increase splicing in of exon 10, as is the case of the intronic mutations.[29,47,49] The N279K mutation (AAT to AAG) in tau creates a purine-rich splice enhancer sequence that explains its effects on exon trapping and soluble four-repeat tau in brain.[22] Similar findings have been obtained with the L284L mutation in exon 10, which is believed to disrupt an exon 10 splicing silencer sequence.[29] The S305N mutation (AGT to AAT) in tau changes the last amino acid in exon 10.[24] This sequence forms part of the predicted stem-loop structure, where the mutation produces a G to A transition at position −1.[46] It is therefore not surprising that the S305N mutation leads to a reduction in the thermodynamic stability of the stem-loop structure and to a marked increase in the splicing in of exon 10.[29,48,49] Like the +3 mutation, the −1 mutation is also expected to lead to increased binding of U1 snRNA to the 5′ splice site. Besides mutations in the intron following exon 10, additional pathogenic mutations may exist in other introns of the *tau* gene. Thus, a G to A transition at position +33 of the intron following exon 9 has been described in a patient with familial frontotemporal dementia.[23] It disrupts one of several (A/T)GGG repeats that may play a role in the regulation of the alternative splicing of exon 10.

NEUROPATHOLOGY

All cases with *tau* mutations that have been examined to date have shown the presence of an abundant filamentous pathology made of hyperphosphorylated tau protein. Strikingly, the morphologies of tau filaments and their isoform compositions appear to be determined by whether tau mutations affect mRNA splicing of exon 10, or whether they are missense mutations located inside or outside exon 10.[50]

Mutations in *tau* that affect splicing in of exon 10 lead to the formation of wide twisted ribbon-like filaments that only contain four-repeat tau isoforms. This has been shown in familial multiple system tauopathy with presenile dementia (MSTD) with the +3 intronic mutation,[13,51] in FTD-Kumamoto with the +12 intronic mutation,[39] as well as in familial progressive subcortical gliosis and Duke family 1684, both with the +16 intronic mutation.[26,34] Similar results have been obtained in pallidopontonigral degeneration with the N279K mutation in exon 10 whose primary effect is at the RNA level.[22,32,35] The same may be true of the families with the L284L and the S305N mutations in exon 10 whose primary effects are also at the RNA level. In all these families, the tau pathology is widespread and present in both nerve cells and glial cells, with an abundant glial component.

Mutations in exon 10 of *tau* that do not affect alternative mRNA splicing lead to the formation of narrow twisted ribbons that contain four-repeat tau isoforms, with a small amount of the most abundant three-repeat isoform. This has been shown in Dutch family 1 and in an American family, both with the P301L mutation.[27,52] Based on electron microscopy of tissue sections, the same also appears to be true of the family with the P301S mutation.[30] At present, no neuropathological information is available for the family with the ΔK280 mutation in exon 10. The P301L, P301S, and ΔK280 mutations all lead to a markedly reduced ability of four-repeat tau to promote microtubule assembly.[23,30,38] The P301L and P301S mutations have no effect on the splicing in of exon 10. By contrast, the ΔK280 mutation leads to reduced splicing in of exon 10,[29] suggesting that its primary effect might be the overproduction of three-repeat tau, and not the reduced ability of four-repeat tau to interact with microtubules. Clarification of this issue must await the availability of frozen brain tissue from an individual with the ΔK280 mutation. In brain tissue from individuals with the P301L and P301S mutations, tau pathology is widespread and present in both nerve cells and glial cells. When compared with mutations that affect the splicing in of exon 10, the glial component appears to be less pronounced.

Coding region mutations located outside exon 10 lead to a tau pathology that is neuronal, without a significant glial component. Some of these mutations lead to the formation of paired helical and straight filaments that contain all six tau isoforms, like the tau filaments of Alzheimer's disease.[53] This has been shown for Seattle family A with the V337M mutation in exon 12 and for a family with the R406W mutation in exon 13.[36,54] In both cases, the morphologies of tau filaments have been found to be indistinguishable from those of Alzheimer's disease. By contrast, the G389R mutation in exon 13 produces tau filament morphologies and a pattern of tau bands that resemble the characteristics of Pick's disease.[38,55,56] Based on light microscopic staining, the G272V mutation in exon 9 leads to the formation of numerous Pick body-like inclusions.[52] These findings indicate that depending on the positions of *tau* missense mutations in exons 9, 12, and 13, and perhaps the nature of these mutations, a filamentous tau pathology ensues that resembles either that of Alzheimer's disease or of Pick's disease.

PATHOGENESIS

The pathway leading from a mutation in the *tau* gene to neurodegeneration is unknown. The likely primary effect of most missense mutations is a reduced ability of mutant tau to interact with microtubules. It may be equivalent to a partial loss of function, with resultant microtubule destabilization and deleterious effects on cellular processes, such as rapid axonal transport. However, in the case of the intronic mutations and the N279K, L284L, and S305N mutations in exon 10, this appears unlikely. The net effect of these mutations is increased splicing in of exon 10, leading to a change in the ratio of three-repeat to four-repeat isoforms, and resulting in the overproduction of four-repeat tau. It is well known that four-repeat tau possesses a greater ability to interact with microtubules than three-repeat tau.[17] It is therefore possible that in cases of FTDP-17 with intronic mutations and those coding region mutations whose primary effect is at the RNA level, microtubules are more stable than in brain from control individuals. Moreover, missense mutations in exon 10 will only affect 20–25% of tau molecules, with 75–80% of tau being normal.

It is possible, however, that a correct ratio of wild-type three-repeat to four-repeat tau is essential for the normal function of tau in human brain. An alternative hypothesis is that a partial loss of function of tau is necessary for setting in motion the mechanisms that will ultimately lead to filament assembly. Earlier work has suggested that three-repeat and four-repeat tau isoforms may bind to different sites on microtubules.[20] Overproduction of tau isoforms with four repeats may result in an excess of tau over available binding sites on microtubules, thus creating a gain of toxic function similar to that of most missense mutations, with unbound excess tau available for assembly into filaments.

Where studied, pathological tau from FTDP-17 brain is hyperphosphorylated.[7,10] Since known mutations in *tau* do not create additional phosphorylation sites (with the possible exception of the P301S mutation in exon 10), hyperphosphorylation of tau must be an event downstream of the primary effects of the mutation and may be a consequence of the partial loss of function. However, some missense mutations may indirectly affect the phosphorylation state of tau. Thus, in transfected cells, tau protein with the R406W mutation displays only little phosphorylation at T231, S396, and S404, in contrast to wild-type tau and tau with the P301L or V337M mutations.[42,57] Hyperphosphorylation of tau probably reinforces the primary effects of the mutations, because it is well established that hyperphosphorylated tau is unable to bind to microtubules and to promote microtubule assembly.[58,59] At present, there is no experimental evidence linking hyperphosphorylation of tau to filament assembly, and it is unclear whether hyperphosphorylation is either necessary or sufficient for assembly.

Sulfated glycosaminoglycans and RNA induce the bulk assembly of nonphosphorylated, recombinant tau protein into Alzheimer-like filaments *in vitro*.[60–64] This work has produced robust methods for the assembly of full-length tau into filaments. However, the mechanisms that lead to assembly of tau into filaments in brain remain to be discovered. It is possible that a reduced ability of tau to interact with microtubules, which could have several different causes, is a necessary step for filament formation. Assembly is an energetically unfavorable, nucleation-dependent process that requires a critical concentration of tau.[60,64] Many cells may have levels of tau below the critical concentration. Other cells may have effective mechanisms for preventing the formation of tau nuclei, or may be able to degrade them once they have formed.

Insufficient protective mechanisms and high tau concentrations may underlie the selective degeneration of nerve cells and glial cells, which is especially striking in FTDP-17, with the characteristic, sometimes unilateral, razor-sharp demarcations between affected and unaffected areas in cerebral cortex. Similar factors may also underpin the late ages of onset of this and other diseases with filamentous protein deposits. Protective mechanisms, such as proteases that degrade nucleation products may be effective throughout much of life. However, as nerve cells age, these mechanisms may become less effective and the balance may tilt in favor of filament formation.

The precise significance of the different filament morphologies observed in FTDP-17 is not clear. It is known that the repeat region of tau forms the densely packed core of paired helical and straight filaments of Alzheimer's disease, with the amino- and carboxy-terminal parts of the molecule forming a proteolytically sensitive coat.[53,65] Also, for filaments assembled *in vitro* in the presence of sulfated glycosaminoglycans, the morphology of the filaments depends on the number of repeats in the tau isoform used.[60] Thus, mutations in the repeat region or a change in the relative amounts of three- and four-repeat isoforms could well influence filament morphology. However, treatment with acid of paired helical filaments, which contain all six tau isoforms, leads to untwisted, ribbon-like filaments like those seen in cases of FTDP-17 with mutations in the intron following exon 10, suggesting a close similarity in packing of tau molecules in the various structures.[66] The most important aspect may be the extended filamentous nature of the assemblies and the deleterious effects that this has on intracellular processes, rather than the detailed morphology of the different filaments.

REFERENCES

 1. PICK, A. 1892. Über die Beziehungen der senilen Hirnatrophie zur Aphasie. Prager Med. Wochenschr. **16:** 765–767.
 2. ALZHEIMER, A. 1911. Über eigenartige Krankheitsfälle des späteren Alters. Z. ges. Neurol. Psychiat. **4:** 356–385.
 3. REWCASTLE, N.B. & M.J. BALL. 1968. Electron microscopic structure of the inclusion bodies in Pick's disease. Neurology **18:** 1205–1213.
 4. POLLOCK, N.J., S.S. MIRRA, L.I. BINDER, L.A. HANSEN & J.G. WOOD. 1986. Filamentous aggregates in Pick's disease, progressive supranuclear palsy, and Alzheimer's disease share antigenic determinants with microtubule-associated protein tau. Lancet **2:** 1211.
 5. PROBST, A., M. TOLNAY, D. LANGUI, M. GOEDERT & M.G. SPILLANTINI. 1996. Pick's disease: hyperphosphorylated tau segregates to the somatoaxonal compartment. Acta Neuropathol. **92:** 588–596.
 6. ALZHEIMER, A. 1907. Über eine eigenartige Erkrankung der Hirnrinde. Allg. Z. Psychiat. Psych. Gerichtl. Med. **64:** 146–148.
 7. SPILLANTINI, M.G. & M. GOEDERT. 1998. Tau protein pathology in neurodegenerative diseases. Trends Neurosci. **21:** 428–433.
 8. WILHELMSEN, K.C., T. LYNCH, E. PAVLOU, M. HIGGINS & T.G. NYGAARD. 1994. Localization of disinhibition-dementia-parkinsonism-amyotrophy complex to 17q21-22. Am. J. Hum. Genet. **55:** 1159–1165.
 9. FOSTER, N.L, K. WILHELMSEN, A.A. SIMA, M.Z. JONES, C.J. D'AMATO & S. GILMAN. 1997. Frontotemporal dementia and parkinsonism linked to chromosome 17: a consensus statement. Ann. Neurol. **41:** 706–715.
10. SPILLANTINI, M.G., T.D. BIRD & B. GHETTI. 1998. Frontotemporal dementia and parkinsonism linked to chromosome 17: a new group of tauopathies. Brain Pathol. **8:** 387–402.
11. POORKAJ, P., T.D. BIRD, E. WIJSMAN, *et al.* 1998. Tau is a candidate gene for chromosome 17 frontotemporal dementia. Ann. Neurol. **43:** 815–825.
12. HUTTON, M., C.L. LENDON, P. RIZZU, *et al.* 1998. Association of missense and 5'-splice-site mutations in *tau* with the inherited dementia FTDP-17. Nature **393:** 702–705.

13. SPILLANTINI, M.G., J.R. MURRELL, M. GOEDERT, M.R. FARLOW, A. KLUG & B. GHETTI. 1998. Mutation in the tau gene in familial multiple system tauopathy with presenile dementia. Proc. Natl. Acad. Sci. USA **95:** 7737–7741.
14. GOEDERT, M., C.M. WISCHIK, R.A. CROWTHER, J.E. WALKER & A. KLUG. 1988. Cloning and sequencing of the cDNA encoding a core protein of the paired helical filament of Alzheimer disease. Proc. Natl. Acad. Sci. USA **85:** 4051–4055.
15. GOEDERT, M., M.G. SPILLANTINI, M.C. POTIER, J. ULRICH & R.A. CROWTHER. 1989 Cloning and sequencing of the cDNA encoding an isoform of microtubule-associated protein tau containing four tandem repeats; differential expression of tau protein mRNAs in human brain. EMBO J. **8:** 393–399.
16. GOEDERT, M., M.G. SPILLANTINI, R. JAKES, D. RUTHERFORD & R.A. CROWTHER. 1989. Multiple isoforms of human microtubule-associated protein tau: sequences and localization in neurofibrillary tangles of Alzheimer's disease. Neuron **3:** 519–526.
17. GOEDERT, M. & R. JAKES. 1990. Expression of separate isoforms of human tau protein: correlation with the tau pattern in brain and effects on tubulin polymerization. EMBO J. **9:** 4225–4230.
18. ANDREADIS, A., M.W. BROWN & K.S. KOSIK. 1992. Structure and novel exons of the human tau gene. Biochemistry **31:** 10626–10633.
19. GUSTKE, N., B. TRINCZEK, J. BIERNAT, E.M. MANDELKOW & E. MANDELKOW. 1994. Domains of tau protein and interaction with microtubules. Biochemistry **33:** 9511–9522.
20. GOODE, B.L. & S.C. FEINSTEIN. 1994. Identification of a novel microtubule binding and assembly domain in the developmentally regulated inter-repeat region of tau. J. Cell Biol. **124:** 769–782.
21. DUMANCHIN, C., A. CAMUZAT, D. CAMPION, *et al.* 1998. Segregation of a missense mutation in the microtubule-associated protein tau gene with familial frontotemporal dementia and parkinsonism. Hum. Mol. Genet. **7:** 1825–1829.
22. CLARK, L.N., P. POORKAJ, Z. WSZOLEK, *et al.* 1998. Pathogenic implications of mutations in the tau gene in pallido-ponto-nigral degeneration and related neurodegenerative disorders linked to chromosome 17. Proc. Natl. Acad. Sci. USA **95:** 13103–13107.
23. RIZZU, P., J.C. VAN SWIETEN, M. JOOSSE. *et al.* 1999. High prevalence of mutations in the microtubule-associated protein tau in a population study of frontotemporal dementia in the Netherlands. Am. J. Hum. Genet. **64:** 414–421.
24. IIJIMA, M., T. TABIRA, P. POORKAJ, *et al.* 1999. A distinct familial presenile dementia with a novel missense mutation in the tau gene. Neuroreport **10:** 497–501.
25. MORRIS, H.R., J. PEREZ-TUR, J.C. JANSSEN, *et al.* 1999. Mutations in the *tau* exon 10 splice site region in familial frontotemporal dementia. Ann. Neurol. **45:** 270–271.
26. GOEDERT, M., M.G. SPILLANTINI, R.A. CROWTHER, *et al.* 1999. *Tau* gene mutation in familial progressive subcortical gliosis. Nature Med. **5:** 454–457.
27. MIRRA, S.S., J.R. MURRELL, M. GEARING, *et al.* 1999. Tau pathology in a family with dementia and a P301L mutation in tau. J. Neuropathol. Exp. Neurol. **58:** 335–345.
28. BIRD, T.D., D. NOCHLIN, P. POORKAJ, *et al.* 1999. A clinical pathological comparison of three families with frontotemporal dementia and identical mutations in the tau gene (P301L). Brain **122:** 741–756.
29. D'SOUZA, I., P. POORKAJ, M. HONG, *et al.* 1999. Missense and silent tau gene mutations cause frontotemporal dementia with parkinsonism-chromosome 17, by affecting multiple alternative RNA splicing regulatory elements. Proc. Natl. Acad. Sci. USA **96:** 5598–5603.
30. BUGIANI, O., J.R. MURRELL, G. GIACCONE, *et al.* 1999. Frontotemporal dementia and corticobasal degeneration in a family with a P301S mutation in *Tau*. J. Neuropathol. Exp. Neurol. **58:** 667–677.
31. NASREDDINE, Z.S., M. LOGINOV, L.N. CLARK, *et al.* 1999. From genotype to phenotype: a clinical, pathological and biochemical investigation of frontotemporal dementia and parkinsonism (FTDP-17) caused by the P301L tau mutation. Ann. Neurol. **45:** 704–715.
32. DELISLE, M.B., J.R. MURRELL, R. RICHARDSON, *et al.* 1999. A mutation at codon 279 (N279K) in exon 10 of the *Tau* gene causes a tauopathy with dementia and supranuclear palsy. Acta Neuropathol. **98:** 62–77.

33. HOULDEN, H., M. BAKER, J. ADAMSON, et al. 1999. Frequency of tau mutations in three series of non-Alzheimer's degenerative dementia. Ann. Neurol. **46:** 243–248.
34. HULETTE, C.M., M.A. PERICAK-VANCE, A.D. ROSES, et al. 1999. Neuropathological features of frontotemporal dementia and parkinsonism linked to chromosome 17q21-22 (FTDP-17): Duke family 1684. J. Neuropathol. Exp. Neurol. **58:** 859–866.
35. YASUDA, M., T. KAWAMATA, O. KOMURE, et al. 1999. A mutation in the microtubule-associated protein tau in pallido-nigro-luysian degeneration. Neurology **53:** 864–868.
36. VAN SWIETEN, J.C., M. STEVENS, S.M. ROSSO, et al. 1999. Phenotypic variation in hereditary frontotemporal dementia with tau mutations. Ann. Neurol. **46:** 617–626.
37. SPERFELD, A.D., M.B. COLLATZ, H. BAIER, et al. 1999. FTDP-17: an early-onset phenotype with parkinsonism and epileptic seizures caused by a novel mutation. Ann. Neurol. **46:** 708–715.
38. MURRELL, J.R., M.G. SPILLANTINI, P. ZOLO, et al. 1999. Tau gene mutation G389R causes a tauopathy with abundant Pick body-like inclusions and axonal deposits. J. Neuropathol. Exp. Neurol. **58:** 1207–1226.
39. YASUDA, M., J. TAKAMATSU, I. D'SOUZA, et al. 2000. A novel mutation at position +12 in the intron following exon 10 of the tau gene in familial frontotemporal dementia (FTD-kumamoto). Ann. Neurol. **47:** 422–429.
40. HASEGAWA, M., M.J. SMITH & M. GOEDERT. 1998. Tau proteins with FTDP-17 mutations have a reduced ability to promote microtubule assembly. FEBS Lett. **437:** 207–210.
41. HONG, M., V. ZHUKAREVA, V. VOGELSBERG-RAGAGLIA, et al. 1998. Mutation-specific functional impairments in distinct tau isoforms of hereditary FTDP-17. Science **282:** 1914–1917.
42. DAYANANDAN, R., M. VAN SLEGTENHORST, T.G. MACK, et al. 1999. Mutations in tau reduce its microtubule binding properties in intact cells and affect its phosphorylation. FEBS Lett. **446:** 228–232.
43. NACHARAJU, P., J. LEWIS, C. EASSON, et al. 1999. Accelerated filament formation from tau protein with specific FTDP-17 missense mutations. FEBS Lett. **447:** 195–199.
44. GOEDERT, M., R. JAKES & R.A. CROWTHER. 1999. Effects of frontotemporal dementia FTDP-17 mutations on heparin-induced assembly of tau filaments. FEBS Lett. **450:** 306–311.
45. ARRASATE, M., M. PEREZ, J. ARMAS-PORTELA & J. AVILA. 1999. Polymerization of tau peptides into fibrillar structures. The effect of FTDP-17 mutations. FEBS Lett. **446:** 199–202.
46. VARANI, L., M. HASEGAWA, M.G. SPILLANTINI, et al. 1999. Structure of tau exon 10 splicing regulatory element RNA and destabilization by mutations of frontotemporal dementia and parkinsonism linked to chromosome 17. Proc. Natl. Acad. Sci. USA **96:** 8229–8234.
47. VARANI, L., M.G. SPILLANTINI, M. GOEDERT & G. VARANI. 2000. Structural basis for recognition of the RNA major groove in the tau exon 10 splicing regulatory element by aminoglycoside antibiotics. Nucleic Acids Res. **28:** 770–779.
48. GROVER, A., H. HOULDEN, M. BAKER, et al. 1999. 5′ Splice site mutations in tau associated with the inherited dementia FTDP-17 affect a stem-loop structure that regulates alternative splicing of exon 10. J. Biol. Chem. **274:** 15134–15143.
49. HASEGAWA, M., M.J. SMITH, M. IIJIMA, T. TABIRA & M. GOEDERT. 1999. FTDP-17 mutations N279K and S305N in tau produce increased splicing of exon 10. FEBS Lett. **443:** 93–96.
50. GOEDERT, M., R.A. CROWTHER & M.G. SPILLANTINI. 1998. Tau mutations cause frontotemporal dementias. Neuron **21:** 955–958.
51. SPILLANTINI, M.G., M. GOEDERT, R.A. CROWTHER, J.R. MURRELL, M.R. FARLOW & B. GHETTI. 1997. Familial multiple system tauopathy with presenile dementia: a disease with abundant neuronal and glial tau filaments. Proc. Natl. Acad. Sci. USA **94:** 4113–4118.
52. SPILLANTINI, M.G., R.A. CROWTHER, W. KAMPHORST, P. HEUTINK & J.C. VAN SWIETEN. 1998. Tau pathology in two Dutch families with mutations in the microtubule-binding region of tau. Am. J. Pathol. **153:** 1359–1363.

53. GOEDERT, M., M.G. SPILLANTINI, N.J. CAIRNS & R.A. CROWTHER. 1992. Tau proteins of Alzheimer paired helical filaments: abnormal phosphorylation of all six brain isoforms. Neuron **8:** 159–168.
54. SPILLANTINI, M.G., R.A. CROWTHER & M. GOEDERT. 1996. Comparison of the neurofibrillary pathology in Alzheimer's disease and familial presenile dementia with tangles. Acta Neuropathol. **92:** 42–48.
55. KATO, S. & H. NAKAMURA. 1990. Presence of two different fibril subtypes in the Pick body: an immunoelectron microscopic study. Acta Neuropathol. **81:** 125–129.
56. MURAYAMA, S., H. MORI, Y. IHARA & M. TOMONAGA. 1990 Immunocytochemical and ultrastructural studies of Pick's disease. J. Neuropathol. Exp. Neurol. **55:** 159–168.
57. MATSUMURA, N., T. YAMAZAKI & Y. IHARA. 1999. Stable expression in Chinese hamster ovary cells of mutated tau genes causing frontotemporal dementia and parkinsonism linked to chromosome 17 (FTDP-17). Am. J. Pathol. **154:** 1649–1656.
58. BRAMBLETT, G.T., M. GOEDERT, R. JAKES, S.E. MERRICK, J.Q. TROJANOWSKI & V.M. LEE. 1993. Abnormal tau phosphorylation at Ser396 in Alzheimer's disease recapitulates development and contributes to reduced microtubule binding. Neuron **19:** 1089–1099.
59. YOSHIDA, H. & Y. IHARA. 1993. Tau in paired helical filament is functionally distinct from fetal tau: assembly incompetence of paired helical filament tau. J. Neurochem. **61:** 1183–1186.
60. GOEDERT, M., R. JAKES, M.G. SPILLANTINI, *et al.* 1996. Assembly of microtubule-associated protein tau into Alzheimer-like filaments induced by sulphated glycosaminoglycans. Nature **383:** 550–553.
61. PEREZ, M., J.M. VALPUESTA, M. MEDINA, E. MONTEJO DE GARCINI & J. AVILA. 1996. Polymerization of tau into filaments in the presence of heparin: the minimal sequence required for tau-tau interactions. J. Neurochem. **67:** 1183–1190.
62. KAMPERS, T., P. FRIEDHOFF, J. BIERNAT, E.M. MANDELKOW & E. MANDELKOW. 1996. RNA stimulates aggregation of microtubule-associated protein tau into Alzheimer-like paired helical filaments. FEBS Lett. **399:** 344–349.
63. HASEGAWA, M., R.A. CROWTHER, R. JAKES & M. GOEDERT. 1997. Alzheimer-like changes in microtubule-associated protein tau induced by sulfated glycosaminoglycans. Inhibition of microtubule binding, stimulation of phosphorylation, and filament assembly depend on the degree of sulfation. J. Biol. Chem. **272:** 33118–33124.
64. FRIEDHOFF, P., M. VON BERGEN, E.M. MANDELKOW, P. DAVIES & E. MANDELKOW. 1998. A nucleated assembly mechanism of Alzheimer paired helical filaments. Proc. Natl. Acad. Sci. USA **95:** 15712–15717.
65. WISCHIK, C.M., M. NOVAK, H.C. THOGERSEN, *et al.* 1988. Isolation of a fragment of tau derived from the core of the paired helical filament of Alzheimer disease. Proc. Natl. Acad. Sci. USA **85:** 4506–4510.
66. CROWTHER, R.A. 1991. Structural aspects of pathology in Alzheimer's disease. Biochim. Biophys. Acta **1069:** 1–9.

Amyloidogenesis in Familial British Dementia Is Associated with a Genetic Defect on Chromosome 13

J. GHISO,[a,d] R. VIDAL,[a] A. ROSTAGNO,[a] L. MIRAVALLE,[a] J.L. HOLTON,[b] S. MEAD,[b] T. RÉVÉSZ,[b] G. PLANT,[c] AND B. FRANGIONE[a]

[a]Department of Pathology, New York University School of Medicine, New York, USA

[b]Department of Neuropathology, Institute of Neurology, London, UK

[c]The National Hospital for Neurology and Neurosurgery, London, UK

ABSTRACT: Familial British dementia (FBD) is a disorder characterized by the presence of amyloid deposits in cerebral blood vessels and brain parenchyma coexisting with neurofibrillary tangles in limbic areas. The amyloid subunit (ABri) is a 4 kDa fragment of a 266 amino acid type II single-spanning transmembrane precursor protein encoded by the *BRI* gene located on chromosome 13. In FBD patients, a single base substitution at the stop codon of this gene generates a larger 277-residue precursor (ABriPP-277). Proteolytic processing by a furin-like enzyme at the C-terminus of the elongated precursor generates the 34 amino acid ABri that undergoes rapid aggregation and fibrillization. ABri is structurally unrelated to all known amyloids including Aβ, the main component of the amyloid lesions in Alzheimer's disease (AD), indicating that cerebral deposition of amyloid molecules other than Aβ can trigger similar neuropathological changes leading to neuronal loss and dementia. These data support the concept that amyloid deposition in the vascular wall and brain parenchyma is of primary importance in the initiation of neurogeneration.

Familial British dementia (FBD) is an autosomal dominant form of cerebral amyloid angiopathy (CAA) clinically characterized by progressive dementia, spastic tetraparesis and cerebellar ataxia, with an age of onset in the fourth to fifth decade. A single extensive pedigree with the disease occurring in multiple generations has been reported.[1] Neuropathologically, there is severe and widespread amyloid angiopathy of the brain and spinal cord with perivascular amyloid plaque formation, periventricular white matter changes resembling Binswanger's leukoencephalopathy, amyloid plaques affecting cerebellum, hippocampus, amygdala, and occasionally cerebral cortex, as well as some neuritic plaques and neurofibrillar degeneration of hippocampal neurons. In spite of the extensive amyloid deposition of the CNS vasculature, intracerebral hemorrhage is not a common feature of the disease.

[d]Address for correspondence: Jorge Ghiso, Ph.D., NYU School of Medicine, 550 First Avenue, Room TH-432, New York, NY 10016. Tel.: (212) 263-7997; fax: (212) 263-6751.
e-mail: ghisoj01@popmail.med.nyu.edu

HISTORY

FBD was first reported in 1933 by Worster-Drought *et al.* in two siblings.[2] The pedigree has been followed and expanded since then,[1] and common ancestors have been identified with separate family case reports by Griffiths *et al.*[3] and Love and Duchen.[4] At present, the Worster-Drought pedigree comprises 343 individuals over nine generations dating back to ~1780. Although this pedigree is large, it is not complete because the descendants of 22 individuals from early generations who were at risk of the disease could not be traced. The family originally lived in South London, but branches have now emigrated around the world. It is likely that the disease has gone unrecognized. Due to the extensive cerebrovascular involvement, the disorder previously had been designated as familial cerebral amyloid angiopathy with non-neuritic plaques[1] and cerebrovascular amyloidosis-British type.[5]

CLINICAL FEATURES

Details of 26 affected individuals in the pedigree are now known, and autopsy findings in five family members have been published.[1,3,6-8] Psychometric assessment early in the course of the disease has shown marked impairment of memory progressing to global dementia. Many of the cases developed personality changes as an early manifestation, either becoming irritable or depressed. The spastic paralysis is far more profound than that seen in Gerstmann-Sträussler-Scheinker or in AD. Pseudobulbar palsy and dysarthria are universal and all patients have progressed to a chronic vegetative state: mute, unresponsive, quadriplegic, and incontinent. Fifty-six members of the family have been identified as at-risk of inheriting FBD. Five affected members of this group, ages between 45 and 50, showed early signs of the disease on the basis of a neurological examination, neuropsychological assessment, and MRI brain scan. All five patients had abnormal imaging. The most consistent finding was a patchy or confluent high signal on T2-weighted scans in the deep white matter located around the frontal and occipital poles of the lateral ventricles and probably represents white matter ischemic changes. Other abnormalities included circumscribed corpus callosum lesions, corpus callosum atrophy, and lacunar infarcts. The neuropsychology was abnormal in four of the five patients. Three had impaired recognition and recall memory, and another had a mild impairment of delayed visual recall. The memory loss is probably related to neuronal loss in the hippocampus. Tests of general intelligence, frontal lobe function, naming, and perception were normal. Neurological signs were found in three of the five individuals with abnormal imaging consisting of gait ataxia and lower limb spasticity. This could be accounted for by cerebellum and spinal cord pathology.

NEUROPATHOLOGY

FBD brains are of normal or slightly reduced overall weight, with leptomeningeal thickening and moderate diffuse atrophy of both the cerebral and cerebellar hemispheres. The cerebral cortex is relatively well preserved whereas the white matter is diffusely discolored and the lateral ventricles enlarged. Brain stem and spinal cord appear normal to the naked eye. One of the main histological findings is severe amyloid deposition in the walls of small leptomeningeal arteries and arterioles as well as of grey and white matter.[1] The affected vessels are usually less than 150 μm in diameter and are seen, with the exception of a few anatomical areas, throughout the neuraxis including the spinal cord. The spread of amyloid in the form of delicate spicules radiating from capillaries into the surrounding neuropil is commonly seen. Occasional small perivascular hemorrhages or collection of inflammatory cells may be present. Parenchymal amyloid plaques on silver impregnations are often nonneuritic and occur in several areas. Ischemic white matter damage is widespread. The numerous hippocampal amyloid plaques are mainly of two varieties: (i) the large plaques (150–200 μm across), sometimes with a central congophilic core with radiating spicules of amyloid and a fine fibrillar peripheral rim, and (ii) small plaques (30–40 μm across) with an appearance similar to the cores of the large plaques without a peripheral rim. A proportion of the plaques appears to be related to a capillary-sized blood vessel. The large plaques are numerous in the dentate fascia, the CA4 and CA3 regions of the hippocampus, presubiculum, and basolateral nucleus of the amygdala. The small plaques are most frequently seen in the CA1 and part of the CA2 regions of the hippocampus. Perivascular amyloid plaques occur chiefly in the cerebral and cerebellar cortex and white matter. That a significant proportion of the hippocampal plaques is associated with dystrophic neurites is better appreciated on tau immunohistochemistry than conventional silver impregnations.[5] The neurofibrillary tangles, which are found in a majority of the remaining pyramidal neurons of the hippocampus, as well as the abnormal neurites associated with the hippocampal amyloid plaques, have ultrastructural features and a tau immunohistochemical profile indistinguishable from those seen in Alzheimer's disease.[5] Neurofibrillary tangles are also present in the subiculum, entorhinal cortex, and amygdala, but only occasionally in the cerebral cortex and in the basal nucleus of Meynert. Ischemic lesions of microscopic size are also scattered in the cerebral cortex while the deep white matter shows patchy myelin loss and cystic infarcts. The deep grey matter nuclei show various degrees of involvement while the cerebellum, including the dentate nucleus, is severely affected with amyloid angiopathy and parenchymal, often perivascular, amyloid plaques. In the cerebellar cortex there is severe diffuse Purkinje cell loss and gliosis. In the medulla, there is a long tract degeneration, especially in the pyramids, amyloid plaques, neuronal loss, and gliosis in the inferior olive. The spinal cord shows the pallor of myelin staining in all columns of white matter with a few large amyloid plaques in grey and white matter and amyloid containing vessels.

The white matter changes may contribute to the dementia and are considered to be secondary to the amyloid deposition in arterioles penetrating through the cortex to supply the white matter. The plaque formation, neurofibrillary tangles, and neuronal cell loss in the hippocampus are sufficient to account for the memory loss; cerebellar plaques and ischemic lesions for the ataxia; and cerebral deep white matter and spinal cord long tract involvement for the spasticity. The explanation for the relative rarity of cerebral hemorrhage in this form of familial CAA, despite the severity of the amyloid angiopathy, is not known. Because of this unusual neuropathology, FBD has been previously interpreted as an atypical form of familial Alzheimer's disease (AD),[9] as an example of spongiform encephalopathy,[10–12] and also regarded as a specific form of primary congophilic angiopathy.[13]

FBD AMYLOID SUBUNIT (ABri)

Since the original description by Worster-Drought, the identity of the amyloid protein subunit has remained elusive. Immunohistochemical attempts to classify the disease using a number of antibodies against known amyloidogenic molecules (cystatin C, Aβ, gelsolin, TTR, amyloid A, PrP, κ and λ light chains, apoA-I, apoA-II, calcitonin, and β2-microglobulin) failed to identify the nature of the amyloid subunit.[14] In addition, C-terminal fragments of α- and β-tubulin were found associated with the amyloid deposits and formed amyloid-like fibrils in *in vitro* experiments.[15] We carried out biochemical studies on amyloid fibrils extracted from leptomeningeal amyloid deposits of a patient with FBD, solubilized in 99% formic acid and further purified by gel filtration chromatography. The main component (Mr 4 kDa on SDS-PAGE) featured pyroglutamate at the N-terminus, which precluded direct sequence analysis. The final amino acid sequence was obtained by combining partial sequence data retrieved from internal peptides generated via trypsin digestion and purified by reverse-phase HPLC, mass spectrometry analysis of the isolated 4 kDa subunit, and homology search in EST data banks. The amyloid subunit (ABri; pEASNC-FAIRHFENKFAVETLICSRTVKKNIIEEN) is composed of 34 amino acids with no sequence identity to any known amyloid protein.[16] Mass spectrometry analysis revealed a mass of 3,935.5 ± 1.0 Da. The peptide is devoid of glycine, methionine, proline, aspartic acid, tryptophane, tyrosine, and glutamine. ABri features two cysteine residues at positions 5 and 22 that may be of importance for polymerization and fibrillization. The predicted pI (7.0) suggests low-solubility properties at physiologic pH. In this sense, synthetic peptides homologous to the full-length ABri spontaneously polymerize in solution and form amyloid-like fibrils *in vitro* (FIG. 1). The experimental molecular mass of the main component isolated from FBD leptomeningeal deposits was 18 Da lower than the expected mass deduced from the cDNA sequence, corroborating a blocked N-terminus. It is interesting to note that pyroglutamate is usually formed by deamination of glutamine; in the case of the ABri amyloid, the nucleotide sequence clearly indicated the presence of glutamic acid at the N-terminus. This finding suggests dehydration as the possible mechanism that results in a blocked ABri. Similar data have been previously published for other amyloids, that is, the peptides derived from the Alzheimer's Aβ.[17–19] A synthetic peptide comprising the last 10 residues of the ABri sequence was used to raise polyclonal antibodies in rabbits. As indicated in FIG. 2, antibody 338 specifically recognized parenchymal and perivascular plaques as well as vascular amyloid deposits. Specificity of the immunostaining was corroborated by absorption of the antibody with a synthetic peptide homologous to the 34-amino acids full-length ABri amyloid. The immunoreactivity co-localized with yellow-green birefringent material observed under polarized light after Congo red staining. No immunoreactivity using antibody 338 was observed in brain sections of sporadic CAA, sporadic AD, Down's syndrome, HCHWA-D, HCHWA-I, Hungarian transthyretin cerebral amyloidosis, and systemic cases of light-chain amyloidosis (kidney), light-chain deposition disease (kidney), and amyloid A (heart).

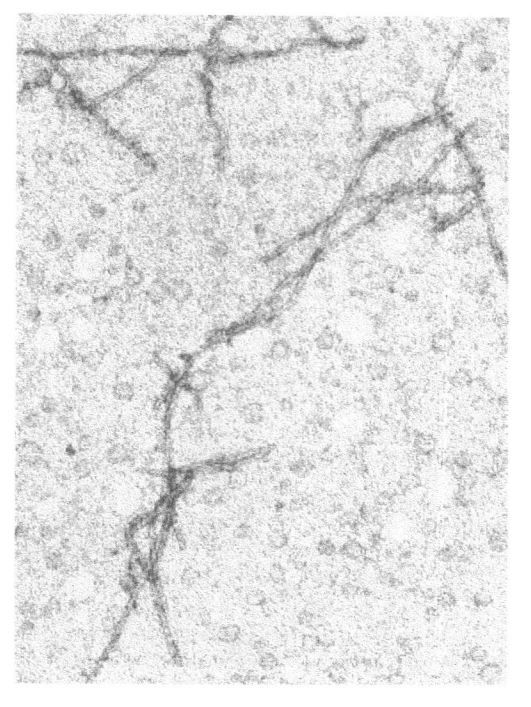

FIGURE 1. Full-length ABri fibril formation *in vitro*. Electron microscopy of ABri amyloid-like fibrils negatively stained with uranyl acetate (×100,000).

ABri PRECURSOR PROTEIN

Since the ABri peptide was not homologous to any known protein and the ESTs databanks indicated the presence of a larger precursor, the gene codifying the precursor molecule of ABri was cloned and sequenced.[16] The gene *(BRI)*, located on the long arm of chromosome 13 (13q14) by FISH analysis, codifies for a 266 amino acids protein with a calculated M_r of 30,329 Da and a theoretical pI of 4.86. Hydropathy analysis indicated the presence of a putative single transmembrane spanning domain at positions 52–74, suggesting that the ABri precursor molecule is a type II integral transmembrane protein with the C-terminal part being extracellular (FIG. 3). A putative single N-glycosylation site was located at asparagine 170. The complete nucleotide sequence of the human transcript[16] was found to be identical to the recently described *ITM2B* cDNA, upregulated during chondro-osteogenic differentiation,[20] and highly homologous to sequences obtained from other EST clones of chicken, rat, mouse, rabbit, and pig origin that had been deposited in the data banks. In fact, the mouse and rat amino acid sequences were 95.5 and 96.2% identical to the human homologue while the chicken sequence exhibited 75.9% homology to the human counterpart.

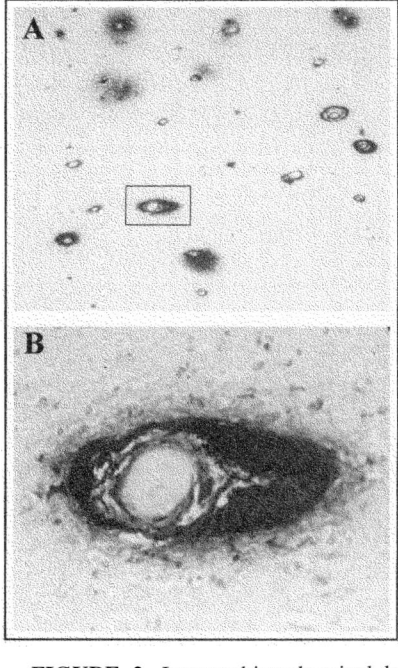

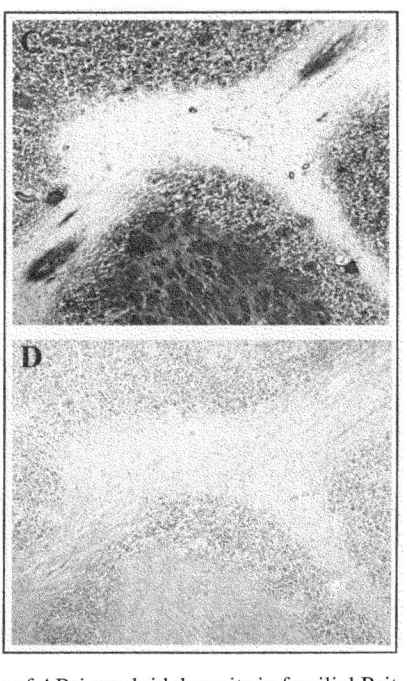

FIGURE 2. Immunohistochemical detection of ABri amyloid deposits in familial British dementia. (**A**) Neocortical perivascular plaques specifically labeled with antibody 338 (anti C-terminal ABri antibody, 1:2,000). (**B**) High-power view of a perivascular amyloid lesion highlighted in panel **A**. (**C**) Amyloid deposits in the cerebellum are immunolabeled with antibody 338, but not detected by the preabsorbed antibody (**D**). Magnification: ×120 (**A**, **C**, and **D**); ×1,200 (**B**).

Nucleotide sequence analysis of the precursor protein from a number of available affected members of FBD revealed a single nucleotide substitution in the stop codon, TGA to AGA at codon 267,[16] resulting in the presence of an arginine residue and an open-reading frame of 277 amino acids instead of 266. The nucleotide substitution creates a *XbaI* restriction site useful to detect asymptomatic carriers. The ABri amyloid peptide is formed by the last 34 amino acids of the mutated precursor protein (FIG. 3). The N- and C-terminal heterogeneity observed in the mass spectrometry analysis of the isolated amyloid is a common finding in almost every type of amyloidosis, regardless of the protein composing the amyloid subunit.[21]

PROCESSING

The mechanism that generates the ABri deposits in patients with FBD remains unknown. The amino acid sequence flanking the cleavage site of the ABri peptide [between amino acids 243 (Arg) and 244 (Glu)] has a classical motif for processing by the so-called subtilisin-like proprotein convertases (SPCs) or more simply

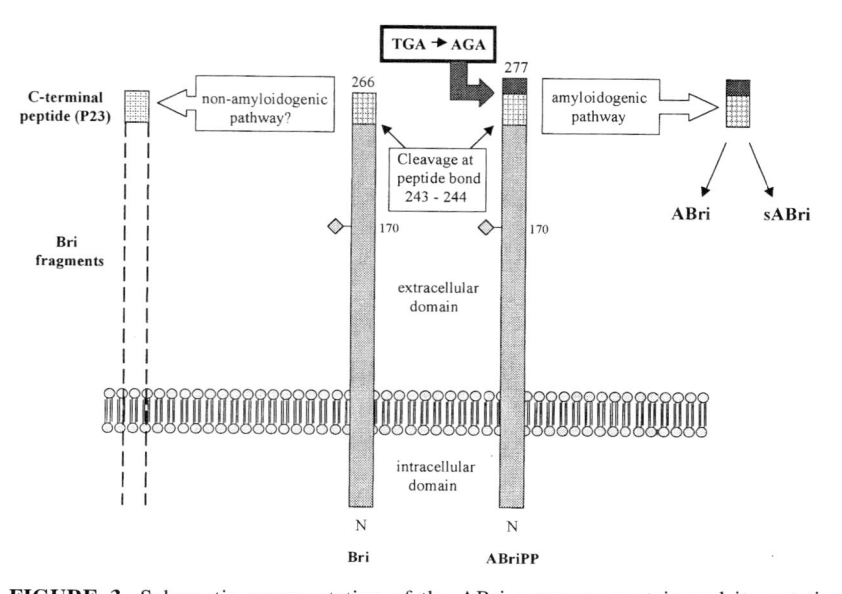

FIGURE 3. Schematic representation of the ABri precursor protein and its putative processing. Soluble ABri (sABri), the 23 amino acids C-terminal peptide (P23) and other Bri fragments are hypothetical, and their existence remains to be investigated.

PCs.[22,23] These are calcium-dependent serine endoproteases related to subtilisin and the yeast processing protease Kex2p, or kexin. The classical motif for processing by these PCs is KR or RR . However, upstream basic residues at the P_4 and/or P_6 position also contribute to substrate recognition. Seven members of this family in mammals, which includes furin, PC2, PC1/PC3, PC4, PACE4, PC5/PC6, LPC/PC7/PC8/SPC7, have now been identified and characterized, some having isoforms generated via alternative splicing. This family has been shown to be responsible for the conversion of precursor of peptide hormones, neuropeptides, and many other proteins into their biologically active forms. Based on their tissue distribution, PCs can be classified into three groups: (i) Furin, PACE4, PC5/PC6, and LPC/PC7/PC8/SPC7 are expressed in a broad range of tissues and cell lines, including the neuroendocrine system, liver, gut, and brain, where their active forms are localized in the *trans*-Golgi network (TGN) and small secretory vesicles of the constitutive pathway. (ii) PC2 and PC1/PC3 expression is limited to neuroendocrine tissues, such as pancreatic islets, pituitary, adrenal medulla, and many brain areas where it is mainly localized in the secretory granules. (iii) Expression of PC4 is highly restricted to testicular spermatogenic cells. Co-expression of furin with a series of prorenin mutants have delineated the following rule that governs the cleavage by furin. (i) An Arg residue is essential at the P_1 position. (ii) In addition to the P_1 Arg, at least two out of the three residues at P_2, P_4, and P_6 are required to be basic for efficient cleavage. (iii) At the P_1' position, an amino acid with a hydrophobic aliphatic side chain is not suitable.[22] Recent studies in transfected cells indicate that both wild-type and mutant BRI are constitutively processed by furin resulting in the secretion of C-terminal peptides that encompass either part or all the ABri sequence.[24] The prediction would be that extracellular carboxyl-terminal fragments of the BRI molecule, and the soluble ABri peptide, would be found in body fluids (FIG. 2). If that is the case, FBD would not be different from other systemic and localized forms of amyloidosis where the soluble precursor of the deposited amyloid fibril is normally found in the circulation. The typical example is the Aβ peptide in Alzheimer's disease that was originally thought to be derived by abnormal processing[25] and was later identified as a normal soluble molecule in body fluids and secreted by cells in culture.[26–29] Whether ABri amyloid deposits will be found outside the brain in FBD cases remain to be investigated.

In summary, our data indicate that FBD is not related to any of the known forms of cerebral or systemic forms of human amyloidosis. Since the stop codon at position 267 was always present in asymptomatic family members ($n = 7$) and normal controls from comparable ethnic origins ($n = 113$) and is conserved in the murine homologues, the nucleotide substitution found in patients with FBD is a pathogenic mutation rather than innocent polymorphism. ABri is structurally unrelated to all known amyloids, including those deposited in the brain; however, immunohistochemical and electron microscopical studies on three cases of FBD demonstrated that the cytoskeletal pathology in these patients is very similar to that seen in patients with Alzheimer's disease.[5,30] Thus, ABri and Aβ cerebral deposition can trigger similar neuropathological changes leading to the same scenario: neuronal loss and dementia. The ABri data support the concept that amyloid deposition in the vascular wall and brain parenchyma may be of primary importance in the initiation of neurodegeneration.

REFERENCES

1. PLANT, G., T. RÉVÉSZ, R. BARNARD, A. HARDING & P. GAUTIER-SMITH. 1990. Familial cerebral amyloid angiopathy with nonneuritic plaque formation. Brain **113:** 721–747.
2. WORSTER-DROUGHT, C., T. HILL & W. McMENEMEY. 1933. Familial presenile dementia with spastic paralysis. J. Neurol. Psychopathol. **14:** 27–34.
3. GRIFFITHS, R., T. MORTIMER, D. OPPENHEIMER & J. SPALDING. 1982. Congophilic angiopathy of the brain: a clinical and pathological report on two siblings. J. Neurol. Neurosurg. Psychiatry **45:** 396–408.
4. LOVE, S. & L. DUCHEN. 1982. Familial cerebellar ataxia with cerebrovascular amyloid. J. Neurol. Neurosurg. Psychiatry **45:** 271–273.
5. RÉVÉSZ, T., J. HOLTON, B. DOSHI, B. ANDERTON, F. SCARAVILLI & G. PLANT. 1999. Cytoskeletal pathology in familial cerebral amyloid angiopathy (British type) with non-neuritic plaque formation. Acta Neuropathol. **97:** 170–176.
6. WORSTER-DROUGHT, C., J.G. GREENFIELD & W. McMENEMEY. 1940. A form of familial presenile dementia with spastic paralysis (including the pathological examination of a case). Brain **63:** 237–254.
7. McMENEMEY, W. 1952. Discussion. *In* Proceedings of the First International Congress of Neuropathology, Rome. Vol. 2: 432–436. Rosemberg and Sellier. Turin.
8. McMENEMEY, W. 1970. Discussion. *In* Alzheimer's Disease and Related Conditions: A Ciba Foundation Symposium. G.EW. Wolstenholme & M. O'Connor, Eds.: 132–133. J. & A. Churchill. London.
9. AIKAWA, H., K. SUZUKI, Y. IWASAKI & R. IIZUKA. 1985. Atypical Alzheimer's disease with spastic paresis and ataxia. Ann. Neurol. **17:** 297–300.
10. MASTERS, C.L., D.C. GAJDUSEK & C.J. GIBBS. 1981. A familial ocurrence of Creutzfeldt-Jacob disease and Alzheimer's disease. Brain **104:** 535–558.

11. BARAISTER, M. 1990. The Genetics of Neurological Disease.: 93, 129, and 284. Oxford Medical Publications. Oxford.
12. COURTEN-MYERS, G. & T.I. MANDYBUR. 1987. A typical Gerstmann-Sträussler syndrome of familial spino cerebellar ataxia and Alzheimer's disease? Neurology **37:** 269–275.
13. VINTERS, H.V. 1987. Cerebral amyloid angiopathy: a critical review. Stroke **18:** 311–324.
14. GHISO, J., G. PLANT, T. RÉVÉSZ, T. WISNIEWSKI & B. FRANGIONE. 1995. Familial cerebral amyloid angiopathy (British type) with nonneuritic amyloid plaque formation may be due to a novel amyloid protein. J. Neurol. Sci. **129:** 74–75.
15. BAUMANN, M.H., T. WISNIEWSKI, E. LEVY, G.T. PLANT & J. GHISO. 1996. C-terminal fragments of α- and β-tubulin form amyloid fibrils *in vitro* and associate with amyloid deposits of familial CAA, British type. Biochem. Biophys. Res. Commun. **219:** 238–242.
16. VIDAL, R., B. FRANGIONE, A. ROSTAGNO, *et al.* 1999. Novel gene BRI mutated at its stop codon causs familial British dementia. Nature **399:** 776–781.
17. MORI, H., K. TAKIO, M. OGAWARA & D. SELKOE. 1992. Mass spectrometry of purified amyloid beta protein in Alzheimer's disease. J. Biol. Chem. **267:** 17082–17086.
18. SAIDO, T., W. YAMAO-HARIGAYA, T. IWATSUBO & S. KAWASHIMA. 1996. Amino- and carboxyl-terminal heterogeneity of beta-amyloid peptides deposited in human brain. Neurosci. Lett. **13:** 173–176.
19. TEKIRIAN, T., T. SAIDO, W. MARKESBERY, *et al.* 1998. N-terminal heterogeneity of parenchymal and cerebrovascular Aβ deposits. J. Neuropathol. Exp. Neurol. **57:** 76–94.
20. PITTOIS, K., W. DELEERSNIJDER & J. MERREGAERT. 1998. cDNA sequence analysis, chromosomal assignment and expression pattern of the gene coding for integral membrane protein 2B. Gene **217:** 141–149.
21. GHISO, J., T. WISNIEWSKI & B. FRANGIONE. 1994. Unifying features of systemic and cerebral amyloidosis. Mol. Neurobiol. **8:** 49–64.
22. NAKAYAMA, K. 1997. Furin: a mammalian subtilisin/Kex2p-like endoprotease involved in processing of a wide variety of precursor proteins. Biochem. J. **327:** 625–635.
23. ZHOU, A., G. WEBB, X. ZHU & D.F. STEINER. 1999. Proteolytic processing in the secretory pathway. J. Biol. Chem. **274:** 20745–20748.
24. KIM, S.-H., R. WANG, D.J. GORDON, *et al.* 1999. Furin mediates enhanced production of fibrillogenic ABri peptides in familial British dementia. Nature Neurosci. **2:** 984–988.
25. SISODIA, S.S., E.H. KOO, K. BEYREUTHER, A. UNTERBECK & D.L. PRICE. 1990. Evidence that beta-amyloid protein in Alzheimer's disease is not derived by normal processing. Science **248:** 492–495.
26. SHOJI, M., T.E. GOLDE, J. GHISO, *et al.* 1992. Production of the Alzheimer amyloid beta protein by normal proteolytic processing. Science **258:** 126–129.
27. GHISO, J., M. CALERO, E. MATSUBARA, *et al.* 1997. Alzheimer's soluble amyloid ß is a normal component of human urine. FEBS Lett. **408:**105–108.
28. HAASS, C., M.G. SCHLOSSMACHER, A.Y. HUNG, *et al.* 1992. Amyloid beta-peptide is produced by cultured cells during normal metabolism. Nature **359:** 322–325.
29. SEUBERT, P., C. VIGO-PELFREY, F. ESCH, *et al.* 1992. Isolation and quantification of soluble Alzheimer's beta-peptide from biological fluids. Nature **359:** 325–327.
30. DICKSON, D. 1997. Neurodegenerative diseases with cytoskeletal pathology: a biochemical classification. Ann. Neurol. **42:** 541–544.

Familial British Dementia: Expression and Metabolism of BRI

SEONG-HUN KIM,[a] RONG WANG,[b] DAVID J. GORDON,[c] JOSEPH BASS,[d]
DONALD F. STEINER,[d] GOPAL THINAKARAN,[a] DAVID G. LYNN,[e]
STEPHEN C. MEREDITH,[e] AND SANGRAM S. SISODIA[a,f]

[a]Department of Neurobiology, Pharmacology and Physiology, University of Chicago, Chicago, Illinois, USA

[b]Laboratory of Mass Spectrometry, Rockefeller University, New York, New York 10021, USA

[c]Medical Scientists Training Program and Department of Biochemistry and Molecular Biology, University of Chicago, Chicago, Illinois, USA

[d]Howard Hughes Medical Institute, University of Chicago, Chicago, Illinois, USA

[e]Department of Pathology, University of Chicago, Chicago, Illinois 60637, USA

ABSTRACT: Vidal et al. (1999. Nature 399: 776–778) discovered that the underlying genetic lesion in familial British dementia (FBD) isa T-A transversion at the termination codon of a membrane protein, termed BRI. The mutation creates an arginine codon; translational read-through generates a novel protein, termed BRI-L, that is extended by 11 amino acids at the carboxyl-terminus. BRI-L is the precursor of the ABri peptide, a component of amyloid deposits in FBD brain. We demonstrate that both BRI and its mutant counterpart are constitutively processed by furin, resulting in the secretion of carboxyl-terminal peptide derivatives that correspond to all, or part of, ABri. Notably, elevated levels of peptides are generated from the mutant BRI precursor, suggesting that subtle conformational alterations at the carboxyl-terminus may influence furin-mediated processing. We have examined BRI/BRI-L processing by other members of the prohormone convertase (PC) family (PACE4, LPC, PC 5/6) and found that these enzymes also process BRI, albeit inefficiently. Moreover, BRI-L processing by the other PC members is severely compromised. Finally, our electron microscopic studies reveal that synthetic ABri peptides assemble into insoluble β-pleated fibrils. Collectively, our results support the view that enhanced furin-mediated processing of mutant BRI generates amyloidogenic peptides that initiate the pathogenesis of FBD.

INTRODUCTION

Familial British dementia (FBD), an autosomal dominant neurodegenerative disorder, is characterized by progressive spastic tetraparesis, cerebellar ataxia, and dementia.[1] The principal pathological hallmarks of FBD include the presence of

[f]Address for correspondence: Sangram S. Sisodia, Ph.D., Department of Neurobiology, Pharmacology and Physiology, University of Chicago, Abbott 316, 947 East 58th Street, Chicago, IL 60637. Tel.: (773) 834-2900; fax: (773) 702-3774.
  e-mail: ssisodia@drugs.bsd.uchicago.edu

nonneuritic plaques and amyloid angiopathy in the cerebellum, hippocampus, amygdala and cerebral cortex, hippocampal neurofibrillary tangles, and ischemic white matter changes.[1–3] The first insight into the biochemical basis of this unusual disorder recently emerged when Vidal et al.[4] described the purification of a peptide, termed ABri, that is a component of highly insoluble amyloid fibrils in leptomeninges and parenchymal deposits from a patient with FBD. Comparison of the sequence obtained from tryptic peptides of ABri to the expressed sequence tag (EST) database revealed the presence of cDNAs encoding a larger, 266 amino acid ABri precursor protein, termed BRI. Unexpectedly, one of the tryptic peptides generated from ABri contained a C-terminal arginine residue that was not predicted from the EST clones; the BRI open reading frame (ORF) typically terminated at this position. Subsequent analysis of BRI cDNA from affected individuals from the FBD pedigree revealed a T to A transversion (TGA–AGA) at the termination codon. As a result, an arginine codon was created and translation of the ORF extended for an additional 10 amino acids, terminating at an ochre codon; the extended ORF encodes a mutant BRI (BRI-L) of 277 amino acids. Indeed, the sequence of one ABri tryptic peptide matched the carboxyl-terminal 6 amino acids of the predicted BRI-L protein.

Matrix-assisted laser desorption time-of-flight mass spectrometry (MALDI-TOF MS) of ABri purified from the leptomeningeal amyloid fraction revealed an M_r of 3,935, suggesting that the peptide was generated following endoproteolytic processing of mutant BRI between arginine 243 and glutamic acid 244.[4] Interestingly, the amino acid sequence of BRI that flanks the predicted cleavage site, ...KGIQKR⇓EA, is highly reminiscent of a consensus sequence required for processing by the prohormone convertase, furin.[5,6] We have demonstrated that BRI adopts the topology of type-II integral membrane proteins. Moreover, both BRI and the mutant variant BRI-L are constitutively processed between Arg243 and Glu244 in transfected mammalian cells, leading to the generation of carboxyl-terminal peptides that are released into the conditioned medium. Furthermore, furin appears to be a critical, if not sole, factor that mediates endoproteolysis of the precursor proteins. Notably, secretion of peptides derived from the mutant BRI-L precursor is enhanced compared to peptides generated from BRI, suggesting that the carboxyl-terminal 11 amino acids in mutant BRI effects furin-mediated proteolysis in a dominant fashion. In addition, electron microscopy (EM) demonstrates that ABri peptides assemble into irregular, tortuous, and short fibrils with an average diameter of ~50 Å.[7] Collectively, our results support the view that enhanced furin-mediated processing of mutant BRI generates amyloidogenic peptides that initiate the pathogenesis in FBD.

RESULTS

Topology and Processing of BRI in Mammalian Cells

To examine the topology of BRI, we generated human BRI cDNA by PCR amplification of adult human brain cDNA; the antisense primer was complementary to sequences encoding the carboxyl-terminal seven amino acids of amyloid precursor-like protein 1 (APLP1). The PCR product was cloned in-frame with sequences encoding a 12 amino acid segment of the c-myc oncoprotein. Secondary structure algorithms, and the presence of a hydrophobic stretch between amino acids 52 and 76, lead to the prediction that BRI is a type II integral membrane protein. To validate this prediction, we transiently transfected myc- and APLP1-tagged *BRI* cDNA into mouse neuroblastoma (N2a) cells, prepared a $100,000 \times g$ postnuclear, membrane fraction and digested this material with increasing amounts of proteinase K (PK). The resulting reactions were subsequently divided, fractionated by SDS-PAGE, and subject to Western blot analysis with 9E10 or CT11 antibodies, specific for the myc- and APLP1-epitope tags, respectively. Approximately 40 kilodalton full-length BRI was detected with either antibody and this molecule was resistant to digestion at 0.25 μg/ml PK. However, N-terminal 9E10-immunoreactivity was markedly reduced at 2.5 μg/ml PK and almost completely abolished at 25 μg/ml PK. Coincident with loss of N-terminal 9E10-immunoreactivity, we detected an ~34 kDa polypeptide using the carboxyl-terminal, CT11 antibody. These studies indicated that the hydrophobic sequence encompassing residues 52 and 76 serves as a transmembrane domain and, in so doing, affords protection of the lumenal domain from PK digestion. Hence, we conclude that the chimeric BRI molecule adopts the topology of a type II integral membrane protein.

To examine the metabolism of BRI and BRI-L, we transiently transfected cDNA encoding these molecules into mammalian cells, and subjected lysates of transfected cells to Western blot analysis using CT11, or 9E10 antibodies. As expected, the CT11 antibody detected ~40 kDa BRI and ~42 kDa BRI-L in lysates of COS-1 or N2a cells. On the other hand, the 9E10 antibody detected a doublet of ~40 kDa and ~37 kDa in lysates of cells expressing BRI, and ~42 kDa and ~37 kDa species in lysates of cells expressing BRI-L. The accumulation of an N-terminal ~37 kDa species derived from either precursor protein strongly suggested that the full-length molecules are being subject to the same carboxyl-terminal truncation event. In parallel, we detected CT11-reactive peptides of ~3 kDa and ~4 kDa in the medium of COS-1 and N2a cells expressing BRI and BRI-L, respectively. To establish the identity of secreted peptides, we immunoprecipitated the peptides from conditioned medium of N2a cells with CT11 antibody, and subjected recovered material to MALDI-TOF MS. These analyses reveal that N2a cells expressing BRI or BRI-L secrete discrete peptides generated by endoproteolytic cleavage of the precursor proteins between Arg243 and Glu244. These data are entirely consistent with the results of the MALDI-TOF MS determination for ABri purified from leptomeninges which also supported *in vivo* endoproteolysis of BRI-L between Arg243 and Glu244.[4]

BRI Processing Is Mediated by Furin

The sequence immediately N-terminal to the BRI cleavage site, …Arg-Gly-Ile-Gln-Lys-Arg, is highly reminiscent to the consensus recognition site for the subtilisin-like, proprotein convertase, furin.[5,8–11] To examine the role of furin in BRI endoproteolysis, we transiently transfected cDNA encoding BRI or BRI-L into Chinese hamster ovary (CHO-K1) cells, or a CHO-K1 derivative, RPE.40, which is furin-deficient.[12–14] Transfected cells were biosynthetically labeled with [^{35}S]-cysteine for 3 h, and detergent lysates of cells and conditioned medium were subject to immunoprecipitation with CT11 antibody. As expected, CT11 antibody detected ~40 kDa BRI and ~42 kDa BRI-L in lysates of transfected CHO-K1. Parallel analysis of the conditioned medium of transfected CHO-K1 cells revealed the presence of ~3 kDa BRI- and ~4 kDa BRI-L C-terminal peptides. However, we failed to detect a CT11-precipitable peptide in medium of RPE.40 cells expressing either BRI or BRI-L, suggesting that endoproteolysis of the precursor proteins required furin. To verify that expression of furin was both necessary and sufficient for processing BRI and BRI-L, we co-transfected *BRI* or *BRI-L* cDNA with cDNA encoding human furin into RPE.40 cells. The ~3 kDa and ~4 kDa CT11-precipitable peptides now appeared in the medium of RPE.40 cells co-expressing furin and BRI or BRI-L, respectively, results that confirm the view that furin mediates endoproteolytic processing of the precursors, resulting in the production of secreted C-terminal peptides.

Enhanced Processing of BRI-L by Furin

While it was apparent that BRI endoproteolysis was mediated by furin, it also became clear that the levels of secreted peptides in medium of CHO-K1 or RPE.40 cells that were derived from the BRI-L precursor were markedly elevated over the peptides generated from the BRI precursor. In order to validate the intriguing observation that the BRI-L precursors were subject to enhanced endoproteolysis, we quantified the levels of BRI- and BRI-L-derived peptides in the medium of N2a cells. N2a cells were transiently transfected with *BRI* or *BRI-L* cDNA, individually, or in combination with *furin* cDNA. Triplicate plates of cells were transfected, biosynthetically labeled with [^{35}S]-cysteine for 3 h, and cellular or secreted BRI derivatives were immunoprecipitated with CT11 antibody. Levels of immunoprecipitated peptides in the conditioned medium were quantified by phosphorimaging. Analysis of cell lysates revealed the presence of both full-length BRI and BRI-L precursors and C-terminal peptides. The latter observation indicated that a fraction of precursor proteins are subject to endoproteolysis in intracellular compartments, a finding consistent with a wealth of information that the preponderant steady-state distribution and activity of furin is within the *trans*-Golgi network (TGN). More importantly, we observed an increase in the levels of secreted peptides generated from the BRI-L precursor, compared to cells expressing BRI, similar to the results obtained in CHO-K1 and RPE.40 cells. These results suggested that the carboxyl-terminal extension present in the BRI-L molecule had a dominant effect on proteolysis at a scissile bond that most likely is mediated by furin.

Electron Microscopy (EM)

Although earlier histological studies indicated that the amyloid deposits in FBD patients exhibit yellow-green birefringence under polarized light after staining with congo red,[4] there are neither ultrastructural analyses of these structures, nor information about the structure of purified ABri fibrils from leptomeninges and parenchyma of FBD patients. In order to examine the assembly of ABri, we generated peptides corresponding to the 34 amino acid peptide purified from FBD patient material and incubated the peptide in PBS at room temperature. EM analysis revealed the formation of fibrils with an average diameter of ~50 Å, though they were irregular and varied from 40 to 75 Å. The fibrils were tortuous and showed occasional branch points or crossing; these fibrils differed from the linear, unbranched 90 Å diameter fibrils generated by Aβ_{1-40}.

DISCUSSION

Recent studies revealed that a mutation at the termination codon of the *BRI* gene is the underlying genetic defect in FBD, an autosomal dominant neurodegenerative disorder.[4] The mutant *BRI* gene encodes BRI-L, the precursor of ~4 kDa ABri peptides that accumulate in leptomeningeal and parenchymal deposits in brains of FBD patients.[4] To these latter efforts, the present report offers several important insights relevant to the structure and metabolism of BRI-L and the nature of ABri fibril assemblies.

First, we have confirmed that BRI and BRI-L adopts the topology of type II integral membrane proteins, and that endoproteolytic cleavage of these proteins between Arg243 and Glu244 generates ~3 kDa and ~4 kDa peptides, respectively, that are released into the conditioned medium. Having confirmed that constitutive endoproteolysis of BRI or BRI-L occurred between Arg243 and Glu244, it also became apparent that the sequence N-terminal to the scissile bond resembled a consensus recognition site for the proprotein convertase, furin. Using somatic cells deficient for furin and furin-complementation strategies, we have demonstrated that furin appears to be both necessary and sufficient for endoproteolytic processing of BRI and BRI-L and the production of secreted, carboxyl-terminal peptides.

While it was apparent that BRI endoproteolysis was mediated by furin, it is also clear that the levels of secreted peptides in medium of CHO-K1, RPE.40 or N2a cells that were derived from the BRI-L precursor were markedly elevated over the peptides generated from the BRI precursor. These results suggested that the carboxyl-terminal extension present in the BRI-L molecule had a dominant effect on proteolysis at the furin site. We favor the notion that the extended peptide introduces subtle conformational transitions within the carboxyl-terminal domain of BRI-L, providing a substrate with enhanced susceptibility to furin proteolysis. However, other models to explain the differences in peptide secretion include differential stability, or intracellular aggregation of wild-type and mutant peptides, notions that are being currently evaluated. We are also struck by the apparently discordant finding that in CHO-K1 and N2a cells, co-expression of human furin had a negligible effect on enhancing the production of secreted peptides derived from either BRI or BRI-L. How do we reconcile these results? At present, we can only offer the speculative model that, in transiently transfected cells, only limiting amounts of BRI and BRI-L are competent for export to late compartments of the secretory apparatus (TGN or plasma membrane) where furin, at saturating levels, is active. In this scenario, transient overexpression of exogenous furin has only a modest effect on the endoproteolysis of the precursor pool that arrives at the TGN or plasma membrane compartments. These hypotheses are now being evaluated in stably transfected cells expressing human BRI and BRI-L.

At present, little information is available pertaining to the cellular distribution or biological function(s) of BRI, or the secreted, carboxyl-terminal peptide derivative, in brain. In this regard, it is notable that *BRI* cDNA is identical to a previously described cDNA encoding integral membrane 2B (ITM2B), a member of a family of proteins identified in a subtraction hybridization screen for markers of chondro-osteogenic differentiation.[15,16] In this regard, subtilisin-like proprotein convertases play critical roles in regulating the turnover and processing of members of the transforming growth factor-β (TGF-β) family of proteins, including TGF-β1, TGF-β2, and TGF-β3, bone morphogenetic proteins (BMP2–7), nodal, activin A and DPP,[17] molecules that are critical for developmental cell fate decisions. It is not inconceivable that BRI may also serve as the precursor of biologically active peptides that play important roles during normal brain development and aging. We have recently raised highly sensitive antibodies to GST fusion proteins encompassing various domains of human BRI, and these reagents are being used to evaluate the cellular and subcellular distribution of the protein in the CNS.

Finally, and despite the strengths of our conclusions relevant to BRI processing, the role of ABri peptides in initiating the clinical syndromes and pathophysiological cascades in patients with FBD is not known. To examine these issues, it will be critical to generate transgenic mice that overexpress human BRI-L in the nervous system, efforts that are ongoing in our laboratory. We anticipate that these mice will recapitulate at least a subset of the histological lesions and behavioral alterations that typify FBD, information that will serve to clarify the processes that lead to neuronal dysfunction and death in this disorder.

ACKNOWLEDGMENTS

This study was supported by National Institute of Health grants AG14248 (S.S.S.) and 5 T32 GM07281 (D.J.G.), The Alzheimer's Association (S.M. and R.W.; IIRG #98 134), and The Stasia Borsuk Memorial Fund (R.W.; RG1-96-070).

REFERENCES

1. PLANT, G.T., T. REVESZ, R.O. BARNARD, A.E. HARDING & P.C. GAUTIER-SMITH. 1990. Familial cerebral amyloid angiopathy with nonneuritic amyloid plaque formation. Brain 113:721–747.
2. WORSTER-DROUGHT, C., J.G. GREENFIELD & W.H. MCMENEMEY. 1940. A form of familial presenile dementia with spastic paralysis (including the pathological examination of a case). Brain 63: 237–254.
3. GRIFFITHS, R.A., T.F. MORTIMER, D.R. OPPENHEIMER & J.M. SPALDING. 1982. Congophilic angiopathy of the brain: a clinical and pathological report on two siblings. J. Neurol. Neurosurg. Psychiatry 45: 396–408.
4. VIDAL, R., B. FRANGIONE, A. ROSTAGNO, S. MEAD, T. REVESZ, G. PLANT & J. GHISO. 1999. A stop-codon mutation in the BRI gene associated with familial British dementia. Nature 399: 776–781.
5. NAKAYAMA, K. 1997. Furin: a mammalian subtilisin/Kex2p-like endoprotease involved in processing of a wide variety of precursor proteins. Biochem. J. 327: 625–635.
6. MOLLOY, S.S., E.D. ANDERSON, F. JEAN & G. THOMAS. 1999. Bi-cycling the furin pathway: from TGN localization to pathogen activation and embryogenesis. Trends Cell Biol. 9: 28–35.
7. KIM, S.H., R. WANG, D.J. GORDON, J. BASS, D.F. STEINER, D.G. LYNN, G. THINAKARAN, S.C. MEREDITH & S.S. SISODIA. 1999. Furin mediates enhanced production of fibrillogenic ABri peptides in familial British dementia. Nat. Neurosci. 2: 984–988.
8. WATANABE, T., T. NAKAGAWA, J. IKEMIZU, M. NAGAHAMA, K. MURAKAMI & K. NAKAYAMA. 1992. Sequence requirements for precursor cleavage within the constitutive secretory pathway. J. Biol. Chem. 267: 8270–8274.
9. WATANABE, T., K. MURAKAMI & K. NAKAYAMA. 1993. Positional and additive effects of basic amino acids on processing of precursor proteins within the constitutive secretory pathway. FEBS Lett. 320: 215–218.

10. MOLLOY, S.S., P.A. BRESNAHAN, S.H. LEPPLA, K.R. KLIMPEL & G. THOMAS. 1992. Human furin is a calcium-dependent serine endoprotease that recognizes the sequence Arg-X-X-Arg and efficiently cleaves anthrax toxin protective antigen. J. Biol. Chem. **267:** 16396–16402.

11. TAKAHASHI, S., K. HATSUZAWA, T. WATANABE, K. MURAKAMI & K. NAKAYAMA. 1994. Sequence requirements for endoproteolytic processing of precursor proteins by furin: transfection and *in vitro* experiments. J. Biochem. (Tokyo) **116:** 47–52.

12. MOEHRING, J.M. & T.J. MOEHRING. 1983. Strains of CHO-K1 cells resistant to Pseudomonas exotoxin A and cross-resistant to diphtheria toxin and viruses. Infect. Immun. **41:** 998–1009.

13. MOEHRING, J.M., N.M. INOCENCIO, B.J. ROBERTSON & T.J. MOEHRING. 1993. Expression of mouse furin in a Chinese hamster cell resistant to Pseudomonas exotoxin A and viruses complements the genetic lesion. J. Biol. Chem. **268:** 2590–2594.

14. SPENCE, M.J., J.F. SUCIC, B.T. FOLEY & T.J. MOEHRING. 1995. Analysis of mutations in alleles of the *fur* gene from an endoprotease-deficient Chinese hamster ovary cell strain. Somat. Cell Mol. Genet. **21:** 1–18.

15. DELEERSNIJDER, W., G. HONG, R. CORTVRINDT, C. POIRIER, P. TYLZANOWSKI, K. PITTOIS, E. VAN MARCK & J. MERREGAERT. 1996. Isolation of markers for chondro-osteogenic differentiation using cDNA library subtraction. Molecular cloning and characterization of a gene belonging to a novel multigene family of integral membrane proteins. J. Biol. Chem. **271:** 19475–19482.

16. PITTOIS, K., W. DELEERSNIJDER & J. MERREGAERT. 1998. cDNA sequence analysis, chromosomal assignment and expression pattern of the gene coding for integral membrane protein 2B. Gene **217:** 141–149.

17. CONSTAM, D.B. & E.J. ROBERTSON. 1999. Regulation of bone morphogenetic protein activity by pro domains and proprotein convertases. J. Cell Biol. **144:** 139–149.

High Frequency of Mutations in Four Different Disease Genes in Early-Onset Dementia

ULRICH FINCKH,[a,i] TOMAS MÜLLER-THOMSEN,[b] ULRIKE MANN,[b] CHRISTIAN EGGERS,[c] JOSEF MARKSTEINER,[d] WOLFGANG MEINS,[e] GIULIANO BINETTI,[f] ANTONELLA ALBERICI,[f] PETER SONDEREGGER,[g] CHRISTOPH HOCK,[h] ROGER M. NITSCH,[h] AND ANDREAS GAL[a]

[a]Department of Human Genetics, University Hospital Eppendorf, University of Hamburg, 22529 Hamburg, Germany

[b]Department of Psychiatry, University Hospital Eppendorf, University of Hamburg, 22529 Hamburg, Germany

[c]Department of Neurology, University Hospital Eppendorf, University of Hamburg, 22529 Hamburg, Germany

[d]Clinic of Psychiatry, University of Innsbruck, 6020 Innsbruck, Austria

[e]Albertinen-Haus, Geriatric Centre, Hamburg, Germany

[f]IRCCS Centro S.Giovanni di Dio, Alzheimer Disease Unit, 25135 Brescia, Italy

[g]Department of Biochemistry, University of Zürich, 8008 Zürich, Switzerland

[h]Department of Psychiatry Research, University of Zürich, 8008 Zürich, Switzerland

ABSTRACT: Heterozygous mutations in the genes for amyloid precursor protein (APP), the presenilins (PS1, PS2), prion protein (PrP), neuroserpin, and tau are associated with early-onset dementia (EOD) with or without neurological signs in the early disease stage. To investigate the proportion of EOD without early neurological signs attributable to known genes we prospectively (i.e., *ante mortem*) screened these six genes for mutations in 36 patients with EOD before age 60. Family history for dementia was positive (PFH) in 16, negative (NFH) in 17, and unknown (UFH) in 3 patients. In 12 patients, we found 5 novel mutations (PS1: F105L; PS2: T122P, M239I; PrP: Q160X, T188K) and 5 previously reported mutations (APP: in three most likely unrelated patients V717I; PS1: A79V, M139V; PrP: P102L, T183A) that all are considered disease causing. Of these 12 patients, 9 had PFH. This indicates a detection rate of 56% (9/16) in patients with PFH. We found 2 mutations (APP V717I) in 2 of the 3 the UFH-patients, and only 1 mutation (PrP T188K) in 1 of the 17 patients with NFH. No mutation was found in tau and neuroserpin genes. To date, three patients died and FAD, predicted by PS mutations in two patients, and prion disease, predicted by a PrP mutation in the third one, were histopathologically confirmed at autopsy. Up to now, mutation findings may be the most specific biomarkers for an *ante mortem* diagnosis of FAD or hereditary prion disease.

[i]Address for correspondence: U. Finckh, Universitätsklinikum Hamburg-Eppendorf, Institut für Humangenetik, Butenfeld 42, 22529 Hamburg, Germany. Tel.: +49 40 42803-4615; fax: +49 40 42803-5138.
e-mail: finckh@uke.uni-hamburg.de

INTRODUCTION

Alzheimer disease (AD) is the most frequent cause of dementia and presents with variable clinical manifestations.[1] Differential diagnosis of early-onset dementia (EOD) may, in addition to familial AD (FAD) associated with mutations in the genes for PS1, PS2, or APP (*PSEN1, PSEN2, APP*),[2–5] include prion disease with mutations in the PrP gene (*PRNP*) but lacking the classic neurological signs of Creutzfeldt-Jakob disease (CJD),[6–8] frontotemporal dementia with mutations in the tau gene (*MAPT*),[9] or other rare dementing disorders, for example, due to mutations in the gene for neuroserpin (*PI12*).[10] The lack of specific and unambiguous clinical or biochemical *ante mortem* diagnostic markers for these entities leads to difficult diagnostic situations in dementia patients without significant neurological signs in the early disease stage, and *post mortem* histopathological evaluation is necessary for confirmation of the clinical diagnosis.

SUBJECTS AND METHODS

DNA was prepared from peripheral blood leukocytes of 36 unrelated German, Austrian, Italian, Hungarian, and Swiss patients with EOD and onset before age 60, and 3 unrelated German patients with late-onset dementia above age 65. None of the patients had significant neurological signs in the early disease stage, and all had a clinical diagnosis of dementia of unknown type or possible or probable AD. Sixteen of the EOD patients had positive family history (PFH) of EOD, whereas the 3 late-onset patients had PFH of late-onset dementia. PFH was assumed if at least one first-degree relative with dementia was reported. Most of the patients seen as outpatients ($n = 15$) and all research-study patients ($n = 24$) underwent full medical and neurological examination, cognitive evaluation, routine blood tests, EEG, and brain CT scans. Clinical diagnosis of possible or probable AD was made according to NINCDS-ADRDA criteria.[11] Ethical approval for this study was obtained from local ethics committees.

Mutation analysis was performed on genomic DNA by direct sequencing of both strands of PCR-amplified coding exons of *PSEN1*, *PSEN2*, exons 16 and 17 of *APP*, the single coding exon of *PRNP*, all coding exons of *PI12*, and exons 9–13 of *MAPT*. Mutation screening was stopped if a known and most likely disease-causing mutation was identified in any patient. All sequence changes were confirmed by restriction enzyme digestion or allele-specific PCR (ASP) (see TABLE 1). *PRNP* haplotypes were determined by selective sequencing of single alleles after restriction digestion at polymorphic codon 129.[12]

RESULTS AND DISCUSSION

In 14 patients, we found a total of 12 different mutations in *PSEN1*, *PSEN2*, *APP*, and *PRNP* (TABLE 1).[13] Five of the 12 mutations were previously undescribed and 7 were known. None of the 5 novel mutations was present on at least 100 control chromosomes. Two (PS1 E318G, PrP del r34) of the 12 mutations reported here are considered nonpathogenic polymorphisms. The 10 remaining mutations, in a total of 12

TABLE 1. Mutations found in 14 patients with early-onset dementia

Patient	Origin[a]	DNA Mutation	Predicted Protein Alteration	Mutation Confirmation[b]	Family History[c]	Onset[d]	Co-Segregation[e]	Histopathological Diagnosis
1	G	GCC→GTC	PS1 A79V	− Hha I	early	~58	n.a.	
2	G	TTT→TTG	PS1 F105L[f]	+ Bst 1107 I	early	~52	n.a.	patient: AD
3	G	ATG→GTG	PS1 M139V	− Nla III	early	32	n.a.	father: AD
4	G	GAA→GGA	PS1 E318G[g]	ASP	negative	53	N.D.	
5	G	GAA→GGA	PS1 E318G[g]	ASP	late	53	n.a.	
6	G	ACG→CCG	PS2 T122P[f]	− Aci I	early	46	+	
6		del 24bp	PrP del r34[h]	sequencing			−	
7	I	ATG→ATA	PS2 M239yf	− Hae III	early	58	+	patient: AD
8	G	GTC→ATC	APP V717I	+ Bcl I	early	~50	n.a.	
9	G	GTC→ATC	APP V717I	+ Bcl I	unknown	53	N.D.	
10	T	GTC→ATC	APP V717I	+ Bcl I	unknown	54	N.D.	
11	G	CCG→CTG	PrP P102L	+ Dde I	early	40	+	brother (1987): AD
12	A	CAA→TAA	PrP Q160X[f]	+ Dde I	early	32	+	
13	G	ACA→GCA	PrP T183A	ASP	early	40	+	spongiform encephalopathy
14	A	ACG→AAG	PrP T188K[f]	ASP	negative	59	N.D.	

[a] G: Germany; T: Thailand; I: Italy; A: Austria.

[b] Confirmation of mutation by restriction endonuclease digestion (+/−, gain/loss of cleavage site, respectively) or allele-specific PCR (ASP).

[c] Early: early-onset dementia; late: late onset dementia reported in first-degree relatives of the index patient; unknown: family history unknown or not informative; negative: family history negative for dementia.

[d] Age of onset of dementia in index patient.

[e] n.a.: no family material available for segregation analysis; N.D.: unknown or negative family history; +: cosegregation; −: no cosegregation of early-onset dementia with the mutation.

[f] Mutation not described previously.

[g] This mutation affects an evolutionarily not conserved residue, and it seems to be a nonpathogenic polymorphism.[28,29]

[h] This in-frame deletion seems to be a nonpathogenic polymorphism.

patients, affect evolutionarily highly conserved residues. No mutation was found in *PI12* and *MAPT* and in the 3 patients with late-onset dementia and PFH for late-onset dementia.

Clinical phenotypes of patients (1, 3, 8–11, and 13 in TABLE 1) and some of their relatives with the previously known mutations PS1 A79V, PS1 M139V, APP V717I, PrP P102L, and PrP T183A were similar to those described in several studies.[2–5,14–20] A novel *PSEN1* mutation predicting F105L in hydrophilic loop 1 (HL1) immediately adjacent to transmembrane domain 1 (TM1) of PS1 was found in a patient (2) with a histopathologically confirmed diagnosis of AD. The two novel missense mutations in *PSEN2* predict T122P and M293I within HL1 and TM5 of PS2, respectively. Both ages of onset of approximately 46 years and the clinical courses were similar in the patient (6) with T122P, her mother, and her maternal grandmother. This suggests a constant pattern of phenotype expression and a higher penetrance of T122P compared to the previously reported *PSEN2* mutations in codons 141 and 239.[3,4] In addition to the T122P mutation, the patient (6) carried a 24-bp in-frame deletion in *PRNP* (del r34). The patient's father, who was not demented at age 81, and who did not have the T122P mutation, also carried M129 in *cis* with del r34. Therefore, del r34 is likely a nonpathogenic polymorphism. In a histopathologically confirmed AD patient (7), we have also identified a novel *PSEN2* mutation that predicts M293I in TM5. In the respective family, 5 siblings carried PS2 M293I, but only 3 of 5 subjects had AD, although the unaffected mutation carriers were at least as old as their affected siblings. This phenotypic variability was similar to that of the previously reported PS2 mutations M239V and N141I in Italian and Volga German kindreds, respectively.[3,4] In 4 patients we identified 3 distinct missense mutations and one nonsense mutation in *PRNP*. A mutation at codon 102 (P102L) was found in 2 siblings, both with disease onset at 40 years. In 1987 one of the siblings had an *ante mortem* biopsy-based histopathological diagnosis of AD. Both siblings shared the Gerstmann-Sträussler-Scheinker disease (GSS) haplotype PrP L102 in *cis* with M129,[17,18] and both were heterozygous for M/V at codon 129. Analysis of the pedigree revealed several relatives with ataxia and largely variable clinical phenotype characteristics for GSS.[18,19] PrP Q160X most likely leads to a premature translation stop, and to the synthesis of C-terminally truncated PrP. This mutation, in *cis* with PrP M129, was found both in a patient (12) with onset of dementia at 32 years, and his elder brother with disease onset at 48 years. Their father, who died at age 60, also had had dementia with an onset at age 48. The wild-type allele of the younger brother encoded M129, that of the elder brother V129. Because the M/V polymorphism at residue 129 is known to modify the phenotype expression of several prion disease alleles,[21–23] it may explain the differences in the age of onset between these two siblings. A premature stop of *PRNP* at the nearby codon 145 was previously found in a patient with a *clinical* diagnosis of AD but with a *post mortem* diagnosis of cerebral PrP amyloid angiopathy.[24,25] The novel missense mutation in *PRNP* codon 188 (T188K) was found in a 59-year old patient (14) with dementia along with dysphasia as the leading initial signs. In this patient the disease was rapidly progressing and reached most severe dementia within less than a year.

Our results, together with those of other authors, suggest that 10 of the 12 different mutations detected in 14 of a total of 36 EOD patients are disease-causing. Our data indicate a high prevalence of pathogenic mutations in *APP, PSEN1, PSEN2*, or

TABLE 2. Frequency of pathogenic mutations detected in 39 unrelated dementia patients grouped according to onset and family history

Clinical Diagnosis of Index Patient	n	Family History	Pathogenic Mutations
Early-onset dementia	16	early-onset dementia	9
	17	negative for early-onset dementia	1
	3	unknown	2
Late-onset dementia	3	late-onset dementia	0

PRNP in patients with onset of dementia before the age of 60 and PFH of EOD. Nine of the 16 patients (56%) with PFH carried pathogenic mutations, whereas only 1 from 17 patients with NFH carried a pathogenic mutation that was in *PRNP* (TABLE 2). This latter patient also has clinical signs atypical of AD, and he most likely has prion disease. The high frequency of mutations in the three known FAD genes of patients with PFH extends the data obtained in Dutch, Japanese, and French FAD studies that reported detection rates of 18%, 20%, and 71%, respectively.[14,26,27] In these studies no mutations in *PSEN2* were found, and *PRNP* was not analyzed. The data from our multinational patient sample suggest both an extensive genetic heterogeneity of FAD and of EOD in general. Furthermore, our data suggest that, in a well-selected group of patients, over 50% of the genetic causes of EOD resembling FAD, or 46% of early-onset FAD, can be readily identified. Our data show the importance of diagnostic sequencing of *APP*, *PSEN1*, *PSEN2*, and *PRNP* in patients with EOD and PFH but without neurological signs in the early phase of the disease and without histopathological analysis. In order not to miss specific treatments of known causes of dementia and for proper clinical and genetic counseling, early and disease-specific diagnosis of EOD is essential.

ACKNOWLEDGMENTS

This work was supported by the Deutsche Forschungsgemeinschaft under Grant FOR 267/2.

REFERENCES

1. MAYEUX, R., Y. STERN & S. SPANTON. 1985. Heterogeneity in dementia of the Alzheimer type: evidence of subgroups. Neurology **35**: 453–461.
2. GOATE, A., M.C. CHARTIER-HARLIN, M. MULLAN, *et al.* 1991. Segregation of a missense mutation in the amyloid protein precursor gene with familial Alzheimer's disease. Nature **349**: 704–709.
3. LEVY-LAHAD, E., W. WASCO, P. POORKAJ, *et al.* 1995. Candidate gene for the chromosome 1 familial Alzheimer's disease locus. Science **269**: 973–977.
4. ROGAEV, E.I., R. SHERRINGTON, E.A. ROGAEVA, *et al.* 1995. Familial Alzheimer's disease in kindreds with missense mutations in a gene on chromosome 1 related to the Alzheimer's disease type 3 gene. Nature **376**: 775–778.
5. SHERRINGTON, R., E.I. ROGAEV, Y. LIANG, *et al.* 1995. Cloning a gene bearing missense mutations in early-onset familial Alzheimer's disease. Nature **375**: 754–760.

6. HALTIA, M., M. VIITANEN, R. SULKAVA, *et al.* 1994. Chromosome 14-encoded Alzheimer's disease: genetic and clinicopathological description. Ann. Neurol. **36:** 362–367.
7. GELDMACHER, D.S. & P.J. WHITEHOUSE, JR. 1997. Differential diagnosis of Alzheimer's disease. Neurology **48**(Suppl. 6): S2–S9.
8. HARDY, J. & K. GWINN-HARDY. 1998. Genetic classification of primary neurodegenerative disease. Science **282:** 1075–1079.
9. HUTTON, M., C.L. LENDON, P. RIZZU, *et al.* 1998. Association of missense and 5′-splice-site mutations in tau with the inherited dementia FTDP-17. Nature **393:** 702–705.
10. DAVIS, R.L., A.E. SHRIMPTON, P.D. HOLOHAN, *et al.* 1999. Familial dementia caused by polymerization of mutant neuroserpin. Nature **401:** 376–379.
11. MCKHANN, G., D. DRACHMAN, M. FOLSTEIN, *et al.* 1984. Clinical diagnosis of Alzheimer's disease: report of the NINCDS-ADRDA group under the auspices of Department of HHS task force on Alzheimer's disease. Neurology **34:** 939–944.
12. OWEN, F., M. POULER, R. LOFTHOUSE, *et al.* 1989. Insertion in prion protein gene in familial Creutzfeldt-Jakob disease. Lancet **1**(8628): 51–52.
13. FINCKH, U., T. MÜLLER-THOMSEN, U. MANN, *et al.* 2000. High prevalence of pathogenic mutations in patients with early-onset dementia detected by sequence analyses of four different genes. Am. J. Hum. Genet. **66:** 110–117.
14. CRUTS, M., C.M. VAN DUIJN, H. BACKHOVENS, *et al.* 1998. Estimation of the genetic contribution of presenilin-1 and -2 mutations in a population-based study of presenile Alzheimer disease. Hum. Mol. Genet. **7:** 43–51.
15. FOX, N.C., A.M. KENNEDY, R.J. HARVEY, *et al.* 1997. Clinicopathological features of familial Alzheimer's disease associated with the M139V mutation in the presenilin 1 gene. Pedigree but not mutation specific age at onset provides evidence for a further genetic factor. Brain **120:** 491–501.
16. HULL, M., B.L. FIEBICH, P. DYKIEREK, *et al.* 1998. Early-onset Alzheimer's disease due to mutations of the presenilin-1 gene on chromosome 14: a 7-year follow-up of a patient with a mutation at codon 139. Eur. Arch. Psychiatry Clin. Neurosci. **248:** 123–129.
17. HSIAO, K., H.F. BAKER, T.J. CROW, *et al.* 1989. Linkage of a prion protein missense variant to Gerstmann-Straussler syndrome. Nature **338:** 342–345.
18. HAINFELLNER, J.A., S. BRANTNER-INTHALER, L. CERVENAKOVA, *et al.* 1995. The original Gerstmann-Straussler-Scheinker family of Austria: divergent clinicopathological phenotypes but constant PrP genotype. Brain Pathol. **5:** 201–211.
19. HAMASAKI, S., S. SHIRABE, R. TSUDA, *et al.* 1998. Discordant Gerstmann-Sträussler-Scheinker disease in monozygotic twins. Lancet **352:** 1358–1359.
20. NITRINI, R., S. OSEMBERG, M.R. PASSOS-BUENO, *et al.* 1997. Familial spongiform encephalopathy associated with a novel prion protein gene mutation. Ann. Neurol. **42:** 138–146.
21. GOLDFARB, L.G., R.B. PETERSEN, M. TABATON, *et al.* 1992. Fatal familial insomnia and familial Creutzfeldt-Jakob disease: disease phenotype determined by a DNA polymorphism. Science **258:** 806–808.
22. BARBANTI, P., G. FABBRINI, M. SALVATORE, *et al.* 1996. Polymorphism at codon 129 or codon 219 of PRNP and clinical heterogeneity in a previously unreported family with Gerstmann-Sträussler-Scheinker disease (PrP-P102L mutation). Neurology **47:** 734–741.
23. YOUNG, K., H.B. CLARK, P. PICCARDO, *et al.* 1997. Gerstmann-Straussler-Scheinker disease with the PRNP P102L mutation and valine at codon 129. Brain Res. Mol. Brain Res. **44:** 147–150.
24. KITAMOTO, T. *et al.* 1993. An amber mutation of prion protein in Gerstmann-Straussler syndrome with mutant PrP plaques. Biochem. Biophys. Res. Commun. **192:** 525–531.
25. GHETTI, B., P. PICCARDO, M.G. SPILLANTINI, *et al.* 1996. Vascular variant of prion protein cerebral amyloidosis with tau-positive neurofibrillary tangles: the phenotype of the stop codon 145 mutation in PRNP. Proc. Natl. Acad. Sci. USA **93:** 744–748.
26. KAMIMURA, K., H. TANAHASHI, H. YAMANAKA, *et al.* 1998. Familial Alzheimer's disease genes in Japanese. J. Neurol. Sci. **160:** 76–81.

27. CAMPION, D., C. DUMANCHIN, D. HANNEQUIN, *et al.* 1999. Early-onset autosomal dominant Alzheimer disease: prevalence, genetic heterogeneity, and mutation spectrum. Am. J. Hum. Genet. **65:** 664–670.
28. PALMER, M.S., S.P. MAHAL, T.A. CAMPBELL, *et al.* 1993. Deletions in the prion protein gene are not associated with CJD. Hum. Mol. Genet. **2:** 541–544.
29. PERRY, R.T., R.C. GO, L.E. HARRELL & R.T. ACTON. 1995. SSCP analysis and sequencing of the human prion protein gene (PRNP) detects two different 24 bp deletions in an atypical Alzheimer's disease family. Am. J. Med. Genet. **60:** 12–18.

Pathological Tau Phenotypes

The Weight of Mutations, Polymorphisms, and Differential Neuronal Vulnerabilities

CHRISTEL MAILLIOT,[a] THIERRY BUSSIÈRE,[b] MALIKA HAMDANE,[a] NICOLAS SERGEANT,[a] MARIE-LAURE CAILLET,[a] ANDRÉ DELACOURTE,[a] AND LUC BUÉE[a,c]

[a]INSERM U422, Place de Verdun, F-59045 Lille Cedex, France

[b]Fishberg Research Center for Neurobiology, Kastor Neurobiology of Aging Laboratories, Mount Sinai School of Medicine, Box1639, One Gustave L. Levy Place, New York, New York 10029, USA

ABSTRACT: In tauopathies, comparative biochemistry of tau aggregates shows that they differ in both phosphorylation and content of tau isoforms. Six tau isoforms are found in human brain that contain either three (3R) or four microtubule-binding domains (4R). In Alzheimer's disease, all six of the tau isoforms are phosphorylated and aggregate into paired helical filaments. They are detected by immunoblotting as a major tau triplet (tau55, 64, and 69). In corticobasal degeneration and progressive supranuclear palsy, only phosphorylated 4R-tau isoforms aggregate and appear as a major tau doublet (tau64 and 69). In Pick's disease, only phosphorylated 3R-tau isoforms aggregate into filaments and are characterized by another major tau doublet (tau55 and 64). Finally, recent findings provide a direct link between a genetic defect in tau and its abnormal aggregation into filaments in frontotemporal dementia with parkinsonism linked to chromosome 17. In the present study, the question of a relationship between tau isoforms and cell morphology is raised. To answer this question, stably transfected human neuroblastoma SY5Y cell lines with either 3R- or 4R-tau isoforms are established. Cell morphology and tau phosphorylation were modified, suggesting that cells undergo profound changes in their metabolism and viability.

INTRODUCTION

Abundant tau-positive neurofibrillary lesions is a neuropathological characteristic of a number of dementing disorders, such as Alzheimer's disease, Pick's disease, progressive supranuclear palsy, corticobasal degeneration, and frontotemporal dementia and parkinsonism linked to chromosome 17. Comparative biochemistry of tau aggregates among these disorders indicates that they exhibit differences that may be related to differential cell vulnerability.

[c]Address for correspondence: Dr. Luc Buée, INSERM U422, Place de Verdun, F-59045 Lille Cedex, France. Tel.: +33/(0) 320 622074; fax: +33/(0) 320 622079.

e-mail: buee@lille.inserm.fr

ALZHEIMER'S DISEASE

Alzheimer's disease (AD) is a progressive neurodegenerative disorder that leads to dementia. The two types of brain lesions observed in AD are amyloid deposits and neurofibrillary tangles (NFTs). NFTs correspond to the accumulation of abnormal fibrils named paired helical filaments (PHFs) and are located in layers II–III and V–VI of the associated areas of the isocortex.[1] The major antigenic components of PHFs are tau proteins, and several groups have reported phosphorylation as the major modification in these proteins.[2,3]

Biochemical characterization by SDS-PAGE and immunoblotting of tau proteins aggregated into PHFs reveals the presence of a triplet of proteins at 55, 64, and 69 kDa (tau55, 64, and 69), and an additional minor 72–74-kDa component. It was shown that tau55 results from the phosphorylation of the shortest isoform (2–, 3–, 10–), tau64 from the phosphorylation of tau variants with one cassette exon (2+, 3, 10– and/or 2–, 3–, 10+), tau69 from the phosphorylation of tau variants with two cassette exons (2+, 3+, 10– and/or 2+, 3–, 10+). Phosphorylation of the longest tau isoform (2+, 3+, 10+) induces the formation of the additional hyperphosphorylated tau74 variant (FIG. 1A).[6] Hyperphosphorylation generates differences that can be visualized by a few phosphorylation-dependent antibodies, such as AT100,[7] AP422,[8] 988,[9] and PHF-27.[10]

PROGRESSIVE SUPRANUCLEAR PALSY AND CORTICOBASAL DEGENERATION

Progressive supranuclear palsy (PSP) is a late-onset atypical parkinsonism disorder described by Steele and coworkers in 1964.[11] Dementia is also a common feature at the end-stage of the disease. Corticobasal degeneration (CBD) is a rare, sporadic, and slowly progressive late-onset neurodegenerative disorder, clinically characterized by cognitive disturbances and extrapyramidal motor dysfunction.[12] There is a clinical and pathological overlap between PSP and corticobasal degeneration. Neuropathologically, PSP and CBD are characterized by neuronal loss, gliosis, and NFT formation, in particular subsets of neurons.[1] Ultrastructural analyses further support differences between AD and PSP, since PHFs are found in AD, while straight filaments are observed in PSP. Ultrastructural studies indicate that tau aggregates in CBD form twisted filaments that differ from PHFs of AD. The electrophoretic profile of aggregated tau proteins in PSP is substantially different from that in AD, as a characteristic doublet is found (tau64 and tau69) instead of the triplet found in AD. A minor 74-kDa band is also detected. In fact, only hyperphosphorylated tau isoforms with sequence encoded by exon 10 (4R-tau isoforms) aggregate into filaments in PSP, whereas tau isoforms without exon 10 (3R-tau isoforms) are not detected (FIG. 1B).[6,13,14] However, most of the phosphorylation sites found in PHF-tau are also encountered in aggregated tau proteins from PSP patients. The electrophoretic profile of tau pathological proteins in CBD is similar to that of PSP.[6,13,14] Although most cases of PSP were usually considered to be sporadic, a recent study of clinical genetics of familial PSP suggests that hereditary PSP is more frequent than previously thought and that the scarcity of familial cases may be related to the lack of rec-

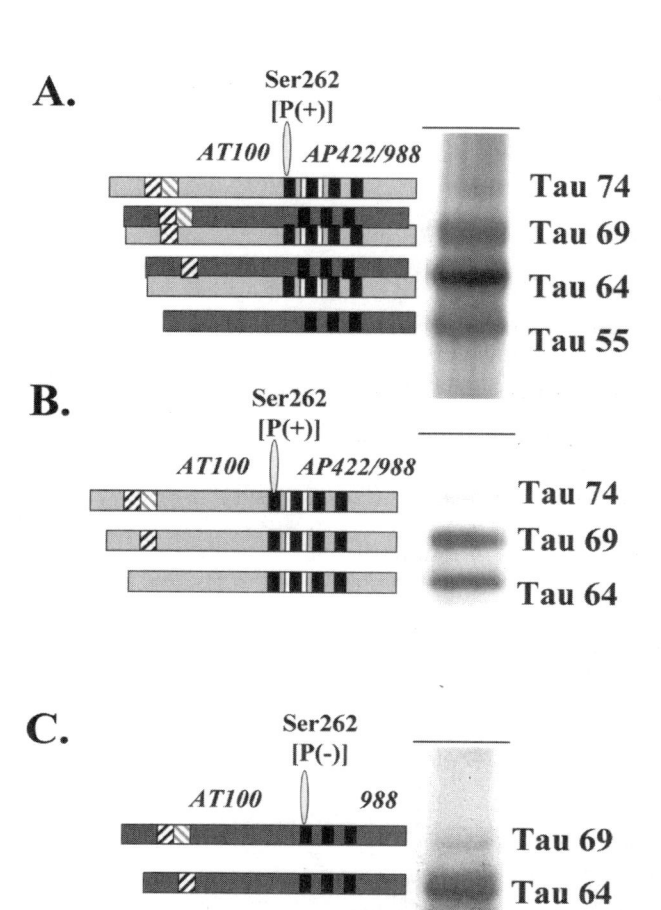

FIGURE 1. Typical Western blots using phosphorylation-dependent monoclonal antibodies exhibiting the electrophoretic tau profiles encountered in AD (**A**), CBD/PSP (**B**), and Pick's disease (**C**). On the *left side* of each blot, a schematic representation of the types of hyperphosphorylated tau isoforms that are found aggregated in filaments is represented. Note that AT100 and AP422/988 label all hyperphosphorylated tau isoforms among tauopathies (A–C). The monoclonal antibody 12E8 (Ser262/356) does not recognize hyperphosphorylated tau isoforms aggregated in Pick bodies (C). Ser262 [P(+)]: phosphorylation at Ser262 and 356. Ser262 [P(+)]: no phosphorylation at Ser262 and 356. Tau isoforms with 3R are *light gray* colored, whereas 4R-tau isoforms are *dark gray*. The *black hatched box* represents exon 2, the *gray hatched box* represents eon 3, and the *white box with a black bar* represents exon 10. *Black bars* are microtubule binding domains.

ognition of the variable phenotypic expression of the disease. Recent data indicate that polymorphisms in the tau gene are probably important in the pathogenesis of PSP. However, it remains to be determined at which level it is involved, that is, as a primary phenomenon or as a secondary one, since in some familial forms of PSP, no linkage to chromosome 17 is observed.[15]

PICK'S DISEASE

Pick's disease is a rare form of neurodegenerative disorder characterized by a progressive dementing process. Early in the clinical course, patients show signs of frontal disinhibition. Neuropathologically, Pick's disease is characterized by prominent frontotemporal lobar atrophy, gliosis, severe neuronal loss, ballooned neurons, and the presence of neuronal inclusions called Pick bodies. The laminar distribution of Pick bodies is clearly different from that of NFTs in AD, CBD, and PSP (for review, see Ref. 1). Ultrastructurally, Pick bodies consist of the accumulation of both random coiled and straight filaments. Biochemically, a major 55- and 64-kDa doublet and a very faint band at 69 kDa are characteristic of Pick's.[16] In fact, only 3R-tau isoforms aggregate into Pick bodies (FIG. 1C), and as expected, Pick bodies and the tau doublet tau55 and tau64 are not labeled with antibodies directed against the sequence encoded by exon 10. Moreover, aggregated tau proteins in Pick's disease cannot be detected by the monoclonal antibody 12E8 raised against phosphorylated residues Ser262 and 356, whereas in other neurodegenerative disorders, this phosphorylation site is always detected.[13,17] Since it was shown that 3R-tau isoforms can be phosphorylated at Ser262/356,[13] the lack of 12E8-immunoreactivity is likely to be related to either a kinase inhibition in neurons that degenerate in Pick's disease or an absence of these kinases within degenerating neurons.[6,13]

FTDP-17

Several families have been described that share both strong clinical features of frontotemporal dementia and pathological hallmarks, and for which there is a linkage with chromosome 17q22-22. These families have been included in a group of pathologies referred to as frontotemporal dementia with parkinsonism linked to chromosome 17 (FTDP-17). One of the most important neuropathological characteristics is the filamentous tau pathology affecting the neuronal cells, or in some cases, both neuronal and glial cells. The absence of amyloid aggregates is usually established. FTDP-17 has been related to mutations on the tau gene. Tau mutations always segregate with the pathology and are not found in the control subjects, suggesting their pathogenic role. The functional effects of the mutations suggest that a reduced ability of tau to interact with microtubules may be upstream of hyperphosphorylation and aggregation (see other chapters of this volume).[6]

These mutations may also lead to an increase in free cytoplasmic tau (especially 4R-tau isoforms), and therefore facilitating their aggregation into filaments. In this respect, we investigated in a neuroblastoma cell line the effects of both 3R- and 4R-tau overexpression.

TAU OVEREXPRESSION IN A CELL MODEL

SY5Y is a human neuroblastoma cell line that can be differentiated using either retinoic acid or NGF. It was previously shown to mainly express the shortest tau isoform. It is a relevant cell model to use in studying tau hyperphosphorylation, since Alzheimer-specific epitopes, including AT100 and AP422, can be induced using okadaic acid (OA). OA, a phosphatase 1 and 2A inhibitor, is a common agent used to induce tau hyperphosphorylation in numerous cell lines, including COS and SY5Y.[13,18] For transfection in SY5Y cells, two tau cDNAs cloned into pcDNA3.1Neo (Invitrogen) were used: "2 + 3 − 10−" encoding a 3R-tau isoform and "2 + 3 − 10+" encoding a 4R-tau isoform. Transfections were performed using *Ex-Gen 500* (Euromedex, France).[13,18] Stably 3R- and 4R-tau transfected cells were characterized at both mRNA and protein levels. Phosphorylation-dependent antibody AD2, directed against phosphorylated Ser396 and 404, was used to characterize tau proteins. M19G is a polyclonal antibody directed against the first 19 amino acids of tau.[6,13,14,16–18]

Different kinds of clones were obtained, depending on their tau levels of expression. Molecular and biochemical analyses were fully correlated. AD2 detected exogenous tau isoforms in both 3R and 4R cell lines. M19G detected both phosphorylated and partially phosphorylated tau isoforms. Interestingly, an increase in MW was observed proportionally to the tau overexpression, suggesting that overexpression of tau proteins leads to their hyperphosphorylation (FIG. 2).

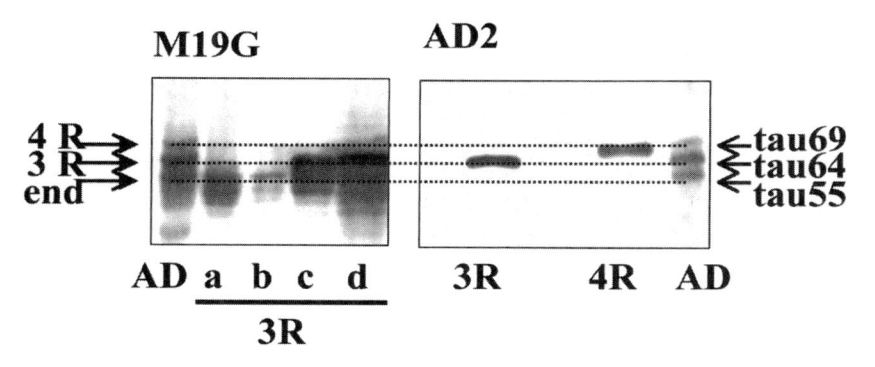

FIGURE 2. Immunoblots of 3R- and 4R-tau transfected SY5Y cells using the antiserum M19G and the AD2 antibody. Both antibodies label the tau triplet in AD (AD). On the *left*, in 3R-tau transfected cell lines, M19G labels both the endogenous (the shortest one) and the overexpressed 3R-tau isoform. It should be noted that low MW 3R-tau variants are detected in cells that exhibit a weak expression (**a** and **b**), whereas high MW 3R-tau variants are detected in cells showing high levels of expression (**c** and **d**). These variations in MW are related to the levels of phosphorylation of the tau isoform. On the *right*, in lysates of tau-transfected cells having the highest level of tau expression, AD2 labels both hyperphosphorylated 3R- and 4R-tau isoforms that migrate at 64 and 69 kDa, respectively. The endogenous tau isoform is poorly detected (not visualized on this blot). 3R and 4R: lysates of stably transfected SY5Y cells with the 2 + 3 − 10− and 2 + 3 − 10+ tau isoform cDNAs, respectively.

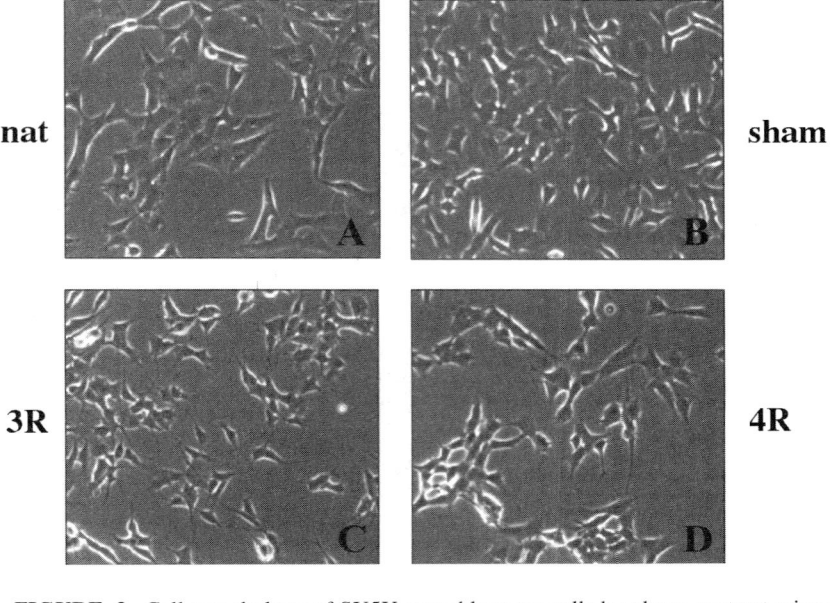

FIGURE 3. Cell morphology of SY5Y neuroblastoma cells by phase-contrast microscopy. (**A**) Normal SY5Y cells (nat). (**B**) Transfected SY5Y cells with the empty pcDNA3.1Neo vector (sham). (**C**) Tau isoform (2 + 3 − 10−)-transfected SY5Y cells (3R). (**D**) Tau isoform (2 + 3 − 10+)-transfected SY5Y cells (4R). There is no striking difference between A and B. There is a lower cell density in C and D compared to A and B. Note the denser neuritic network in C compared to A, B, and D. 3R-tau transfected cells exhibit longer neurites and present more ramifications (C).

In order to better mimic the pathology from a morphological point of view, we have chosen to work with the cell lines expressing the highest levels of exogenous tau. Tau overexpression, as previously shown, induces neuritic extension in human neuroblastoma SY5Y cells (FIG. 3). Surprisingly, however, neurites of 3R-tau expressing cell lines (FIG. 3C) seem to be longer and present more ramifications than neurites of 4R stably transfected cells (FIG. 3D), and thus form a denser neuritic network. Moreover, since the 3R cells are more differentiated, they grow more slowly than 4R cells.

Altogether, these data indicate that particular sets of tau isoforms (3R-, 4R-, or all of the six tau isoforms) aggregate in subpopulations of neurons and explain the specific electrophoretic tau profiles observed among these disorders. In our model of 3R- or 4R-tau stably transfected human neuroblastoma SY5Y cells, tau overexpression leads to hyperphosphorylation and modifications of the cytoskeleton. Interestingly, weak differentiation was observed in 4R-tau transfected cell lines compared to the 3R ones, suggesting that 4R-tau overexpression may interfere with the dynamics of microtubules.

ACKNOWLEDGMENTS

This work was sponsored by the Institut de la Santé et de la Recherche Médicale, the Centre National de la Recherche Scientifique, Aventis (to L.B.), and Conseil Régional Nord Pas-de-Calais (Pôle Neurosciences) (to L.B.). C.M. is a recipient of a scholarship from the French Research Ministry. T.B. and N.S. are supported by fellowships from the Philippe Foundation and Société de Secours des Amis des Sciences, respectively. AD2 was developed through collaboration between INSERM and UMR9921 CNRS-Sanofi Diagnostics Pasteur. The authors thank Dr. Michel Goedert (Cambridge, UK) for tau isoform cDNAs, and Drs. Eugeen Vanmechelen (Innogenetics) and Dale Schenk (Elan Pharmaceutical) for AT and 12E8 antibodies, respectively.

REFERENCES

1. HOF, P.R. *et al.* 1999. Cortical neuropathology in aging and dementing disorders: neuronal typology, connectivity, and selective vulnerability. *In* Cerebral Cortex, Vol. 14, A. Peters and J.H. Morrison, Eds.: 175–312. Kluwer Academic Plenum. New York.
2. TROJANOWSKI, J.Q. & V.M. LEE. 1995. Phosphorylation of paired helical filament tau in Alzheimer's disease neurofibrillary lesions: focusing on phosphatases. FASEB J. **9:** 1570–1576.
3. DELACOURTE, A. & L. BUÉE. 1997. Normal and pathological tau proteins as factors for microtubule assembly. Int. Rev. Cytol. **171:** 167–224.
4. SPILLANTINI, M.G. & M. GOEDERT. 1998. Tau protein pathology in neurodegenerative diseases. Trends Neurosci. **21:** 428–433.
5. GOEDERT, M. *et al.* 1989. Cloning and sequencing of the cDNA encoding an isoform of microtubule-associated protein tau containing 4 tandem repeats—Differential expression of tau protein messenger RNAs in human brain. EMBO J. **8:** 393–399.
6. BUÉE, L. & A. DELACOURTE. 1999. Comparative biochemistry of tau in progressive supranuclear palsy, corticobasal degeneration, FTDP-17 and Pick's disease. Brain Pathol. **9:** 681–693.
7. ZHENG-FISCHHÖFFER, Q. *et al.* 1998. Sequential phosphorylation of tau by glycogen synthase kinase-3beta and protein kinase A at Thr212 and Ser214 generates the Alzheimer-specific epitope of antibody AT100 and requires a paired-helical-filament-like conformation. Eur. J. Biochem. **252:** 542–552.
8. HASEGAWA, M. *et al.* 1996. Characterization of mAb AP422, a novel phosphorylation-dependent monoclonal antibody against tau protein. FEBS Lett. **384:** 25–30.
9. BUSSIÈRE, T. *et al.* 1999. Phosphorylated serine422 on tau proteins is a pathological epitope found in several diseases with neurofibrillary degeneration. Acta Neuropathol. **97:** 221–230.
10. HOFFMANN, R. *et al.* 1997. Unique Alzheimer's disease paired helical filament specific epitopes involve double phosphorylation at specific sites. Biochemistry **36:** 8114–8124.
11. STEELE, J.C. *et al.* 1964. Progressive supranuclear palsy. A heterogeneous degeneration involving brain stem, basal ganglia and cerebellum with vertical gaze and pseudobulbar palsy, nuchal dystonia and dementia. Arch. Neurol. **10:** 333–359.
12. REBEIZ, J.J. *et al.* 1968. Corticodentatonigral degeneration with neuronal achromasia. Arch. Neurol. **18:** 20–33.
13. MAILLIOT, C. *et al.* 1998. Phosphorylation of specific sets of tau isoforms explains different neurodegeneration processes. FEBS Lett. **433:** 201–204.
14. SERGEANT, N. *et al.* 1999. Neurofibrillary degeneration in progressive supranuclear palsy and corticobasal degeneration: tau pathologies with exclusively "exon 10" isoforms. J. Neurochem. **72:** 1243–1249.

15. ROJO, A. *et al.* 1999. Clinical genetics of familial progressive supranuclear palsy. Brain **122:** 1233–1245.
16. BUÉE-SCHERRER, V. *et al.* 1996. Hyperphosphorylated tau proteins differentiate corticobasal degeneration and Pick's disease. Acta Neuropathol. **91:** 351–359.
17. DELACOURTE, A. *et al.* 1998. Vulnerable neuronal subsets in Alzheimer's and Pick's disease are distinguished by their tau isoform distribution and phosphorylation. Ann. Neurol. **43:** 193–204.
18. MAILLIOT, C. *et al.* 1998. Alzheimer-specific epitope of AT100 in transfected cell lines with tau: toward an efficient cell model of tau abnormal phosphorylation. Neurosci. Lett. **255:** 13–16.

Coexistent Tau and Amyloid Pathology in Hereditary Frontotemporal Dementia with Tau Mutations

S.M. ROSSO,[a] W. KAMPHORST,[b] R. RAVID,[c] AND J.C. VAN SWIETEN[a,d]

[a]Department of Neurology, Erasmus University Rotterdam, Rotterdam, the Netherlands

[b]Department of Pathology, Vrije Universiteit, Amsterdam, the Netherlands

[c]Netherlands Brain Bank, Amsterdam, the Netherlands

ABSTRACT: Hereditary frontotemporal dementia with Parkinsonism linked to chromosome 17 (FTDP-17) is associated with different mutations in the microtubule-associated protein (MAP) tau gene. Pathological changes consist of accumulation of hyperphosphorylated tau protein in frontal and temporal cortex, hippocampus, and some subcortical nuclei. We describe the neuropathological findings in five patients with P301L mutation, and in two affected sibs with R406W mutation. The P301L brains all showed a pretangle-type tauopathy of the frontal and temporal cortices. One of these patients, however, also showed an Alzheimer-type tauopathy with neurofibrillary tangles (NFT), neuritic plaques, and amyloid angiopathy of the temporoparietal cortex. Three tau bands (64, 68, and 72 kDa) were seen in the frontal cortex, while the temporal cortex revealed four bands (60, 64, 68, and 72 kDa), containing all six tau isoforms. The first R406W brain showed many NFT in affected regions with only a few diffuse amyloid plaques. The second R406W brain contained a much higher density of NFT in affected regions, and an extensive amyloid deposition consisting of both diffuse and neuritic plaques with dense cores. An intriguing question is whether the FTD and Alzheimer disease changes are concomitant, or whether there is an interaction between tau and amyloid pathology. An acceleration of NFT formation due to amyloid deposition has been observed in nondemented aging and preclinical AD. The question whether this mechanism occurs in FTD with tau mutations remains to be elucidated.

INTRODUCTION AND METHODS

The term frontotemporal dementia (FTD) covers a group of presenile dementias with progressive behavioral changes and often frontal or temporal atrophy on neuroimaging.[1] Several mutations in the tau gene have been found in families with hereditary frontotemporal dementia and parkinsonism linked to chromosome 17q21–22 (FTDP-17).[2–8] These mutations explain the accumulation of hyperphosphorylated tau protein in neurons and glial cells in the cortex, hippocampus, and subcortical nuclei. Tau pathology shows considerable variation in the type and distribution of tau

[d]Address for correspondence: Dr. John C. van Swieten, University Hospital Dijkzigt, Dr. Molenwaterplein 40, 3015 GD Rotterdam, the Netherlands. Tel.: 00-31-10-4633274; fax 00-31-10-4633208.

e-mail: vanswieten@neur.azr.nl

TABLE 1. Cortical distribution of tau and amyloid depositions

		Tau Deposition			Amyloid Deposition			
Brain	Age	Type	Localization	Density^a	Type	Localization	Density^b	Angiopathy
P301L 1	65	pretangles	F, T, P	++	none	–	–	–
P301L 2	66	pretangles	F, T, P	++	none	–	–	–
P301L 3	53	pretangles	F, T, P	++	none	–	–	–
P301L 4	76	pretangles	F, T, P	+++	neuritic	T, O	++	–
P301L 5	64	pretangles	F, T	++	neuritic	T, P, O	+	+
		NFT	T, P	+				
R406W 1	69	NFT	F, T	+	diffuse	F, O	+	–
R406W 2	70	NFT	F, T, P	++	neuritic	F, T, P, O	++	+

ABBREVIATIONS: F, frontal cortex; T, temporal cortex; P, parietal cortex; O, occipital cortex; NFT, neurofibrillary tangles.
^{a}Mean tangle density (both NFT and pretangles; number per mm^2): – = 0/mm^2, + = 1–50/mm^2, ++ = 50–100/mm^2, +++ = 100 or more/mm^2.
^{b}Mean plaque density (both diffuse and neuritic; number per mm^2): – = 0/mm^2, + = 1–5/mm^2, ++ = 5–10/mm^2, +++ = 10 or more/mm^2.

deposits, the physical structure of filaments, and tau isoform composition between the different FTDP-17 families.[8–14]

We have investigated tau and amyloid pathology in five P301L and two R406W patients (see TABLE 1). All brains showed moderate to severe atrophy of frontal and anterior temporal lobes. Sections from different cortical regions, hippocampus, substantia nigra, and other subcortical nuclei were processed for routine staining and for immunohistochemistry using phosphorylation-dependent [AT8, AT180, AT100, PHF1, 12 E8 and E10], phosphorylation-independent anti-tau [BR133, BR134, BR304, BR189], anti-β-amyloid (βA4), and ubiquitin antibodies. Tissue sections were pretreated with 90% formic acid for 5 min before immunohistochemistry with antibody against βA4 was performed. Sarkosyl-insoluble tau was extracted from fresh-frozen cortices and hippocampus, dephosphorylated as previously described, and run on 10% SDS-PAGE and blotted onto immobilon P [Millipore].[15,16] Blots were incubated overnight at 4°C with antisera [BR133 and BR134] and stained using the biotin-avidin Vectastain system (Vector Laboratories). Sarkosyl-soluble tau was extracted using 2.5% perchloric acid. Aliquots of sarkosyl-insoluble tau were processed for EM.[17]

RESULTS

P301L Brains

Neuronal loss and gliosis were moderate to severe in the frontotemporal cortex. The substantia nigra showed severe loss of pigmented cells. Tau deposits of the pretangle type were found in the frontal and temporal cortex, and to a lesser degree in the parietal cortex, the granular cells of dentate gyrus, and substantia nigra. In the first three P301L brains, no amyloid staining was observed, while in P301L brain 4, some diffuse plaques were seen, mainly in the temporal and occipital cortex; no neuritic plaques or amyloid angiopathy were found. In P301L brain 5, many neurofibrillary tangles (NFT), some extracellular, and many diffuse and neuritic plaques with dense amyloid cores were present in all cortices, subiculum, and hippocampus, whereas some tau-positive glial cells were additionally found in grey and white matter.

Immunoblots of sarkosyl-insoluble tau from P301L brain 5 showed two major bands (64 and 68 kDa) and a minor band of 72 kDa in frontal cortex, and four bands of 60, 64, 68, and 72 kDa in temporal cortex and hippocampus. Electron microscopy (EM) study of sarkosyl-insoluble tau preparations from P301L brain 5 showed tau-containing filaments in hippocampal formation, which were structurally similar to paired helical filaments (PHFs) in AD, and slender twisted filaments in frontal cortex, similar to the other P301L family that we have recently described.

R406W Brains

In the first R406W brain, neuronal loss and gliosis were of variable intensity in frontal and temporal cortex. NFT were abundant in the frontal and temporal cortex, pyramidal layer of the hippocampus, and gyrus parahippocampalis. Substantia nigra showed only a few NFT and neuropil threads. Occasional tau-positive glial cells were seen in the grey and white matter. A few diffuse plaques and occasional classic plaques (stained by βA4 antibody) were present. The antibody against ubiquitin showed staining of numerous neurons and dystrophic neurites in cortices and hippocampus. The second R406W brain showed severe neuronal loss and gliosis in the frontal, temporal, and parietal cortex. Many NFT and extracellular tangles were present in all cortices (except for occipital), hippocampus, gyrus parahippocampalis, amygdala, and hypothalamus. The NFT density in this brain was much higher than that in the R406W brain 1. Many diffuse and neuritic plaques with dense cores (stained by anti-βA4 antibody) were present in all cortices with moderate deposition of β-amyloid in blood vessels.

Immunoblots of sarkosyl-insoluble tau from the R406W brain 2 showed four bands of 60, 64, 68, and 72 kDa, and after alkaline phosphatase treatment six immunoreactive bands corresponding to the six tau isoforms in Alzheimer's disease (AD). The pattern of soluble tau was similar to that from control brains.

EM of sarkosyl-insoluble tau preparations from the R406W brain 2 showed tau-containing filaments in the frontal and temporal cortices and hippocampal formation, which were structurally similar to PHFs in AD, with a diameter of 8–20 nm and a crossover spacing of approximately 80 nm. A minority of filaments consisted of straight filaments (SFs) of about 12 nm.

DISCUSSION

All seven brains of patients with tau mutations (five P301L, two R406W mutations) showed NFT and/or tau deposits of pretangle type. However, large numbers of neuritic plaques and amyloid angiopathy were present in P301L brain 5 and in R406W brain 2. There are at least two other reports of diffuse or classic plaques in patients with presenile dementia and P301L or splice donor mutations.[9,18]

Tau-positive pretangles (mainly perinuclear deposits) were seen in the frontal and temporal cortex, and dentate gyrus of the P301L brains, and this is similar to the Dutch family (HFTD1) with this mutation.[11] This P301L pathology is also supported by the presence of slender twisted filaments, two major bands of 64 and 68 kDa, and a minor band of 72 kDa of sarkosyl-insoluble tau from the frontal cortex, which is consistent with the pattern in other P301L families.[8,12,13] However, NFT, diffuse and senile plaques, PHFs and a pattern of four bands (60, 64, 68, and 72 kDa) of sarkosyl-insoluble tau from the temporal cortex and hippocampus of the P301L brain 5 is consistent with the pathological diagnosis AD. This is further supported by the presence of all six tau isoforms following treatment with alkaline phosphatase. This implies that two different types of tau pathology coexist in the same brain, but were differently distributed in some brain regions.

The presence of NFT in nerve cells with occasional tau deposits in glial cells in both R406W brains is in agreement with studies carried out in another R406W family.[19] NFT, extracellular NFT, PHFs, and SFs are found when all six tau isoforms are mutated, as in cases with mutations in exons 12 and 13. The R406W brain 2 showed a higher density of NFT and a higher number of diffuse and neuritic plaques than the R406W brain 1.

An intriguing question is whether the FTD and AD changes are concomitant, or whether there is an interaction between tau and amyloid pathology. An acceleration of NFT formation due to amyloid deposition has recently been observed in nondemented aging and preclinical AD.[20] The question, therefore, whether this mechanism occurs in FTD with tau mutations remains to be elucidated in future studies.

REFERENCES

1. NEARY, D., J.S. SNOWDEN, L. GUSTAFSON, et al. 1998. Frontotemporal lobar degeneration. A consensus on clinical diagnostic criteria. Neurology **51:** 1546–1554.
2. FOSTER, N.L., K. WILHELMSEN, A.A.F. SIMA, et al. 1997. Frontotemporal dementia and parkinsonism linked to chromosome 17: a consensus statement. Ann. Neurol. **41:** 706–715.
3. POORKAJ, P., TH. BIRD, E. WIJSMAN, et al. 1998. Tau is a candidate gene for chromosome 17 frontotemporal dementia. Ann. Neurol. **43:** 815–825.
4. HUTTON, M., C.L. LENDON, P. RIZZU, et al. 1998. Coding and splice-donor site mutations in tau cause inherited dementia (FTDP-17). Nature **393:** 702–705.
5. SPILLANTINI, M.G., J.R. MURRELL, M. GOEDERT, et al. 1998. Mutation in the tau gene in familial multiple system tauopathy with presenile dementia. Proc. Natl. Acad. Sci. USA **95:** 7737–7741.
6. GOEDERT, M., M.G. SPILLANTINI, R.A. CROWTHER, et al. 1999. Tau gene mutation in familial progressive subcortical gliosis. Nature Med. **5:** 454–457.
7. BUGIANI, O., J.L. MURRELL, G. GIACCONE, et al. 1999. Frontotemporal dementia and corticobasal degeneration in a family with a P301S mutation in tau. J. Neuropathol. Exp. Neurol. **58:** 667–677.
8. CLARK, L.N., P. POORKAJ, Z. WSZOLEK, et al. 1998. Pathogenic implications of mutations in the tau gene in pallido-ponto-nigral degeneration and related neurodegenerative disorders linked to chromosome 17. Proc. Natl. Acad. Sci. USA **95:** 13103–13107.
9. D'SOUZA, I., P. POORKAJ, M. HONG, et al. 1999. Missense and silent tau gene mutations cause frontotemporal dementia with parkinsonism, chromosome 17 type, by affecting multiple alternative RNA splicing regulatory elements. Proc. Natl. Acad. Sci. USA **96:** 5598–5603.

10. SPILLANTINI, M.G., M. GOEDERT, R.A. CROWTHER, J. MURRELL, M.J. FARLOW & B. GHETTI. 1997. Familial multiple system tauopathy with presenile dementia: a disease with abundant neuronal and glial tau filaments. Proc. Natl. Acad. Sci. USA **94:** 4113–4118.
11. SPILLANTINI, M.G., R.A. CROWTHER, W. KAMPHORST, P. HEUTINK & J.C. VAN SWIETEN. 1998. Tau pathology in two Dutch families with mutations in the microtubule-binding region of tau. Am. J. Pathol. **153:** 1359–1363.
12. BIRD, TH.D., D. NOCHLIN, P. POORKAI, *et al.* 1999. A clinical pathological comparison of three families with frontotemporal dementia and identical mutations in the tau gene (P301L). Brain **122:** 741–756.
13. MIRRA, S.S., J.R. MURRELL, M. GEARING, *et al.* 1999. Tau pathology in family with dementia and a P301L mutation in tau. J. Neuropathol. Exp. Neurol. **58:** 335–345.
14. VAN SWIETEN, J.C., M. STEVEN, S.M. ROSSO, *et al.* 1999. Phenotypic variation in hereditary frontotemporal dementia with tau mutations. Ann. Neurol. **46:** 617–626.
15. GOEDERT, M., M.G. SPILLANTINI, N.J. CAIRNS & R.A. CROWTHER. 1992. Tau proteins of Alzheimer paired helical filaments: abnormal hyperphosphorylation of all six isoforms. Neuron **119:** 961–975.
16. GOEDERT, M. & R. JAKES. 1990. Expression of separate isoforms of human tau: correlation with tau pattern in brain and tubulin polymerization. EMBO J. **9:** 4225–4230.
17. CROWTHER, R.A. 1991. Straight and paired helical filaments in Alzheimer disease have a common structural unit. Proc. Natl. Acad. Sci. USA **88:** 2288–2292.
18. DARK, F. 1997. A family with autosomal dominant non-Alzheimer's presenile dementia. Aust. N. Z. J. Psychiatry **31:** 706–715.
19. REED, L.A., TH.J. GRABOWSKI, M.L. SCHMIDT, *et al.* 1997. Autosomal dominant dementia with widespread neurofibrillary tangles. Ann. Neurol. **42:** 564–572.
20. PRICE, J.L. & J.C. MORRIS. 1999. Tangles and plaques in nondemented aging and preclinical Alzheimer disease. Ann. Neurol. **45:** 358–368.

The Clinical Spectrum of Guam ALS and Parkinson-Dementia Complex: 1997–1999

DOUGLAS GALASKO,[a,c] DAVID SALMON,[a] ULLA-KATRINA CRAIG,[b] AND WIGBERT WIEDERHOLT[a]

[a]Department of Neurosciences, University of California, San Diego, San Diego, California, USA, and [b]University of Guam, Guam

Neurology, VA Medical Center, V127, 3350 La Jolla Village Drive, San Diego, California 92161, USA

BACKGROUND

Amyotrophic lateral sclerosis (ALS)[1] was characterized among Chamorros, the native inhabitants of Guam, in the early 1950s, and Parkinson-dementia complex (PDC)[2] was described in the 1960s. Over the next three decades, the prevalence of ALS and, to a lesser extent, PDC decreased,[3] age at onset of both disorders increased, and a pure dementia syndrome was reported. ALS and PDC are of interest for many reasons. The neuropathology of these disorders consists of neurofibrillary tangles (NFT) that are morphologically and biochemically identical to those found in Alzheimer's disease (AD). There is minimal or no accompanying amyloid deposition. The etiology and high prevalence of these disorders on Guam has not been explained. The shifts in prevalence and age at onset suggest that environmental factors are important,[5] although none has been proven to be causative. Through the years, attention has shifted between putative environmental factors such as ingestion of toxins released during the preparation of flour from local cycads, or neurotoxicity related in some way to the unusual mineral content of the water on Guam or to aluminum, but evidence for these has not been conclusive. Genetic influences may be important because familial clustering of cases occurs to an extent, but does not follow an obvious pattern of inheritance.[6-8] It is conceivable that an interaction between genetic predisposition and environment may predispose to developing neurologic disease.

Patients on Guam have been evaluated by a number of research teams during more than four decades of research, with varying approaches to clinical assessment. From 1997–1999, we have carried out standardized medical, neurologic, and psychometric examination of patients on Guam, to re-evaluate the contribution of the environment and to collect detailed family information and DNA on patients to search for genetic predisposition. We have found that ALS continues to decline, PDC is relatively common though the age at onset continues to rise, and a late-life dementia syndrome is becoming increasingly more common.

[c]Address for correspondence: Douglas Galasko, M.D., Neurology, VAMC, 127, 3350 La Jolla Village Drive, San Diego, CA 92161.

CASE FINDING AND EVALUATION, 1997–1999

Cases are referred by several pathways. Many patients are recognized by medical providers on Guam to have a neurologic disease of interest or were diagnosed by a previous research team. We also screen subjects over the age of 60 or first-degree relatives of patients identified as having ALS or PDC in previous registries or studies. A trained research assistant obtains a screening history and brief examination, and tests cognition with the Cognitive Abilities Screening Instrument (CASI).[9] We have pilot tested the CASI on Guam to ensure cultural fairness, assess the extent of variation due to age and education, and develop cutoff points for screening. All subjects who fail the CASI or whose history or brief examination suggests neurologic disease undergo detailed evaluation. Information is collected on risk factors, family history, medication use, medical and neurologic history, cognitive and motor symptoms, and functional performance (of activities of daily living). A neurologist examines mental status and performs a structured neurologic examination that includes the Unified Parkinson's Disease Rating Scale (UPDRS). A psychometrist administers a standardized test battery for which normative data have been obtained from elderly Chamorro subjects, who lacked significant medical or neurologic diagnoses.

Consensus diagnoses are made by three neurologists, who review all clinical information. Diagnoses are made at two levels: descriptive syndromes (such as dementia, parkinsonism, ALS, stroke or other conditions) and suspected etiologic diagnosis (such as ALS or PDC). We use standard clinical diagnostic criteria wherever possible. Parkinsonism arising after neuroleptic exposure or in very severe stages of dementia is considered to be secondary. PDC requires the insidious onset and gradual progression of primary parkinsonism and dementia. Modifying factors such as stroke or other brain diseases are taken into account. Dementia is diagnosed using DSM-IV criteria (American Psychiatric Association, 1994).[10] The pure dementia syndrome on Guam resembles AD clinically and many patients meet standard criteria for probable AD.[11] Clinico-pathological studies of patients with this syndrome are in progress, and will help to decide whether the substrate is AD or tangle-only pathology. It will be referred to as dementia in this paper.

GENERAL FINDINGS IN 1997–1999 COMPARED TO PRIOR STUDIES

In surveys in the early 1950s, the prevalence of **ALS** among Chamorros was estimated as over 400 per 100,000. ALS has decreased markedly since then, but new cases are still seen. Detailed early descriptions of Guam ALS[1,12,13] noted that it resembled classic ALS in its insidious onset and clinical features, combining upper and lower motor neuron findings. Dysarthria and bulbar palsy occur in about one-third of patients. The age at onset ranges widely, from 20 to70. From 1950–1979, ALS was about twice as common in men than in women, but more recently it appears to be evenly divided.[2] Most patients have pure ALS, while about 5–10% also show parkinsonism or dementia. Non-Chamorros on Guam rarely develop ALS. Nine cases were documented from 1962–1977 in Filipino immigrants to Guam, all men.[14] From 1997–1999, we have diagnosed seven new patients as having ALS: five Chamorros, one Filipino, and one long-term Caucasian resident of Guam. This represents a much lower incidence than that typical of the 1950s. ALS has decreased among Chamorros, but has not disappeared.

Surveys of Guam conducted in the 1950s found that PDC was about as common as ALS. With the dramatic decline in the number of ALS cases, the number of PDC cases now greatly exceeds that of ALS. The clinical picture typically includes both parkinsonism and dementia; a minority of patients have isolated parkinsonism.[15] The mean age at onset of PDC increased: from 1950 to 1979, it increased from 55 to 59 years in men and 51 to 59 years in women.[2] PDC was noted to be 2–3 times more common in men than women. Parkinsonism is the usual presenting feature of PDC. It is accompanied by cognitive decline either at onset or within the next two to three years.[15,16] In about 30% of patients, cognitive decline precedes parkinsonism. The parkinsonism seen in PDC shares many features with typical idiopathic PD. Bradykinesia, affecting axial movements, gait, or both, and increased muscle tone are common. They are usually symmetrical and affect the arms more than the legs. Dysarthria, hypophonic speech, loss of facial expression and of associated movements, and decreased blinking are common. Action or postural tremor is more common than rest tremor, which occurs in about 30–40% of patients. Gait difficulty is extremely common, with slowing and short steps and an overall slow, apraxic pattern. Festination and marked shuffling are uncommon. Patients with PDC respond to some extent to L-dopa or dopaminergic agonists.[17] Recent studies have shown olfactory impairment in PDC. This is also common in PD and Alzheimer's disease. Autonomic dysfunction can be shown in many patients with PDC by sensitive laboratory testing, but symptomatic orthostatic hypotension is rare.[18]

The dementia syndrome of PDC usually begins with forgetfulness and disorientation. Difficulty with calculation and problem-solving are also common, but language abilities generally are preserved until late in the course. In advanced dementia, patients become bed-bound, with limited language output or mutism. Behavioral or neuropsychiatric symptoms are not prominent in PDC. Major depression is rare, but apathy or decreased initiative is common, together with increased daytime drowsiness or sleep.[16] Agitation and aggressive behavior may occur as the dementia progresses. The psychometric picture of PDC has not been reported, and it is not clear whether a cortical or subcortical pattern should be expected.

From 1997–1999, we have diagnosed 73 patients as having PDC. Some were seen at advanced stages of dementia, but could still be diagnosed as PDC from the history supplemented by review of medical records. In patients with late-life dementia, who developed parkinsonism only after a long course and at a stage of severe dementia, we have clinically diagnosed dementia rather than PDC. The mean age at onset for PDC was 66 years, which represents a further increase compared to that seen in the 1970s. We continue to find that PDC is more common in men than women (1.7:1). On the motor section of the UPDRS, the mean score for PDC patients was 34 points, indicating widespread findings. Findings were usually symmetrical, and about 45% of patients had a rest tremor. Additional neurologic features, such as supranuclear palsy or simultaneous ALS, were rare occurring in fewer than 5% of patients. Responses to L-dopa or dopaminergic agonists are variable. The clinical profile in our patients is similar to that documented by previous studies.

A "pure dementia syndrome" has recently been recorded in elderly Chamorros. Neuropathologic findings in a small number of patients have varied. Some showed

TABLE 1. Selected psychometric test scores in controls and patients with neurologic disorders among Chamorros on Guam

	Normal Controls	PDC	Dementia	Parkinson's Disease
n	35	30	52	10
Age	69 ± 5.4	71 ± 6.3	$77 \pm 6.8^{*\#+}$	67 ± 9.3
CASI (0–100)	87.1 ± 7.7	$53.8 \pm 20.3^{*\#}$	$56.4 \pm 12.1^{*\#}$	82.8 ± 9.5
Attention: digit span	11.3 ± 2.2	$7.8 \pm 3.5^{*}$	$7.4 \pm 2.7^{*\#}$	10.1 ± 2.6
Memory: CERAD list				
Trial 3 (0–10)	8.5 ± 1.9	$3.4 \pm 2.0^{*\#}$	$3.7 \pm 1.8^{*\#}$	7.3 ± 1.8
Delayed recall (0–10)	7.4 ± 2.5	$1.9 \pm 2.2^{*\#}$	$1.3 \pm 1.6^{*\#}$	6.1 ± 1.5
Language: Boston Naming Test (0–15)	14.4 ± 0.9	$11.3 \pm 3.3^{*\#}$	$11.2 \pm 3.3^{*\#}$	14.0 ± 1.4
Executive function: trails A (seconds)	66 ± 34	$127 \pm 37^{*}$	$118 \pm 46^{*}$	99 ± 32
Construction: clock drawing				
Copy (0–3)	2.9 ± 0.3	$1.6 \pm 1.1^{*\#}$	$1.7 \pm 1.0^{*\#}$	2.8 ± 0.4
Command (0–3)	2.8 ± 0.4	$1.2 \pm 0.9^{*\#}$	$1.2 \pm 0.8^{*\#}$	2.3 ± 1.0
Psychomotor speed: grooved pegboard (seconds)	99 ± 34	$157 \pm 53^{*}$	$149 \pm 50^{*}$	$160 \pm 30^{*}$

NOTE: PDC, Parkinson's-dementia complex; CASI, Cognitive Abilities Screening Instrument. For each psychometric test listed, the range or units of measurement are given.

Data were compared between groups by ANOVA, followed by Tukey's test for post-hoc comparisons. * Different from normal controls ($p < 0.05$); # different from PD ($p < 0.05$); + different from PDC ($p < 0.05$). The PDC and dementia patients showed similar extents of deficits on memory, language, attention, executive functions, visuospatial abilities, and psychomotor speed, indicating a global dementia.

widespread tangles in a topographic distribution consistent with that found in PDC, with amyloid deposition, the extent of which did not meet criteria for AD; others have shown AD pathology.[19,20] The frequency and clinical characteristics of pure dementia have not been well documented.

We have examined over 70 patients with "pure" dementia, in institutional and community settings. The high level of family support given to demented patients allows for continued care at home even in severe dementia. Pending further neuropathological studies, we have called the diagnosis Marianas dementia, recognizing that the syndrome is highly suggestive of AD. The mean age at onset, 75, is older than that of PDC and is compatible with AD. Women exceed men by over 2:1 among demented patients. As mentioned above, clinical cognitive testing reveals deficits in multiple areas of brain function. Memory impairment is usually the initial and most prominent symptom. Patients may show apathy and withdrawal, but are rarely depressed. With progression of dementia, other areas of cognition are involved, including calculation, abstract reasoning, language function, and visuospatial and constructional abilities. Behavioral symptoms are more common in pure dementia cases than in PDC: 29% of patients had hallucinations and 36% delusions. Physical or verbal agitation may occur as the dementia progresses. The UPDRS is generally normal in patients with pure dementia until advanced stages, when cognitive dysfunction precludes meaningful testing. Some patients show questionable or minimal parkinsonism at an early stage, for example, hypophonic speech and slowed speed of movement. The duration of the dementia varies from about 4–10 years. In advanced stages, patients become totally dependent, lose the ability to walk, and have greatly reduced language output.

PSYCHOMETRIC PROFILES OF PDC AND DEMENTIA

Among patients with PDC and pure dementia who were adequately testable—that is, defined as able to complete the CASI meaningfully and comply with testing—psychometric evaluation showed deficits in all areas of intellectual function, namely, orientation, recall, language, visuospatial and constructional tests, and frontal-executive tasks. This pattern indicated the presence of a global dementia. Selective impairment of frontal-subcortical cognitive abilities was not seen in PDC. Patients with PDC did show relatively severe slowing on timed tests involving motor speed compared to patients with pure dementia. Cognitive deficits in PDC therefore appear to follow a pattern similar to those in AD, with prominent memory dysfunction followed by more widespread impairment of other areas of cognition. NFT in PDC are found in the hippocampus and cortex, which perhaps outweighs the contribution of nigral-subcortical impairment in producing dementia.

CONCLUSIONS

Patterns of neurodegenerative disorders on Guam have changed over the past 40 years. The incidence of ALS has declined markedly, although new cases continue to be identified. The prevalence of PDC has declined slightly, and age at its onset continues to increase. With gains in life expectancy on Guam and systematic assessment of many elderly Chamorros, dementia is being diagnosed with increased frequency. PDC and pure dementia syndromes may show considerable clinical overlap, and PDC does not fit a pattern of subcortical dementia. A key research question that will need careful clinicopathologic study is to determine the pathologic basis of dementia among the many cases now being encountered among elderly individuals on Guam.

We are conducting molecular genetic studies of PDC, ALS, and dementia, supplementing earlier pedigree information collected on Guam with follow-up of children of the generation documented to have PDC from 1950–1980. To date, the tau gene has been sequenced in Chamorro patients and controls, and no mutations or polymorphisms have been associated with neurologic disease. Of interest, the apolipoprotein E e4 allele frequency among Chamorros is low, ranging from 3–6%, in controls as well as patients with PDC and pure dementia. If the later-life dementia among Chamorros does represent AD, then the APO-E e4 allele is not a susceptibility gene, and it may prove worthwhile to search for new genes related to dementia in this population.

ACKNOWLEDGMENT

This work was supported by NIA Grant AG14382.

REFERENCES

1. KURLAND, L.T. & D.W. MULDER. 1954. Epidemiological investigations of ALS. 1. Preliminary reports on geographic distribution, with special reference to the Mariana Islands, including clinical and pathological observations. Neurology **4**: 335–378.
2. HIRANO, A. *et al.* 1961. Parkinson-dementia complex: an endemic disease of the island of Guam. I. Clinical features. Brain **84**: 642–661.
3. GARRUTO, R.M., R. YANIGIHARA & D.C. GAJDUSEK. 1985. Disappearance of high-incidence amyotrophic lateral sclerosis and parkinsonism-dementia on Guam. Neurology **35**:193–198.
4. RODGERS-JOHNSON, P., R.M. GARRUTO, R. YANAGIHARA, *et al.* 1986. ALS and PDC on Guam: a 30-year evaluation of clinical and neuropathologic trends. Neurology **36**: 7–13.
5. REED, W. & J.A. BRODY. 1975. ALS and PD on Guam, 1945–1972. I. Descriptive epidemiology. Am. J. Epidemiol. **101**: 287–301.
6. PLATO, C.C., D.M. REED, T.S. ELIZAN & L.T. KURLAND. ALS/PDC of Guam. IV. Familial and genetic investigations. 1967. Am. J. Hum. Genet. **19**: 617-632.
7. PLATO, C.C., M.T. CRUZ & L.T. KURLAND. 1969. ALS/PDC of Guam. IV. Further genetic investigation. Am. J. Hum. Genet. **21**: 133–141.
8. REED, W., J. TORRES & J.A. BRODY. 1975. ALS and PD on Guam, 1945–1972. II. Familial and genetic studies. Am. J. Epidemiol. **101**: 302–310.
9. TENG, E.L., K. HASEGAWA, A. HOMMA, *et al.* 1994. The Cognitive Abilities Screening Instrument (CASI): a practical test for cross-cultural epidemiological studies of dementia. Int. Psychogeriatr. **6**: 45–58.
10. AMERICAN PSYCHIATRIC ASSOCIATION. 1994. Diagnostic and Statistical Manual of Mental Disorders. 4th edit. American Psychiatric Association. Washington, DC.
11. MCKHANN, G., D. DRACHMAN, M. FOLSTEIN, *et al.* 1984. Clinical diagnosis of Alzheimer's disease: Report of the NINCDS-ADRDA Work Group under the auspices of Department of Health and Human Services Task Force on Alzheimer's Disease. Neurology **4**: 939–944.
12. KOERNER, D.R. 1952. ALS on Guam: a clinical study and review of the literature. Ann. Int. Med. **37**: 1204–1220.
13. HIRANO, A., N. ARUMUGASAMY & H.M. ZIMMERMAN. 1967. Amyotrophic lateral sclerosis. A comparison of Guam and classical cases. Arch. Neurol. **16**: 357–363.
14. GARRUTO, R.M., D.C. GAJDUSEK & K.M. CHEN. 1981. Amyotrophic lateral sclerosis and parkinsonism-dementia among Filipino migrants to Guam. Ann. Neurol.**10**: 341–350.
15. ELIZAN, T.S., A. HIRANO, B.M. ABRAMS, *et al.* 1966. Amyotrophic lateral sclerosis and parkinsonism-dementia complex of Guam. Neurological re-evaluation. Arch. Neurol. **14**: 356–368.
16. CHEN, K.M. & T.N. CHASE. 1986. Parkinsonism-dementia complex. *In* Handbook of Clinical Neurology, Vol. 49. Extrapyramidal Disorders. P.J. Vinken, G.M. Bruyn & H.I. Klawans, Eds.: 167–183. Elsevier Science. New York.
17. DOI, H., K.M. CHEN, T.N. CHASE, *et al.* 1983. Effect of L-dopa on clinical duration and quality of life in PDC of Guam. Clin. Neurol. (Jpn.) **23**: 935–942.
18. LOW, P.A., J.E. AHLSKOG, R.C. PETERSEN, *et al.* 1997. Autonomic failure in Guamanian neurodegenerative disease. Neurology **49**: 1031–1034.
19. SUENAGA, T., A. HIRANO & J.F. LLENA. 1990. Cerebellar senile plaques in a Chamorro patient with senile dementia. Neurol. Med. **33**: 523–524.
20. PERL, D.P., *et al.* 1994. Neuropathologic studies of a pure dementing syndrome (Marianas dementia) among the inhabitants of Guam, a form of ALS/parkinsonism-dementia complex. Brain Pathol. **4**: 529.

In Vivo Analysis of Wild-type and FTDP-17 Tau Transgenic Mice

J. GÖTZ,[a,d] R. BARMETTLER,[a] A. FERRARI,[a] M. GOEDERT,[b] A. PROBST,[c] AND R.M. NITSCH[a]

[a]*Department of Psychiatry Research, University of Zürich, August Forel Str.1, 8008 Zürich, Switzerland*

[b]*MRC Laboratory of Molecular Biology, Cambridge, CB2 2QH, England, UK*

[c]*Institute of Pathology, University of Basel, 4003 Basel, Switzerland*

ABSTRACT: Mutations in the coding and intronic regions of the tau gene cause frontotemporal dementia and parkinsonism linked to chromosome 17 (FTDP-17). Some of these mutations lead to an overproduction of tau isoforms with four microtubule-binding repeats, followed by the development of fibrillary lesions and selective cell death. In order to analyze the development of these neurofibrillary lesions in transgenic mice, the longest four-repeat human brain tau isoform was expressed under control of two different neuron-specific promoters. In a first model, utilizing the human Thy1 promoter, transgenic tau was hyperphosphorylated and abnormally localized to cell bodies and dendrites. In a second model, which made use of a human Thy1.2 expression vector, transgenic expression levels were much higher, and an additional phenotype was observed: Large numbers of pathologically enlarged axons containing neurofilament- and tau-immunoreactive spheroids were present, especially in spinal cord. Signs of Wallerian degeneration and neurogenic muscle atrophy were observed. Behaviorally, transgenic mice showed signs of muscle weakness. Our data show that overexpression of human four-repeat tau in itself is sufficient to lead to nerve cell dysfunction and amyotrophy. We have now extended our initial studies by introducing exonic mutations including G2*t* 2V and PS01L into the tau gene in order to achieve a more advanced FTDP-17 associated phenotype.

INTRODUCTION

Abundant neurofibrillary and glial fibrillary lesions composed of hyperphosphorylated microtubule-associated tau protein constitute the major cellular pathology of a number of common neurodegenerative diseases, the so-called tauopathies. These include Alzheimer's disease (AD), Pick's disease, progressive supranuclear palsy, corticobasal degeneration and frontotemporal dementia, and parkinsonism linked to chromosome 17 (FTDP-17) and others.

Tau is an axonal phosphoprotein in normal adult brain, and phosphorylation is developmentally regulated. In AD and other tauopathies, brain tau is hyperphosphory-

[d]Address for correspondence: Dr. Jürgen M. Götz, Department of Psychiatry Research, University of Zürich, August Forel Str. 1, 8008 Zürich, Switzerland. Tel.: +41-1-63-48873; fax: +41-1-63-48874.

e-mail: goetz@bli.unizh.ch

lated and is found not only in axons, but also in cell bodies and dendrites of affected nerve cells.[1] Tau has microtubule-binding and tubulin-polymerizing activities *in vitro*, and it establishes short crossbridges between axonal microtubules. In addition, it controls intracellular trafficking.[2] In adult human brain, six tau isoforms are produced from a single gene by alternative mRNA splicing. They differ by the presence or absence of one or two short inserts in the amino-terminal half and an additional microtubule-binding repeat in the carboxy-terminal half. The other three isoforms have three repeats each. In contrast to humans, mice express only four-repeat isoforms.[3]

AD is characterized by a good correlation between the presence of tau pathology and the degree of cognitive impairment, indicating a close link between the development of tau pathology and nerve cell degeneration. The formation of neurofibrillary lesions may predate amyloid plaque formation, a histopathological hallmark of Alzheimer's disease. The recent discovery of mutations in coding and intronic regions in the tau gene in FTDP-17 has firmly established that dysfunction of tau can cause neurodegeneration, and lead to dementia.[4]

Mutations in the tau gene in FTDP-17 result either in the reduced ability of tau to interact with microtubules, or to quantitative changes in the splicing-in of exon 10. The primary effect of the intronic mutations located close to the splice-donor site of the intron following exon 10 is a change of the normally existing ratio of four-repeat (4R) to three-repeat (3R) tau, resulting in the net overproduction of 4R tau isoforms. These observations strongly suggest that overproduction of four-repeat tau is sufficient to cause frontotemporal dementia. Therefore, overproduction of 4R tau in transgenic mice may help in the development of an animal model for FTDP-17.

EXPRESSION OF HUMAN 4R WILD-TYPE TAU IN TRANSGENIC MICE: THE ALZ 7 LINE

Expression of the longest human four-repeat tau isoform under the control of the human Thy1 promoter along with a polyadenylation/splice cassette derived from the β-globin gene (ALZ 7 construct, see TABLE 1) resulted in the presence of hyperphosphorylated tau not only in axons, but also in nerve cell bodies and dendrites. Furthermore, tau was phosphorylated at sites that are known to be phosphorylated in paired helical filaments, the principal filamentous component of neurofibrillary lesions including neurofibrillary tangles, neuropil threads, and dystrophic neurites.[5] A similar phenotype was also reported in mice with neuronal expression of the shortest human tau isoform.[6] In summary, these mouse strains showed early changes associated with the development of neurofibrillary lesions in AD and related tauopathies, but they failed to produce neurofibrillary tangles.

EXPRESSION OF HUMAN 4R WILD-TYPE TAU IN TRANSGENIC MICE: THE ALZ 17 LINE

Because the amyloid plaque in transgenic mice expressing FAD mutations of human APP (amyloid precursor protein) was directly correlated with the expression level of the transgene,[7] we chose a stronger mouse Thy1.2 expression vector for tau

TABLE 1. Expression constructs to establish a transgenic mouse model for FTDP-17

Group	Construct	Encoding	Correlated phenotype in humans
I	ALZ7	hThy-htau40 (4Rtau)	"intronic mutation"
	ALZ17	mThy1.2-htau40 (4Rtau)	
II	pR3	tetOp-TA-tetOp-htau40 (G272V) (mated with PrP-TA, CaMKII-TA)	G272V (exon 9), all isoforms affected, straight filaments, predominantly neuronal phenotype
	pR8	mThy1.2-NLS.htau40 (G272V)	
	pAF4	PrP-htau40 (G272V)	
III	pR5	mThy1.2-htau40 (P301L)	P301L (exon10), 4-repeat isoforms mutated, narrow, twisted ribbons, rope-like filaments, neuronal and glial pathology
	pR7	mThy1.2-NLS.htau40 (P301L)	
	pAF3	PrP-htau40 (P301L)	
IV	pAF1	GFAP-htau40 (P301L)	restricted to glial compartment
	pAF2	GFAP-htau40 (G272V)	
V	T.P301S	mThy1.2-htau46 (P301S)	age of onset: 27 years, single or paired straight bundles, most severe tau pathology observed so far
	T.P301E	mThy1.2-htau46 (P301E)	
	P.P301S	MoPrPXho-htau46 (P301S)	
	P.P301E	MoPrPXho-htau46 (P301E)	

NOTE: (a) Group I (human 4-repeat wild-type tau) resembles the intronic mutations described in some FTDP-17 families, (b) group II carries the exonic G272V mutation, (c) group III carries the exonic P301S mutation, (d) group IV expresses both mutations under control of an astrocyte-specific promoter, and (e) group V expresses the P301S mutation both with and without a change of proline into glutamate (P301E) in order to mimic the potential phosphorylation introduced by the P301S mutation.

expression. Two lines with high expression levels of the longest human 4R tau isoform were established[8] (ALZ 17 construct, see TABLE 1). Tau mRNA levels were approximately fivefold higher than in the previously described ALZ 7 line.[5] We found in brains of these mice transgenic tau that reacted with a number of phosphorylation-dependent anti-tau antibodies including AT8, AT180, AT270, and AD2. To determine the solubility of tau, spinal cords from up to 12 month-old mice were extracted in high-salt RAB buffer, RIPA buffer, and formic acid buffers to allow for the extraction of increasingly insoluble proteins. Unlike tau from control mice, a substantial amount of transgenic tau was also present in the RIPA-soluble fraction, and a small amount in the formic acid-soluble fraction. These findings indicate a markedly reduced solubility of tau from ALZ 17 mice relative to tau from control animals. This is, again, similar to pathological tau extractable from brains of patients with AD or other tauopathies.

In brains of homozygous mice of the ALZ 17 line, strong tau immunoreactivity of nerve cell bodies and dendritic processes was observed with the phosphorylation-dependent anti-tau antibodies AT8, AT180, and PHF1, and with the human-specific phosphorylation-independent antibody T14. Tau-positive nerve cells were observed in cerebral cortex and the hippocampus, including CA1, dendate gyrus, as well as in the entorhinal cortex. Gallyas silver impregnations[9] failed to identify classical neurofibrillary lesions.

Tau-immunoreactive neurons and axonal spheroids (see below) were already present in 3-week-old mice, and their number slightly increased with age. When brain sections were stained with anti-neurofilament antibodies, multiple spheroids with 7–10 μm in diameter were evident. Spheroids consisted of focal dilatations of axons and were found in neocortical areas with many AT8-positive neurons.

The spinal grey matter from homozygous mice of the ALZ 17 line contained large numbers of nerve cell bodies that were strongly immunostained by phosphorylation-dependent antibodies. In contrast to axonal spheroids in the cerebral cortex, the majority of spinal cord spheroids was strongly immunoreactive with a number of anti-tau antibodies. Axonal spheroids similar to those described here are a neuropathological characteristic of the majority of cases of sporadic and familial amyotrophic lateral sclerosis (ALS), where they are believed to impair slow axonal transport.[10]

Evidence for axonal degeneration, including axonal breakdown and segmentation of myelin into ellipsoids (so-called digestion chambers) was obtained in anterior spinal roots. Only few AT8-positive axons were detected in interfascicular nerve bundles of skeletal muscle. However, clear evidence of neurogenic muscle atrophy, with groups of small angular muscle fibers, was present in the hindleg musculature of transgenic, but not control, mice.

Electron microscopy studies revealed that axonal spheroids were surrounded by a thin myelin sheath made of only few myelin leaflets. The axoplasm was filled with loosely arranged 10 μm thick filaments and microtubules, with only few mitochondria in between. In spinal cord, in addition to axonal spheroids, there was evidence of axonal degeneration with collapsed and fragmented myelin sheaths.

Transgenic mice appeared to be normal during the first few weeks of postnatal life. Then, progressively, they showed signs of neurological malfunction. When lifted by the tail, normal mice extend their hindlimbs and spread their toes. At 1–3 months, homozygous ALZ 17 mice extended their legs, but retracted their paws, in marked contrast to control mice. At ages of 8–16 months, the same mice were unable to extend their hindlimbs when lifted by the tail. On the rotarod test, ALZ 17 mice showed abnormal motor co-ordination.[8]

The major difference between the ALZ 17 line and the histopathology of FTDP-17 was the absence of abundant tau filaments and overt nerve cell loss in the transgenic mice. It appears likely that the formation of tau filaments is necessary for the massive loss of nerve cells that is observed in FTDP-17.

EXPRESSION OF HUMAN FTDP-17 MUTANT TAU IN TRANSGENIC MICE

In order to develop a more advanced model of FTDP-17, we chose four alternative approaches (for a list of constructs, see TABLES 1 and 2):

1. To achieve sufficiently high expression levels, we chose an autoregulatory tetracycline-dependent transactivator (TA) system as initially described by Shockett *et al.*[11] This system combines two transgenic lines, one expressing the tetracycline-dependent TA under the control of a murine PrP promoter (cosmid) that directs ex-

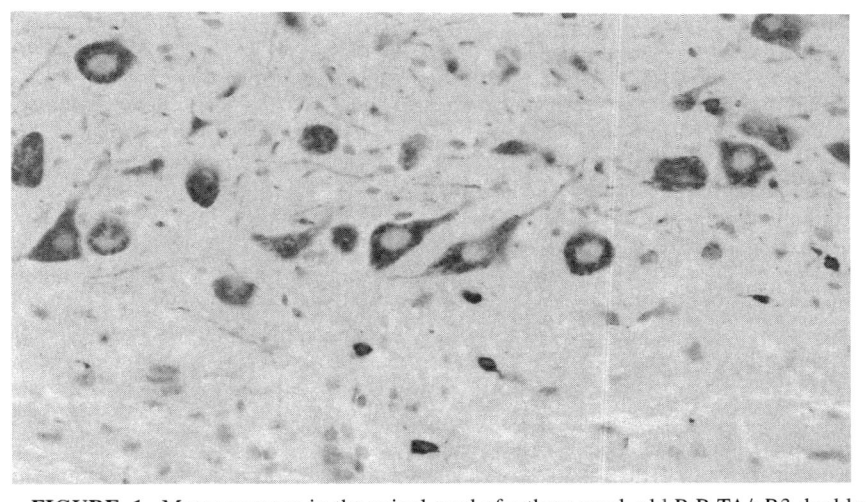

FIGURE 1. Motor neurons in the spinal cord of a three week old PrP-TA/pR3 doubly transgenic mouse stained with the human tau specific monoclonal antibody HT7 (Innogenetics, SA, Belgium). Control mice are negative when stained with this antibody.

pression of the tetracycline-dependent TA to both neuronal and glial cells. The second line (construct pR3) contained two tetOp motifs, one upstream of a TA gene, the other upstream of a tau cDNA encoding an FTDP-17-linked exonic mutation (G272V). We expected that interbreeding of these two transgenic lines would lead to very high expression levels of G272V tau in the subset of neurons and glial cells in which the PrP-TA transgene is active. In doubly transgenic mice, we found massive, clod-like, pre-tangle-type accumulations of tau in the somatodendritic compartment. These were already obvious in 3-week-old mice (FIG. 1).

2. A second approach is based on the finding that incubation of recombinant tau with either sulfated glycosaminoglycans or RNA results in bulk assembly of tau into Alzheimer-like filaments.[12] Sulfated glycosaminoglycans and RNA share a repeat sugar backbone and negative charges in the form of sulfates or phosphates. Binding of heparin or RNA to tau may induce or stabilize a conformation of tau that brings the microtubule-binding repeats of individual tau molecules into close proximity, creating sites which favor polymerization into filaments.

Because of the highly compartmentalized concentration of RNA in nuclei, and because of the absence of its physiological binding partner, the microtubules, we designed two constructs (pR7 and pR8, TABLE 1) that target expression of transgenic tau to the nucleus. A small fraction of tau is reportedly found in the nucleus under physiological conditions.[13]

Our approach was based on the fact that RNA concentrations used in the *in vitro* assembly experiments of tau into paired helical filaments were in the range of 100 µg/ml,[12] and that the average cellular contents of RNA are 25 pg, of which 14%, or 3.5 pg, resides in the nucleus. Cells used in our study have a nuclear volume of around 1.5×10^{-7} µl. The total RNA concentration in the nucleus under physiological conditions is approximately 0.02 µg/ml, orders of magnitude lower than those

TABLE 2. Expression constructs designed to decrease protein phosphatase 2A (PP2A) activity and to interfere with tau phosphorylation in neurons of transgenic mice

Construct	Encoding	Comments
DOM0	mThy1.2-HA.PP2ACα	wild-type control
DOM1	mThy1.2-HA.PP2ACα.2512	overexpression of wt PP2ACα reverses mutant phenotype, point mutation
DOM2	mThy1.2-HA.PP2ACα.266	overexpression of wt PP2ACα does not reverse mutant phenotype, C-terminal truncation
DOM3	mThy1.2-HA.PP2ACα.216	overexpression of wt PP2ACα does not reverse mutant phenotype, C-terminal truncation
DOM5	mThy1.2-HA.PP2ACα.DYFL309A	reduced to no binding of regulatory B subunit
DOM6	mThy1.2-HA.PP2ACα.DYFL309Δ	reduced to no binding of regulatory B subunit

NOTE: All cDNAs are equipped with an HA-tag at the N-terminus.

used in the above *in vitro* experiments. Considering the actual exclusion volume, the nucleosolic RNA concentration may be considerably higher. Most of the RNA synthesized in a cell is hnRNA; it is rapidly exported from the nucleus upon splicing. In addition, it is difficult to predict the free concentrations of RNA in the nucleus. We anticipate that targeting of tau protein to the nucleus may result in its self-aggregation due to the presence of negatively charged polymers with a sugar backbone (RNA) but also due to the absence of microtubules, the natural "binding partner" of tau. Nuclear filamentous inclusions have been described for other neurodegenerative diseases: Ataxin-1 develops nuclear inclusions in spinocerebellar ataxia-1,[14] and mice transgenic for huntingtin display nuclear fibrillar structures.[15] It remains to be seen whether tau, localized to the nucleus, is stable, and if so, whether tangle formation can be induced in the nuclear compartment.

    3. The third approach is based on the possibility that murine neurons may not allow tangle formation. Therefore, expression was targeted to astrocytes by using either the GFAP promoter (constructs pAF1, pAF2) or the PrP promoter (constructs pAF3, pAF4, P-P301S, P-P301E). The PrP vectors do confer additional expression to neuronal cells. We are currently analyzing mice which have been generated with these constructs.

    4. Careful staging of brains has shown that tau phosphorylation precedes filament formation.[16] *In vitro*, phosphorylated tau fails to assemble into PHF-like filaments. On the other hand, sulfated glycosaminoglycans stimulate tau phosphorylation at lower concentrations than those required for filament formation.[12] Several kinases and phosphatases have been suggested to play a role in tau phosphorylation *in vivo*. Among the phosphatases which dephosphorylate tau *in vitro*, protein phosphatase 2A (PP2A) has been shown to be associated with microtubules.[17] Targeted disruption of the catalytic subunit of PP2A resulted in embryonic lethality,[18,19] making it necessary either to target regulatory subunits of PP2A or to

express dominant negative mutant forms of PP2A[20] in order to obtain both a more subtle phenotype and to interfere with tau phosphorylation *in vivo*. Transgenic mice with a neuron-specific expression of dominant negative mutant forms of the catalytic subunit of PP2A (TABLE 2) will be interbred with FTDP-17 mutant mice in order to determine the role of phosphorylation in the FTDP-17-associated pathology.

OUTLOOK

The identification of the FTDP-17 mutations provided a direct link between genetic lesions of tau and the formation of tau filaments. These mutations are suited to test *in vivo* whether the presence of tau filaments causes degeneration of neurons in tauopathies or whether filament formation is only a mere consequence of a more general degenerative process. By analogy, in α1-antitrypsin-associated liver disease hepatocyte loss and cirrhosis is clearly a consequence of abnormal deposits and not of a loss of function, because cirrhosis develops only with a conformationally unstable variant, but not with mutations that cause "null" suppressions of synthesis (discussed in Ref. 21). Mice lacking tau appeared to be immunohistologically normal, suggesting that other microtubule-binding proteins including MAP-1A can functionally compensate for the loss as shown by intact axonal elongation in cultured neurons. But in some small-caliber axons, microtubule stability was decreased, and microtubule organization was significantly changed.[22] Together, these data are compatible with the view that neurofibrillary lesion formation is causative for the disease process in FTDP-17 and related tauopathies. It remains to be determined whether filament formation can be achieved in mice, and whether formation of neurofilaments leads to neuronal cell death. Based on the effort put into transgenic tau models in several laboratories around the world, it is plausible that this question will be answered soon.

[Note added in proof: Since the writing of this article, filament formation has been achieved in two P301L tau transgenic mouse models.[23,24]]

ACKNOWLEDGMENTS

This work was supported in part by funds from the Swiss National Science Foundation (SNF), the Bayer Alzheimer Research Network (BARN), and the Kanton Zürich. We thank Claudia Mistl, Daniel Schuppli, and Yves Santini for excellent technical assistance.

REFERENCES

1. GOEDERT, M., M.G. SPILLANTINI, R. JAKES, *et al.* 1995. Molecular dissection of the paired helical filament. Neurobiol. Aging **16:** 325–334.
2. TRINCZEK, B., A. EBNETH, E.M. MANDELKOW & E. MANDELKOW. 1999. Tau regulates the attachment/detachment but not the speed of motors in microtubule-dependent transport of single vesicles and organelles. J. Cell. Sci. **112:** 2355–2367.
3. GOEDERT, M. & R. JAKES. 1990. Expression of separate isoforms of human tau protein: correlation with the tau pattern in brain and effects on tubulin polymerization. EMBO J. **13:** 4225–4230.

4. HUTTON, M., C.L. LENDON, P. RIZZU, *et al.* 1998. Association of missense and 5'-splice-site mutations in tau with the inherited dementia FTDP-17. Nature **393**: 702–705.
5. GÖTZ, J., A. PROBST, M.G. SPILLANTINI, *et al.* 1995. Somatodendritic localization and hyperphosphorylation of tau protein in transgenic mice expressing the longest human brain tau isoform. EMBO J. **14**: 1304–1313.
6. BRION, J.P., G. TREMP & J.N. OCTAVE. 1999. Transgenic expression of the shortest human tau affects its compartmentalization and its phosphorylation as in the pretangle stage of Alzheimer's disease. Am. J. Pathol. **154**: 255–270.
7. STURCHLER-PIERRAT, C., D. ABRAMOWSKI, M. DUKE, *et al.* 1997. Two amyloid precursor protein transgenic mouse modsels with Alzheimer disease-like pathology. Proc. Natl. Acad. Sci. USA **94**: 13287–13292.
8. PROBST, A., J. GÖTZ, K.H. WIEDERHOLD, *et al.* Axonopathy and amyotrophy in mice transgenic for human four-repeat tau protein. Submitted.
9. GALLYAS, F. 1971. Silver staining of Alzheimer's neurofibrillary changes by means of physical development. Acta Morphol. Acad. Sci. Hung. **19**: 1–8.
10. ROULEAU, G.A., A.W. CLARK, K. ROOKE, *et al.* 1996. SOD1 mutation is associated with accumulation of neurofilaments in amyotrophic lateral sclerosis. Ann. Neurol. **39**: 128–131.
11. SHOCKETT, P., M. DIFILIPPANTONIO, N. HELLMAN & D.G. SCHATZ. 1995. A modified tetracycline-regulated system provides autoregulatory, inducible gene expression in cultured cells and transgenic mice. Proc. Natl. Acad. Sci. USA **92**: 6522–6526.
12. HASEGAWA, M., R.A. CROWTHER, R. JAKES & M. GOEDERT. 1997. Alzheimer-like changes in microtubule-associated protein Tau induced by sulfated glycosaminoglycans. Inhibition of microtubule binding, stimulation of phosphorylation, and filament assembly depend on the degree of sulfation. J. Biol. Chem. **272**: 33118–33124.
13. BRADY, R.M., R.P. ZINKOWSKI & L.I. BINDER. 1995. Presence of tau in isolated nuclei from human brain. Neurobiol. Aging **16**: 479–486.
14. SKINNER, P.J., B.T. KOSHY, C.J. CUMMINGS, *et al.* 1997. Ataxin-1 with an expanded glutamine tract alters nuclear matrix-associated structures. Nature **389**: 971–974.
15. DAVIES, S.W., M. TURMAINE, B.A. COZENS, *et al.* 1999. From neuronal inclusions to neurodegeneration: neuropathological investigation of a transgenic mouse model of Huntington's disease. Philos. Trans. R. Soc. Lond. B. Biol. Sci. **354**: 981–989.
16. BRAAK, H. & E. BRAAK. 1995. Staging of Alzheimer's disease-related neurofibrillary changes. Neurobiol. Aging **16**: 271–284.
17. SONTAG, E., V. NUNBHAKDI-CRAIG, G.S. BLOOM & M.C. MUMBY. 1995. A novel pool of protein phosphatase 2A is associated with microtubules and is regulated during the cell cycle. J. Cell Biol. **128**: 1131–2244.
18. GÖTZ, J., A. PROBST, E. EHLER, B. HEMMINGS & W. KUES. 1998. Delayed embryonic lethality in mice lacking protein phosphatase 2A catalytic subunit Calpha. Proc. Natl. Acad. Sci. USA **95**: 12370-12375.
19. GÖTZ, J. & W. KUES. 1999. The role of protein phosphatase 2A catalytic subunit Calpha in embryogenesis: evidence from sequence analysis and localization studies. Biol. Chem. **380**: 1117–1120.
20. EVANS, D.R., T. MYLES, J. HOFSTEENGE & B.A. HEMMINGS. 1999. Functional expression of human PP2Ac in yeast permits the identification of novel C-terminal and dominant-negative mutant forms. J. Biol. Chem. **274**: 24038–24046.
21. DAVIS, R.L., A.E. SHRIMPTON, P.D. HOLOHAN, C. BRADSHAW, *et al.* 1999. Familial dementia caused by polymerization of mutant neuroserpin. Nature **401**: 376–379.
22. HARADA, A., K. OGUCHI, S. OKABE, *et al.* 1994. Altered microtubule organization in small-calibre axons of mice lacking tau protein. Nature **369**: 488–491.
23. LEWIS, J., E. MCGOWAN, J. ROCKWOOD, H. MELROSE, P. NACHARAJU, *et al.* 2000. Neurofibrillary tangles, amyotrophy and progressive motor disturbance in mice expressing mutant (P301L) tau protein [In Process Citation]. Nat. Genet. **25**: 402–405.
24. GÖTZ, J., F. CHEN, R. BARMETTLER & R.M. NITSCH. 2000. Tau filament formation in transgenic mice expressing P301L tau. J. Biol. Chem. In press. (Accidentally added into database as Goetz *et al.*)

Pathogenic Mechanisms of Alzheimer's Disease Analyzed in the APP23 Transgenic Mouse Model

CHRISTINE STURCHLER-PIERRAT AND MATTHIAS STAUFENBIEL[a]

Nervous System Research, Novartis Pharma Inc., CH-4002 Basel, Switzerland

ABSTRACT: APP23 transgenic mice overexpress human APP with the Swedish double mutation. The mice start to develop amyloid plaque pathology at about six months of age, followed somewhat later by vascular amyloid deposits. Plaques are mostly of the compact type and increase exponentially during aging. Female mice show a slightly more rapid Aβ plaque deposition than do male animals. Associated with the amyloid are inflammatory reactions, neuritic and synaptic degeneration as well as tau hyperphosphorylation. Older mice have a reduced cholinergic fiber length and a reduced neuron number in the hippocampal CA1 region. Crossbreeding with transgenic mice expressing human presenilin 1 carrying Alzheimer's disease-linked mutations lead to an enhancement of the pathology. The APP23 line is a suitable model to analyze the contribution of APP, Aβ, and amyloid to the pathogenesis of Alzheimer's disease.

INTRODUCTION

Alzheimer's disease (AD) is etiologically heterogeneous, and genetic as well as ill-defined environmental factors contribute to the risk of developing the disease.[1] Several susceptibility genes have been identified, most notably the apolipoprotein allele e4, which increase the chance of getting the disease.[2] In addition, a number of autosomal dominant mutations were found, which are rare, but show a very high penetrance. These include mutations in the amyloid precursor protein (APP) gene and two related genes encoding the presenilins 1 and 2 (PS1, PS2).[3–7] Because these mutations always lead to AD if the carrier reaches a certain age, they seem well suited for model generation. This is particularly true for the APP mutations because this protein is the precursor of Aβ, the peptide deposited as amyloid in the brains of all AD patients. Obviously, with this strategy a rare cause of AD is used for the generation of a model that should reflect all forms of the disease. This relies on the notion that AD is a single disorder and the pathogenic mechanisms merge into a common part even though they start at different points. We have generated transgenic mice expressing mutated APP as well as PS1. Some of these mice are described below.

[a]Address for correspondence: Matthias Staufenbiel, Novartis Pharma Inc., WSJ-386.806, CH-4002 Basel, Switzerland. Tel.: +41 61 324 9642; fax: +41 61 324 5524.
e-mail: Matthias.Staufenbiel@Pharma.Novartis.Com

MOLECULAR CHARACTERISTICS OF THE APP23 MOUSE LINE

After testing various promoters, we have selected a mouse Thy-1 gene fragment to overexpress human proteins in mouse brain.[8,9] This promoter is neuron-specific and leads to high levels of transgene derived protein. It is primarily expressed in the cerebral cortex and the hippocampus, but also in most other brain regions including cerebellum although at lower levels. In the APP23 mouse line, human APP751 carrying the Swedish double mutation[4] is overexpressed sevenfold over the endogenous mouse APP. The mice were generated in a C57Bl/6xDBA2 background and were backcrossed into C57Bl/6.

AMYLOID FORMATION IN APP23 MICE

The first $A\beta$ plaques are found at about six months of age in this mouse line.[9] Plaque formation starts in the frontal cortex and the subiculum and rapidly extends to the entire neocortex and hippocampus. In mice about a year of age, the thalamus and amygdala become affected, while deposits in striatum and basal forebrain are rare. In very old mice (2 to 3 years) most or all brain regions contain at least some plaques; the only obvious exception is the cerebellum. Plaques are also formed in white matter such as the corpus callosum and the fimbria fornix. In addition, amyloid deposition is found in the cerebral vasculature in mice beyond the age of one year.[10] This is remarkable since cells of the vasculature do not express detectable amounts of APP nor can $A\beta$ be measured in the plasma. The $A\beta$ deposited must originate from APP made in brain neurons. These data, therefore, do not support the vascular origin of the amyloid deposits in AD.

The vast majority of the amyloid deposits is fibrillar in nature in APP23 mice. Almost all plaques appear compact, and are Thioflavin S fluorescent and Congo red birefringent.[9] A significant amount of diffuse $A\beta$ deposits only become discernible at old age.[11] In young mice, plaques are small but already compact, while small and very large plaques coexist in the brains of old animals. This argues in favor of a continuous formation of new plaques. No evidence for plaque maturation could be obtained in the APP23 or any other APP transgenic mouse line we generated. This is in contrast to hypotheses for human AD brain, postulating a maturation of diffuse plaques into compact ones.

KINETICS OF $A\beta$ DEPOSITION AND PLAQUE FORMATION

The plaque load in the cerebral cortex increases exponentially with age and reaches 10 to 15% of the total cortical area in heterozygous APP23 animals at two years of age. A more rapid increase is found in homozygous animals. The plaque load varies substantially among different animals. Similar data are obtained when $A\beta$ is quantified using Western blotting of SDS-gels, which separate $A\beta_{1-40}$ and $A\beta_{1-42}$. Small and about equal amounts of both major $A\beta$ peptides are present in young animals before plaques can be detected histologically. As plaque formation commences, the $A\beta$ levels increase exponentially. Interestingly, the ratio of $A\beta_{1-42}$ to $A\beta_{1-40}$ changes with age, such that more $A\beta_{1-40}$ is found in the brains of old mice with more deposits. Similar observations have been made in humans. A considerable variation in Aβ deposited is found among different animals of the same age. This is not due to methodological variations because the data correlate very well with the plaque load determined histologically for the same mice.

Analyses of the mice separated by gender show that female animals deposit more Aβ than do male animals. This gender difference, however, explains only part of the variation. There must be other factors that influence Aβ deposition and plaque formation in the brains of these mice. Based on the fact that the mice have a C57Bl/6 background, genetic factors may not be a likely explanation. An alternative possibility could be the nature of the Aβ fibril formation, which is a nucleation-dependent event following nonlinear kinetics.

INFLAMMATORY PROCESSES

The formation of plaques as well as vascular amyloid deposits is accompanied by inflammatory reactions. Gliosis can be detected as early as the first small deposits become discernible.[12] Hypertrophic astrocytes and reactive microglia cells are present around the deposits.[9,12,13] While microglia activation is largely restricted to the plaques, hypertrophic astrocytes are found also at a distance, but only in plaque-containing brain regions. Both glia cell types are always associated with compact amyloid, but are not found at diffuse deposits.

Plaque-associated microglia cells show increased staining for MAC-1 or F4/80 indicative of activation.[13] This is further supported by ultrastructural analyses, which in addition demonstrates their intimate association with the amyloid deposits.[12] Evidence for a phagocytic state of these cells comes from an increased expression of macrosialin and Fc receptor.[13] These cells may phagocytose Aβ or other plaque-associated material such as dystrophic neurites, but more direct evidence for this notion needs to be obtained. A subpopulation of the plaque-associated microglia cells displays elevated levels of MHC class II antigens, the function of which is not clear. As in AD brain, no evidence is found for a cell-based immune response because neither T- nor B-lymphocytes could be detected in the brains of these mice.

PLAQUE-ASSOCIATED NEURONAL DYSTROPHY

Degenerative processes are obvious around compact amyloid plaques. Abundant neuritic spheroids are present, and visualized by silver impregnation or neurofilament staining.[9,14] Plaque-associated dystrophic structures are also strongly labeled by ubiquitin antibodies. These swollen, dystrophic structures are closely associated with the plaque periphery. Of note, the most dramatic effect is on the axons and their connections, because peripheral staining of plaques is found for axonal and synaptic markers such as synaptophysin or APP.[14,15] Little or no labeling with the dendritic marker MAP-2 is obtained. The enlarged dystrophic boutons visible show light and electron microscopic characteristics of axonal terminals. It appears that axons in the vicinity of the plaques grow toward and make contact with the plaques, thereby forming dystrophic structures. Ectopic, aberrant terminal formation is also observed around white matter plaques and vascular Aβ deposits, locations where synaptic terminals are not normally found.

To study these processes better, the axonal projections from the entorrhinal cortex were analyzed after anterograde tracing using *Phaseolus vulgaris* leucoagglutinin (PHAL) injections.[15] These studies demonstrate that axons actively grow toward Aβ deposits and form dystrophic boutons in ectopic locations outside their normal termination zone. Many of the dystrophic terminals can be labeled by the growth-associated protein GAP-43, indicating aberrant sprouting. These data are in agreement with the concept that the neurotrophic effect of amyloid leads to the formation of the ectopic terminals.

The plaques formed in the APP23 mice are compact structures, which exclude most other material. Consequently, they lead to a local distortion of neurites. In older mice with a heavy plaque load, a distortion of the laminar cytoarchitecture is apparent. This is most obvious in the hippocampus as well as in the cortex. It can be expected that these processes together strongly affect neuronal connectivity.

LOSS OF CHOLINERGIC FIBERS

To assess the effect of Aβ plaque formation on neurites more globally, we chose to analyze cholinergic fibers since this system has been shown to be affected in AD.[16,17] Staining for acetylcholinesterase (AChE) revealed a distortion of the cholinergic fibers in regions containing plaques. Often the homogeneous distribution of fibers as seen in the controls was lost, suggestive of an overall reduction. In addition, a strong labeling of plaques was visible as known from human AD brain, indicating an association of AChE itself or of AChE-containing dystrophic neurites with the amyloid plaques.[9]

NEURON LOSS IN THE CA1 REGION OF THE HIPPOCAMPUS

Using modern stereological methods, neuron loss has been found in the CA1 region of the hippocampus in brains from AD patients.[18,19] No global neuron loss was detected in the neocortex of these patients although it is clear that there is a reduction in neuron number in distinct regions such as the entorrhinal cortex. Using the same methods, we made similar observations in the brains of APP23 mice.[11] The hippocampal CA1 region showed a significant neuron loss, which was correlated with the plaque load. In animals with the highest plaque load, the number of neurons was reduced by about 25%. No reduction in neuron number was found for the neocortex of the APP23 mice. Nevertheless, visual inspection indicated a reduced neuron number, for example, in entorrhinal cortex. These data indicate that the formation of amyloid plaques is sufficient to induce neuron loss in APP transgenic mice.

TAU HYPERPHOSPHORYLATION

Neurofibrillary pathology is a prominent feature of AD. Analyzing the APP23 mice with a number of phosphorylation-specific antibodies, we found that all compact deposits are labeled.[9,14] Examples are the antibodies AT8 and PHF-1, which reveal fiber-like, distorted structures surrounding the core of the amyloid plaques.

Often spherical enlargements can be seen. Immunoreactivity is also found with the Alz50 antibody recognizing an epitope on tau that is generated by a conformational change associated with the assembly into filaments. However, attempts to stain paired helical filaments using the Gallyas silver impregnation failed. It seems that the APP23 mice develop plaque-associated early neurofibrillary pathology, but lack true paired helical filaments.

PRESENILIN TRANSGENIC MICE CARRYING AD-LINKED MUTATIONS ENHANCE PLAQUE FORMATION IN APP23 MICE

We have also used the mouse Thy-1 promoter to generate transgenic mice over-expressing PS1 carrying AD-linked mutations.[20] These mice do not form Aβ plaques nor did we detect any gross pathological abnormalities in their brains. Line PS35, which carries the H163R familial AD mutation, has been crossed with the APP23 mouse line. The resulting bigenic mice show a considerably enhanced plaque formation starting already at about three months of age. An enhancement is also observed with presenilin transgenics carrying other AD-linked mutations. The intensity of the effect varies with the mutation used.

APP23 MICE: A MOUSE MODEL OF ALZHEIMER'S DISEASE

The APP23 transgenic mouse line shows a robust formation of amyloid plaques as well as vascular amyloid, both of which are largely of the compact type. Associated with these deposits are inflammatory processes and neuronal degeneration including a region-specific neuron loss. While hyperphosphorylated tau can be detected in structures at the Aβ deposits, no paired helical filaments seem to be formed. This is in line with the notion that neuronal degeneration is mostly axonal with little dendritic involvement. The APP23 mice show a learning impairment in the Morris water maze and a passive avoidance paradigm that have not been described here. An important feature is that the alterations mentioned are progressing with age. In summary, the APP23 transgenic mouse line is well suited for study of the role of APP, Aβ, and amyloid in the pathogenesis of AD.

REFERENCES

1. St George-Hyslop, P., J.L. Haines, L.A. Farrer, et al. 1990. Genetic linkage studies suggest that Alzheimer's disease is not a single homogeneous disorder. Nature 347: 194–197.
2. Corder, E.H., A.M. Saunders, W.J. Strittmatter, et al. 1993. Gene dose of apolipoprotein E type 4 allele and the risk of Alzheimer disease in late onset families. Science 261: 921–923.
3. Goate, A., M.C. Chartier-Harlin, M. Mullan, et al. 1991. Segregation of a missense mutation in the amyloid precursor protein gene with familial Alzheimer's disease. Nature 349: 704–706.
4. Mullan, M., F. Crawford, K. Alexman, et al. 1992. A pathogenic mutation for probable Alzheimer's disease in the APP gene at the N-terminus of beta-amyloid. Nature Genet. 1: 345–347.

5. SHERRINGTON, R., E.I. ROGAEV, Y. LIANG, *et al.* 1995. Cloning of a gene bearing missense mutations in early-onset familial Alzheimer's disease. Nature **375:** 754–760.
6. LEVY-LAHAD, E., W. WASCO, P. POORKAJ, *et al.* 1995. Candidate gene for the chromosome 1 familial Alzheimer's disease locus. Science **269:** 973–977.
7. ROGAEV, E.I., R. SHERRINGTON, E.A. ROGAEV, *et al.* 1995. Familial Alzheimer's disease in kindreds with missense mutations in a gene on chromosome 1 related to the Alzheimer's disease type 3 gene. Nature **376:** 775–778.
8. ANDRÄ, K., D. ABRAMOWSKI, M. DUKE, *et al.* 1996. Expression of APP in transgenic mice: a comparison of neuron-specific promoters. Neurobiol. Aging **17:** 183–190.
9. STURCHLER-PIERRAT, C., D. ABRAMOWSKI, M. DUKE, *et al.* 1997. Two amyloid precursor protein transgenic mouse models with Alzheimer disease-like pathology. Proc. Natl. Acad. Sci. USA **94:** 13287–13292.
10. CALHOUN, M.E., P. BURGERMEISTER, A.L. PHINNEY, *et al.* 1999. Neuronal overexpression of mutant amyloid precursor protein results in prominent deposition of cerebrovascular amyloid. Proc. Natl. Acad. Sci. USA **96:** 14088–14093.
11. CALHOUN, M.E., K.H. WIEDERHOLD, D. ABRAMOWSKI, *et al.* 1998. Neuron loss in APP transgenic mice. Nature **395:** 755–756.
12. STALDER, M., A. PHINNEY, A. PROBST, B. SOMMER, M. STAUFENBIEL & M. JUCKER. 1999. Association of microglia with amyloid plaques in brains of APP23 transgenic mice. Am. J. Pathol. **154:** 1673–1684.
13. BORNEMANN, K.D. & M. STAUFENBIEL. 2000. Transgenic mouse models of Alzheimer's disease. Ann. N. Y. Acad. Sci. **908:** 260–266.
14. STAUFENBIEL, M., C. STURCHLER-PIERRAT, D. ABRAMOWSKI, *et al.* 1997. Pathological features in APP transgenic mice resembling those of Alzheimer's disease. *In* Alzheimer's Disease II: Exploiting Mechanisms for Drug Development and Diagnosis. E. Friedman & L.M. Savage, Eds.: 4.2.1–4.2.12. IBC Library Series, International Business Communications, Southborough, MA.
15. PHINNEY, A.L., T. DELLER, M. STALDER, *et al.* 1999. Cerebral amyloid induces aberrant axonal sprouting and ectopic terminal formation in amyloid precursor protein transgenic mice. J. Neurosci. **19:** 8552–8559.
16. TAGO, H., P.L. MCGEER & E.G. MCGEER. 1987. Acetycholinesterase fibers and the development of senile plaques. Brain Res. **406:** 363–369.
17. GEULA, C. & M. MESULAM. 1989. Cholinesterases and the pathology of Alzheimer's disease. Neuroscience **33:** 469–481.
18. WEST, M.J., P.D. COLEMAN, D.G. FLOOD & J.C. TRONCOSO. 1994. Differences in the pattern of hippocampal neuron loss in normal ageing and Alzheimer's disease. Lancet **344:** 769–772.
19. REGEUR, L., G.B. JENSEN, H. PAKKENBERG, S.M. EVANS & B. PAKKENBERG. 1994. No global neocortical nerve cell loss in brains from patients with senile dementia of Alzheimer's type. Neurobiol. Aging **15:** 347–352.
20. ZHANG, Z., H. HARTMANN, V.M. DO, *et al.* 1998. Destabilization of β-catenin by mutations in presenilin-1 potentiates neuronal apoptosis. Nature **395:** 698–702.

Prions: Pathogenesis and Reverse Genetics

ADRIANO AGUZZI,[a] MICHAEL A. KLEIN, FABIO MONTRASIO,
VLADIMIR PEKARIK, SEBASTIAN BRANDNER, HISAKO FURUKAWA,
PASCAL KÄSER, CHRISTIANE RÖCKL, AND MARKUS GLATZEL

Institute of Neuropathology, University Hospital Zurich, CH-8091 Zurich, Switzerland

ABSTRACT: Spongiform encephalopathies are a group of infectious neurodegenerative diseases. The infectious agent that causes transmissible spongiform encephalopathies was termed *prion* by Stanley Prusiner. The prion hypothesis
states that the partially protease-resistant and detergent-insoluble prion
protein (PrP^{Sc}) is identical with the infectious agent, and lacks any detectable
nucleic acids. Since the latter discovery, transgenic mice have contributed
many important insights into the field of prion biology. The prion protein
(PrP^c) is encoded by the *Prnp* gene, and disruption of *Prnp* leads to resistance
to infection by prions. Introduction of mutant PrP^c genes into PrP^c-deficient
mice was used to investigate structure-activity relationships of the PrP^c gene
with regard to scrapie susceptibility. Ectopic expression of PrP^c in PrP^c knockout mice proved a useful tool for the identification of host cells competent for
prion replication. Finally, the availability of PrP^c knockout and transgenic
mice overexpressing PrP^c allowed selective reconstitution experiments aimed
at expressing PrP^c in neurografts or in specific populations of hemato- and
lymphopoietic cells. The latter studies helped in elucidating some of the mechanisms of prion spread and disease pathogenesis.

RECENT HISTORY OF PRION DISEASES

The prototype of all prion diseases, scrapie in sheep and goats, has been known
for more than two centuries. A recent form of animal prion disease designated bovine spongiform encephalopathy (BSE) has since its first recognition in 1986 developed into an epizootic, which fortunately has been receding since 1992.[1–3] The
emergence of a new variant form of Creutzfeldt-Jakob disease (vCJD) in young people in the UK has raised the possibility that BSE has spread to humans by dietary
exposure.[4,5] This scenario has recently been supported by experimental evidence
claiming that the agent causing BSE is indistinguishable from the vCJD agent.[6–10]

THE NATURE OF THE INFECTIOUS AGENT

Prion diseases are caused by a novel type of pathogen, the "prion," which differs
from known bacteria and viruses in major respects. For one, prions are extremely resistant to heat. Even prolonged heating to 100°C (212°F) and disinfection by most
of the commonly used disinfectants does not lead to inactivation.[11] Prions are not

[a]Address for correspondence: Adriano Aguzzi, Institute of Neuropathology, Schmelzberg-
strasse 12, CH-8091 Zurich, Switzerland. Tel.: +41 1 2552869; fax: +41 1 2554402.
e-mail: Adriano@pathol.unizh.ch

easily biodegradable.[12] Purification of the infectious agent has led to the identification of a protein (denominated prion protein) which is intimately associated with infectivity. Although the exact physical nature of the transmissible agent is controversial, a very large body of experimental data supports the "protein only" hypothesis which postulates that the agent is devoid of nucleic acid and consists solely of an abnormal conformer of a cellular protein called PrP^c.[13,14] Accumulation of an abnormal isoform (PrP^{Sc} or PrP-res) of the host encoded prion protein (PrP^c or PrP-sen)[15–17] in the central nervous system (CNS) is a hallmark of prion diseases.

Because of its location at the outer surface of cells, anchored by phosphatidyl-inositol glycolipid,[18] PrP^c is a candidate for a signaling, cell adhesion or perhaps even for some transport functions. PrP^c is expressed on many cell types, including neurons,[19] astrocytes,[20] and lymphocytes[21] and appears to be developmentally regulated during mouse embryogenesis.[22] Although PrP^c is predominantly found in brain tissue, high levels are also present in heart, skeletal muscle, and kidney, whereas it is barely detectable in the liver.[23] Several candidate proteins that bind PrP^c have been reported. Among them is the amyloid precursor-like protein 1 (APLP1) which is a member of the amyloid precursor protein gene family. This opens up new questions in the light of its relevance to Alzheimer's disease.[24] Other possible PrP^c binding proteins are the human laminin receptor precursor, which serves as a cell surface receptor for infectious agents,[25,26] and an uncharacterized 66-kDa membrane protein.[27] Interaction of the PrP^c with Bcl-2, a protein that can rescue neurons, points towards a possible role of the prion protein in neuronal cell survival.[28] However, evidence that any of these interactions is physiologically significant is still missing.

PrP KNOCKOUT MICE AND THEIR PHENOTYPES

The "protein only" hypothesis states that PrP^c is a substrate for the PrP^{Sc}-mediated conversion of PrP^c into new PrP^{Sc} molecules. As a consequence of this hypothesis, an organism lacking PrP^c should be resistant to scrapie and unable to propagate the infectious agent. The mice generated by Büeler and colleagues[29] carry a targeted disruption of the *Prnp* gene. This was achieved by homologous recombination in embryonic stem cells. In the disrupted *Prnp* allele, 184 codons of the *Prnp* coding region (which consists of 254 codons) were replaced by a drug-resistance gene as selectable marker. A second line of PrP^c knockout mice was generated by Manson and co-workers[30] by inserting a selectable marker into a unique *Kpn*I site of the PrP^c open reading frame, thereby disrupting—but not deleting—the *Prnp* coding region. In a third PrP^c knockout line created by Sakaguchi and colleagues the whole PrP^c ORF and about 250 bp of the 5′ intron and 452 bp of 3′ untranslated sequences were replaced with a drug-resistance gene.[31] Both the Büeler and Sakaguchi mice were on a mixed genetic (129/Sv × C57BL) background whereas the Manson mice were bred on a pure 129/Ola background. According to the terminology which has become customary in the literature, and by which we abide in this manuscript, the Zurich mice have been designated *Prnp*$^{o/o}$ while the Edinburgh and the Japanese mice are termed *Prnp*$^{-/-}$.

Although it was proposed that PrP^c, which is an ubiquitously expressed neuronal protein, may have housekeeping function,[32] the homozygous PrP^c knockout mice

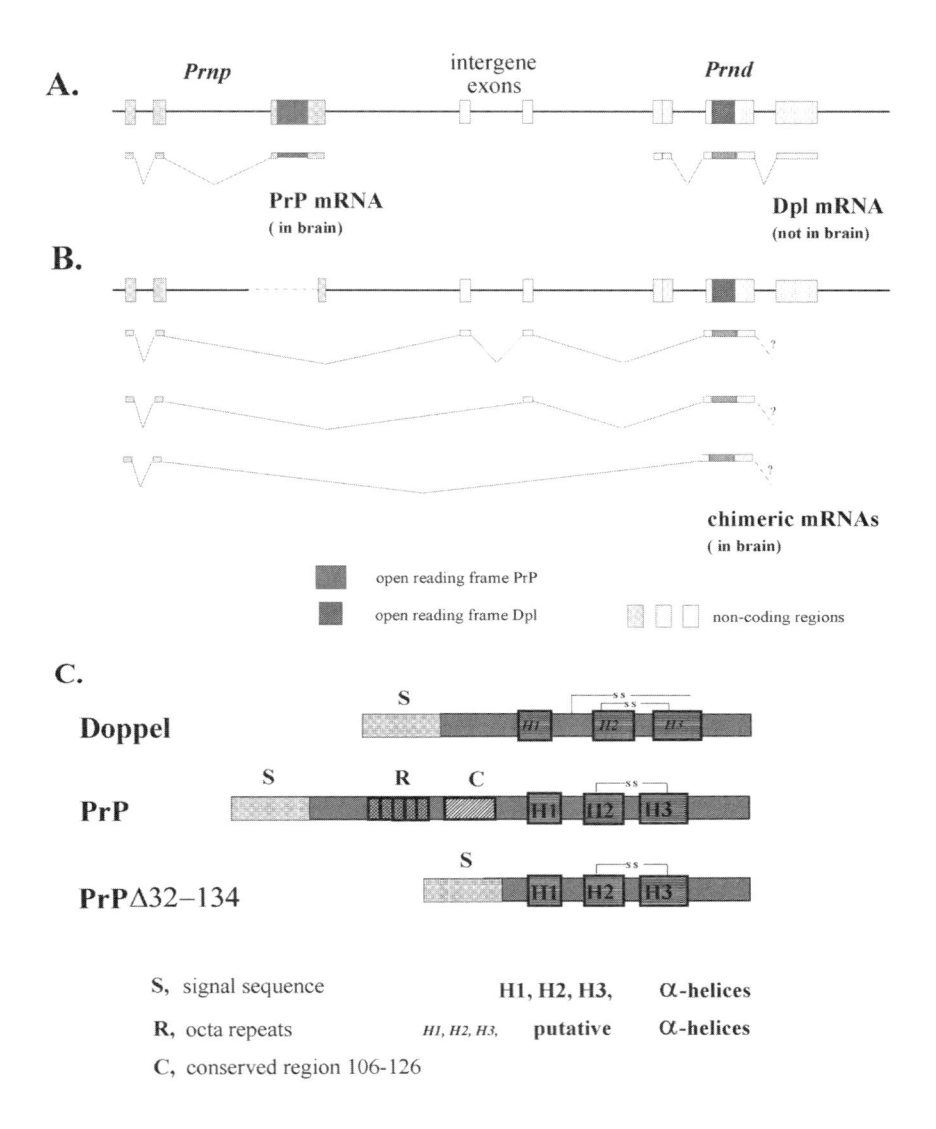

FIGURE 1. (**A**) The Prnp and Prnd loci and expression of the PrP^c and Dpl mRNAs and proteins that they encode. Coding and noncoding exons of *Prnp*, *Prnd*, and intergenic exons of unknown function. (**B**) Deletion of the exon of *Prnp* containing an open reading frame and its flanking regions results in the formation of several chimeric mRNAs that comprise the first two exons of *Prnp* , which are spliced directly or indirectly to the exon encoding Dpl. (**C**) Comparison of predicted domains of Dpl with full-length PrP^c and with PrP^c in which amino acid residues 32–134 have been deleted.

generated by Büeler[29] and Manson[30] were viable with no behavioral impairment and showed no overt phenotypic abnormalities, suggesting that PrP^c does not play a crucial role in development or function of the nervous system.[29,30] Although there was no overt phenotype, detailed analysis revealed electrophysiological defects such as weakened GABA-A receptor-mediated fast inhibition and impaired long-term potentiation in the hippocampus for these two lines of PrP^c knockout mice when compared to their corresponding wild-type counterparts, indicating that PrP^c might play a role in synaptic plasticity.[33] Tobler *et al.*[34] reported altered sleep patterns and rhythms of circadian activity in the Büeler and Manson mice.

Instead the PrP^c null mice derived by Sakaguchi *et al.*[31] developed severe progressive ataxia starting from 70 weeks of age. Analysis of the brains of affected animals revealed extensive loss of cerebellar Purkinje cells.[35] Because no such phenotype was observed in the other two lines of PrP^c knockout mice, it seems likely that this phenotype is not due to the lack of PrP^c but rather to the deletion of flanking sequences. Interestingly, a Purkinje cell-specific enhancer was proposed to be contained within the second intron of *Prnp*.[36] The report that expression of a *Prnp* transgene can rescue this phenotype argues against the hypothesis that the phenotype was caused by deletion of a regulatory element rather than of the *Prnp* reading frame.[37] Recently evidence has been forthcoming that the phenotype observed in the Sakaguchi mice is caused by upregulation of a second *Prnp*-like gene located 16 kb downstream of the *Prnp* gene (FIG. 1).[38] The exact mechanism of this process is still under discussion.[39]

NO SCRAPIE IN PrP NULL MICE

One of the milestones in scrapie research was the inoculation of PrP^c null mice with mouse-adapted scrapie strains. All three PrP^c null mouse lines were resistant to scrapie. The $Prnp^{o/o}$ mice generated by Büeler *et al.* inoculated with the RML isolate of mouse-adapted prions remained healthy for their whole life span and did not show any signs of scrapie typical neuropathology.[40] This observation was confirmed using different PrP^c null mice with different mouse-adapted scrapie inocula.[31,41] Mice hemizygous for the disrupted *Prnp* gene ($Prnp^{o/+}$) showed partial resistance to scrapie infection as manifested by prolonged incubation times of about 290 days as compared to about 160 days in the case of $Prnp^{+/+}$ mice. The incubation times until the first scrapie symptoms appear seem to correlate with levels of PrP^c in the host, whereas the severity of the disease in terms of neuropatholgical changes in the brain and levels of prion infectivity were not dependent on the PrP^c level.[41,42] The amount of PrP^c present in the brain seems to be the rate-limiting step in the development of the disease. Therefore therapeutic efforts aimed to reduce the amount of PrP^c may be effective.

STRUCTURE AND IMPLICATIONS ABOUT FUNCTION OF THE PrP GENE

When PrP^{Sc} undergoes limited proteolysis, the N terminus is cleaved off and a fragment termed PrP$^{27-30}$ is left. This portion of PrP^{Sc} is still infectious meaning that the last 60 amino-proximal residues of PrP^{Sc} are not required for infectivity.[16,43]

PrP^c lacking residues 23–88 can be converted into protease-resistant PrP^c in scrapie-infected neuroblastoma cells.[44] An important question arising from these experiments is the question whether N-terminally truncated PrP^c molecules can support prion replication in mice. Transgenic mice expressing N-terminal deletions of the prion protein on a PrP^c null background were established. These mutant PrP^c mice with amino-proximal deletions of residues 32–80 and 32–93 corresponding to truncations of 49 and 63 residues restore scrapie susceptibility, prion replication, and formation of truncated PrP^{Sc} in PrP^c-deficient mice.[45]

These experiments demonstrate that the octapeptide region encompassing residues 51–90 of murine PrP^c is dispensable for scrapie pathogenesis. This is remarkable in view of the fact that additional octapeptide repeats instead of the normal 5 segregate with affected individuals in families with inherited CJD,[46] and that expression of a mutant PrP^c with a pathological number of octarepeats induces a neurodegenerative disease in transgenic mice.[47]

PHENOTYPE IN MICE EXPRESSING TRUNCATED PrP^c

The three-dimensional structure determination using NMR revealed a highly flexible amino terminal tail that lacks ordered secondary structures extending from residue 23 to 121 within full-length mature PrP^c, whereas the carboxy terminal part of PrP^c consists of a stably folded globular domain.[48,49] The flexible tail, part of which is protease-sensitive in PrP^{Sc}, comprises the most conserved region of PrP^c across all species examined.[50] The possibility that the flexible tail may play a role in the conformational transition of PrP^c to PrP^{Sc} by initiating the structural rearrangements from α-helices to β-sheets was proposed.[48,51] To further analyze the importance of the flexible tail in regard to scrapie susceptibility, Shmerling and colleagues generated amino-proximal deletions of residues 32–121 and 32–134 and expressed them as transgenes in PrP^c-deficient mice. Mice overexpressing these transgenes developed severe ataxia and neuronal death limited to the granular layer of the cerebellum, as early as 1–3 months of age. No pathological phenotype was observed in transgenic mice with shorter deletions encompassing residues 32–80, 32–93 and 32–106. The selective degeneration of granule cells in the cerebellum argues against an unspecific toxic effect elicited by the truncated PrP^c. Another argument for a specific effect is the fact that neurons in the cortex and elsewhere express truncated PrP^c at similar levels but do not undergo cell death by apoptosis. If just one copy of a wild-type *Prnp* allele was introduced in these mice, the phenotype was abolished. These results are consistent with a model in which truncated PrP^c acts as dominant negative inhibitor of a functional homologue of PrP^c, with both competing for the same putative PrP^c ligand.[45]

A different spontaneous neurologic phenotype was reported in mice carrying PrP^c transgenes with internal deletions corresponding to either of the two carboxy-proximal α-helices. Two transgenic mouse lines generated on the *Prn*$^{po/o}$ background expressing mutant PrP^c with deletions of residues 23–88 and either residues 177–200 or 201–217 developed CNS dysfunction and neuropathological changes characteristic of a neuronal storage disease.[52] Since deletion of residues 23–88 alone did not lead to a spontaneous phenotype, it was concluded that ablation of either of

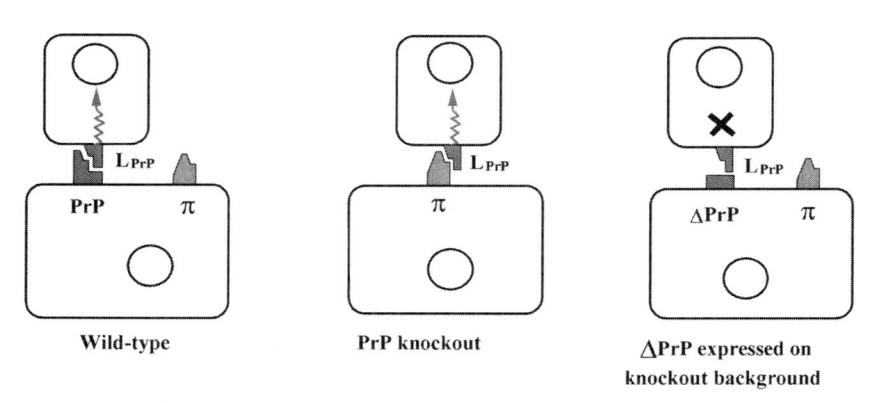

Wild-type   PrP knockout   ΔPrP expressed on
                   knockout background

FIGURE 2. According to a hypothesis advanced by C. Weissmann, in wild-type mice PrP^c binds to its receptor (L) to elicit an essential signal. In the absence of PrP^c a PrP^c-like molecule (π) with a lower binding affinity can fulfill the same function. In PrP^c knockout mice with the truncated PrP^c, the truncated PrP^c can interact with the receptor, but without eliciting the signal which leads to the observed phenotype.

the two carboxy-terminal α-helices is sufficient to cause this novel CNS illness. Ultrastructural studies indicated extensive proliferation of the endoplasmic reticulum and revealed accumulation of mutant PrP^c within cytoplasmic inclusions in enlarged neurons. Since both Asn-linked glycosylation sites are located within residues 177–200, it is conceivable that aberrant glycosylation affects processing of the mutant PrP^c. However, it is unlikely that altered glycosylation of PrP^c is sufficient to account for neuronal storage disease, because transgenic mice expressing hamster PrP^c with point mutations that block Asn-linked glycosylation did not show this spontaneous disease phenotype.[53]

A completely new light is shed on all these studies by the discovery of a PrP^c-like gene named Dpl (Doppel, German for double) located 16 kb downstream of the murine *Prnp* gene (FIG. 1).[38] Dpl is overexpressed in certain strains of PrP^c knockout mice that develop neurological symptoms. The fact that the mice with a truncated *Prnp* transgene lacking the amino terminus which are devoid of the conserved 106–126 amino acid region develop granule cell degeneration which can be rescued by introduction of single intact PrP^c allele led to the hypothesis that PrP^c interacts with a ligand to produce an essential signal. In PrP^c knockout mice a PrP^c like molecule with a lower binding affinity could substitute the role of PrP^c. In the amino-terminated transgenic mice the truncated PrP^c could bind the ligand with high affinity without eliciting the survival signal. Dpl could act in a similar way and produce its effects through a competition with PrP^c for the PrP^c ligand thus blocking an important signal (FIG. 2).[38,39]

NEUROGRAFTS IN PRION RESEARCH

The fact that *Prnp*$^{o/o}$ mice show normal development and behavior,[29,30] has led to the hypothesis that scrapie pathology may come about because PrP^{Sc} deposition is neurotoxic,[54] rather than by depletion of cellular PrP^c.[33] If the depletion of cellular PrP^c is really the reason for scrapie pathology, lack of PrP^c might result in embryonic or perinatal lethality, especially since PrP^c is encoded by a unique gene for which no related family members have been found. Until now there is no stringent mouse model where PrP^c can be depleted in an acute fashion. In this case the depletion of PrP^c may be much more deleterious than its lack throughout development, since the organism may then not have the time to enable compensatory mechanisms.

In order to study the question of neurotoxicity, we exposed brain tissue of $Prnp^{o/o}$ mice to a continuous source of PrP^{Sc}. This was achieved by grafting neural tissue overexpressing PrP^c into the brain of PrP^c-deficient mice using well-established protocols.[55–57] Following intracerebral inoculation with scrapie prions, neuroectodermal grafts accumulated high levels of PrP^{Sc} and infectivity, and developed severe histopathological changes characteristic for scrapie (FIG. 3). At later timepoints, substantial amounts of graft-derived PrP^{Sc} migrated into the host brain, and even in areas distant from the grafts, substantial amounts of infectivity were detected (FIG. 3).[36,58] Nonetheless, even 16 months after transplantation and infection with prions, no pathological changes were detected in the PrP^c-deficient tissue, not even in the immediate vicinity of the grafts or the PrP^c deposits. These results clearly suggest that PrP^{Sc} is inherently nontoxic, and PrP^{Sc} plaques found in spongiform encephalopathies may be an epiphenomenon rather than a cause of neuronal damage.[59] Maybe the PrP^{Sc}-containing plaques have to be formed and localized intracellularly in order to act neurotoxic. If this is the case, plaques that are localized extracellularly might not be toxic. This would explain the absence of pathological changes outside the PrP^c-containing grafts.

Because the host mice harboring a chronically scrapie-infected neural graft did not develop any sign of disease, they not only enabled us to study the effects of prions on the surrounding tissue but also were an ideal model to assess all changes occurring during the progression of scrapie disease in neuroectodermal tissue. The possibility of studying extremely late timepoints after infection with the scrapie agent was useful in order to observe phenomena that cannot be seen in PrP^c-containing mice, because these mice develop clinical symptoms eventually leading to death earlier. With increasing length of the incubation time, grafts underwent progressive astrogliosis and spongiosis which was accompanied by loss of neuronal processes within the grafts and subsequent destruction of the neuropil. The latest studied timepoint was 435 days after inoculation. Grafts showed an increase of cellular density probably due to astroglial proliferation and a complete loss of neurons. Intriguingly, with *in vivo* imaging with magnetic resonance imaging using gadolinium as a contrast-enhancing medium, a progressive disruption of the blood-brain barrier in scrapie-infected grafts was detected during the course of the disease.[60] These findings confirmed several predictions about the pathogenesis of spongiform encephalopathies, mainly that scrapie leads to selective neuronal loss while astrocytes and perhaps other neuroectodermal cells, while being affected by the disease, can survive and maintain their phenotypic characteristics for very long periods of time.

In other experimental models as experimental hamster scrapie, disruption of the blood-brain barrier was also visible,[61] yet no such observations were made in human spongiform encephalopathies. The localized blood-brain barrier disruption in chronically infected grafts might contribute to the spread of prions from grafts to the sur-

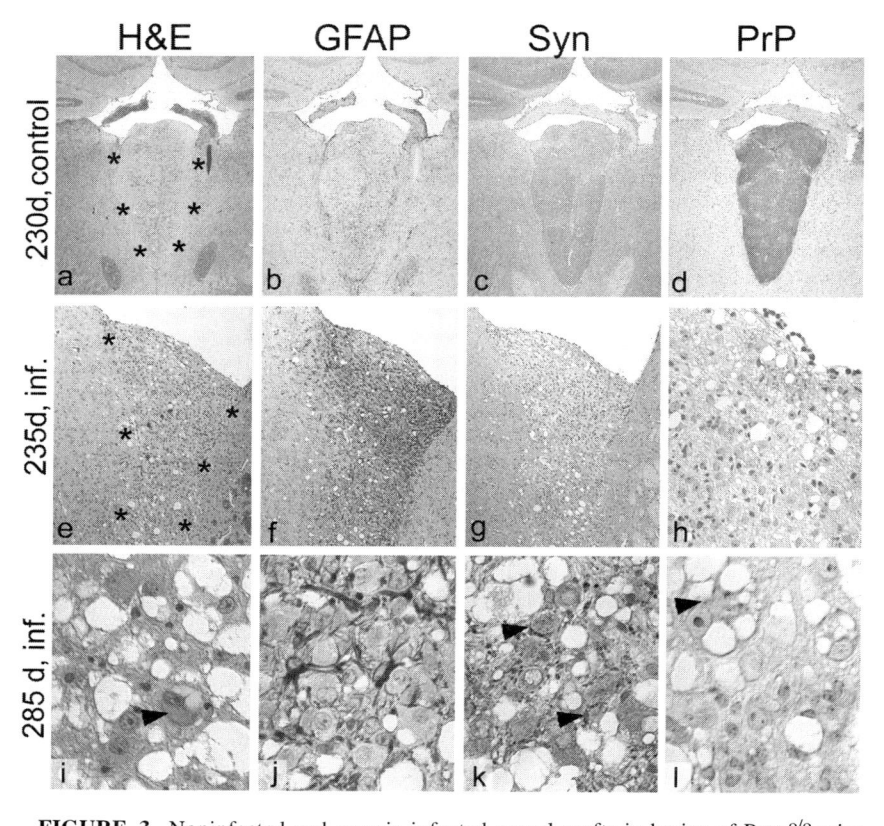

FIGURE 3. Noninfected and scrapie-infected neural grafts in brains of Prnp^o/o mice. *Upper row* (**a, b, c, d**): healthy control graft 230 days after mock inoculation. The graft is located in the third ventricle of the recipient mouse (a, see *asterisks*, hematoxylin-eosin), and shows no spongiform change, little gliosis (b, immunostain for GFAP), and strong expression of synaptophysin (c) and of PrP^c (d). *Middle row* (**e, f, g, h**): scrapie-infected graft 235 days after inoculation with increased cellularity (e), brisk gliosis (f), and a significant loss of synaptophysin (g) and PrP^c (h) staining intensity is shown. *Bottom row* (**i, j, k, l,**): high magnification of a similar graft shows characteristic pathological changes in a chronically infected graft. (i) Appearance of large vacuoles and ballooned neurons (*arrow*). In the GFAP immunostain (j), astrocytes appear wrapped around densely packed neurons. Granular deposits and intracytoplasmic accumulation of synaptophysin (k) and PrPrP^c PC immunoreactivity (l) in the cytoplasm of neurons.

rounding brain, as described previously.[58] It may also account for the accumulation pattern of protease-resistant PrP^c within the white matter and in brain areas surrounding the grafts. The accumulation of PrP^Sc in nonaffected neuropil surrounding the graft could also be explained through vasogenic diffusion from the affected graft towards the host brain.

SPREAD OF PRIONS IN THE CENTRAL NERVOUS SYSTEM

Scrapie can be transmitted by injecting scrapie-infected brain homogenate into suitable recipients by a number of different inoculation routes. Intracerebral inoculation is the most effective method for transmission of spongiform encephalopathies and may even facilitate circumvention of the species barrier. Other modes of transmission are oral uptake of the agent,[2,62,63] intravenous and intraperitoneal injection,[64] as well as conjunctival instillation,[65] implantation of corneal grafts,[66] and intraocular injection.[67] Intraocular injection is an elegant way of studying the neural spread of the agent, since the retina is a part of the CNS and intraocular injection does not produce direct physical trauma to the brain, which may disrupt the blood-brain barrier and impair other aspects of brain physiology. The assumption that spread of prions within the CNS occurs axonally rests mainly on the demonstration of diachronic spongiform changes along the retinal pathway following intraocular infection.[67]

It has been repeatedly shown that expression of PrP^c is required for prion replication[40,68] and for neurodegenerative changes to occur.[58] To investigate whether spread of prions within the CNS is dependent on PrP^c expression in the visual pathway, PrP^c-producing neural grafts were used as sensitive indicators of the presence of prion infectivity in the brain of an otherwise PrP^c-deficient host.

Following inoculation with prions into the eye of grafted $Prnp^{o/o}$ mice, none of the grafts showed signs of spongiosis, gliosis, synaptic loss, or PrP^{Sc} deposition. In one instance, the graft of an intraocularly inoculated mouse was assayed and found to be devoid of infectivity. Therefore, it was concluded that infectivity administered to the eye of PrP^c-deficient hosts cannot induce scrapie in a PrP^c-expressing brain graft.[69]

One problem that is encountered while conducting work with PrP^c-containing grafts in $Prnp^{o/o}$ mice is the fact that PrP^c-producing tissue might lead to an immune response to PrP^c [70] and possibly to neutralization of infectivity. Indeed, analysis of sera from grafted mice revealed significant anti-PrP^c antibody titers,[69] and it was shown that PrP^c presented by the intracerebral graft (rather than the inoculum or graft-borne PrP^c) was the offending antigen. In order to definitively rule out the possibility that prion transport was disabled by a neutralizing immune response, the experiments were repeated in mice tolerant to PrP^c, namely, the $Prnp^{o/o}$ mice transgenic for the PrP^c coding sequence under the control of the lck-promoter. These mice overexpress PrP^c on T lymphocytes, but were resistant to scrapie and did not replicate prions in brain, spleen, or thymus after intraperitoneal inoculation with scrapie prions.[71] Upon grafting with PrP^c-overexpressing neuroectoderm these mice do not develop antibodies to PrP^c presumably due to clonal deletion of PrP^c-immunoreactive lymphocytes. As before, intraocular inoculation with prions did not provoke scrapie in the graft, supporting the conclusion that lack of PrP^c, rather than immune response to PrP^c, prevented prion spread.[69] Therefore, PrP^c appears to be necessary for the spread of prions along the retinal projections and within the intact CNS.

These results indicate that intracerebral spread of prions is based on a PrP^c-paved chain of cells, perhaps because they are capable of supporting prion replication. When such a chain is interrupted by interposed cells that lack PrP^c, as in the case described here, no propagation of prions to the target tissue can occur. Perhaps prions require PrP^c for propagation across synapses: PrP^c is present in the synaptic region,[72] and certain synaptic properties are altered in $Prnp^{o/o}$ mice.[33,73] Perhaps transport of prions within (or on the surface of) neuronal processes is PrP^c-dependent. These findings support the "domino-stone" model in which spreading of scrapie prions in the CNS occurs *per continuitatem* through conversion of PrP^c by adjacent PrP^{Sc}.[74]

SPREAD OF PRIONS FROM EXTRACEREBRAL SITES TO THE CNS

From an epidemiological point of view oral uptake of prions may be more relevant than intracerebral transmission, because it is thought to be responsible for the BSE epidemic and for transmission of BSE to a variety of species including humans.[8,9] Prions can find their way through the body to the brain of their host, yet histopathological changes have not been identified in organs other than the CNS. One of the main characteristics of prion diseases is the long incubation time. This incubation time can be explained by multiplication of prions in "reservoirs." A likely candidate that could constitute this reservoir is the lymphoreticular system (LRS). This is supported by the finding that prion replication in lymphoid organs always precedes prion replication in the CNS, even if infectivity is administered intracerebrally (FIG. 4).[75] Prions may multiply silently in "reservoirs" during the incubation phase of the disease. Infectivity can accumulate in all components of the LRS, including lymph nodes and intestinal Peyer's patches, where prions replicate almost immediately after oral administration of prions to mice.[76] Recently, it was shown that vCJD prions accumulate in the lymphoid tissue of tonsils in such large amounts that PrP^{Sc} can easily be detected with antibodies on histological sections.[77]

A wealth of early studies points to the importance of prion replication in lymphoid organs, yet little is known about which cells support prion propagation in the LRS. Whole-body ionizing radiation studies in mice[78] after intraperitoneal infection have suggested that the critical cells are long-lived. The follicular dendritic cell (FDC) would be a prime candidate, and indeed PrP^{Sc} accumulates in such cells of wild-type and nude mice (which have a selective T-cell defect).[79] In addition when mice with severe combined immunodeficiency (SCID) whose FDCs are thought to be functionally impaired are challenged with the scrapie agent intraperitoneally, they do not develop the disease nor is there any replication of prions in the spleen.[80] Upon reconstitution of SCID mice with wild-type spleen cells, susceptibility to scrapie is restored after peripheral infection.[81] These findings suggest that components of the immune system are required for efficient transfer of prions from the site of peripheral infection to the CNS.

To study the role of the immune system in more detail we used a panel of immune-deficient mice which were inoculated intraperitoneally with prions. We found that defects affecting T cells had no apparent effect, but that all mutations that disrupted the differentiation of B cells prevented the development of clinical scrapie.[82] From these results, one can conclude that B cells are important for the development of scrapie after peripheral infection. Do B cells physically transport prions all the way from the periphery to the CNS? This possibility seems very unlikely, since lymphocytes do not normally cross the blood-brain barrier unless they have a specific reason to do so (e.g., during an inflammatory reaction). Furthermore, up to 30% of B-cell-deficient mice contain prions in their brains despite no signs of clin-

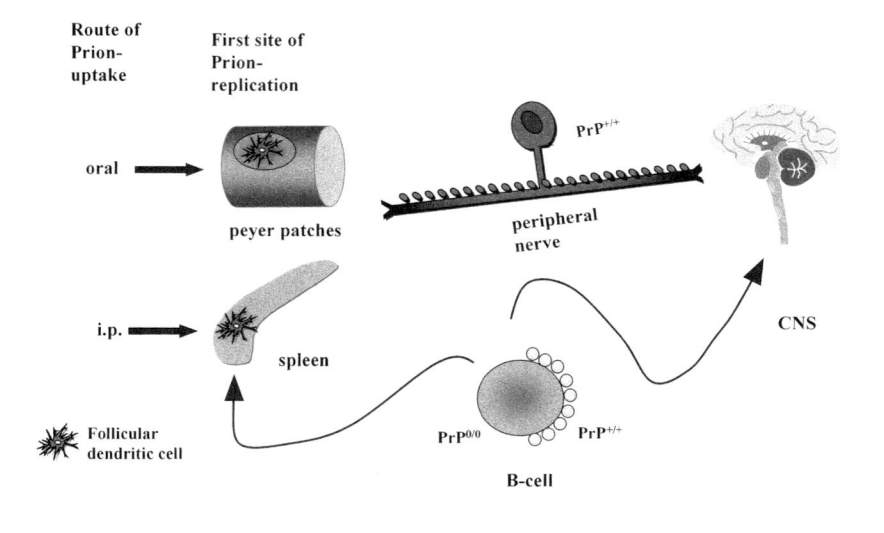

FIGURE 4. Neuroinvasion of prions. Depending on the route of administration of the infectious agent, the first site of replication is probably in the lymphoid tissue of the gut or in the spleen. From there neuroinvasion is most likely accomplished via the PNS. The presence of B cells is crucial for neuroinvasion. The precise mode of action of B cells is still unclear.

ical disease.[83] How is the spread of prions accomplished within the body? Perhaps, prions administered to peripheral sites are first brought to lymphatic organs by mobile immune cells such as B cells. Once infection has been established in the LRS, prions invade peripheral nerve endings.[84,85] How the neuroinvasion from cells belonging to the lymphoreticular system to peripheral nerves is accomplished, is still a matter of discussion (FIG. 4). Access to peripheral nerves may perhaps be facilitated if myelination of the nerves is reduced or absent.[86] Considering this, the mantle zone of the lymph follicles which is innervated by terminal unmyelinated nerve fibers could be the entry point of the scrapie agent into the PNS. It is also here that processes belonging to FDCs are in close contact with nerve fibers. Along the peripheral nerves the scrapie agent reaches the CNS where further spread occurs trans-synaptically and along fiber tracts.[87,88] Is PrP^c also required for the spread of prions from peripheral sites to the CNS? Indirect evidence points in this direction: PrP^c-expressing neurografts in *Prnp*$^{o/o}$ mice did not develop scrapie histopathology after intraperitoneal or intravenous inoculation with prions and no infectivity was detectable in the spleen. Following reconstitution of the host lymphohemopoietic system with PrP^c-expressing cells, prion titers in the spleen were restored to wild-type levels but, surprisingly, PrP^c-expressing grafts failed to develop scrapie upon intraperitoneal or intravenous infection with prions (FIG. 5).[89] These findings suggest that transfer of infectivity from the spleen to the CNS is crucially dependent on the expression of PrP^c in a tissue compartment interposed between the LRS and the CNS that cannot be reconstituted by bone marrow transfer. Several studies suggest that this compartment may comprise part of the peripheral nervous system.[86,90]

Host	Prnp$^{o/o}$	tg20	wt	Prnp$^{o/o}$	Prnp$^{o/o}$
Graft	---	---	---	tg20	tg20
B.Marrow	---	---	---	wt	wt
Inoculation	---	---	i.p.	i.c.	i.p.

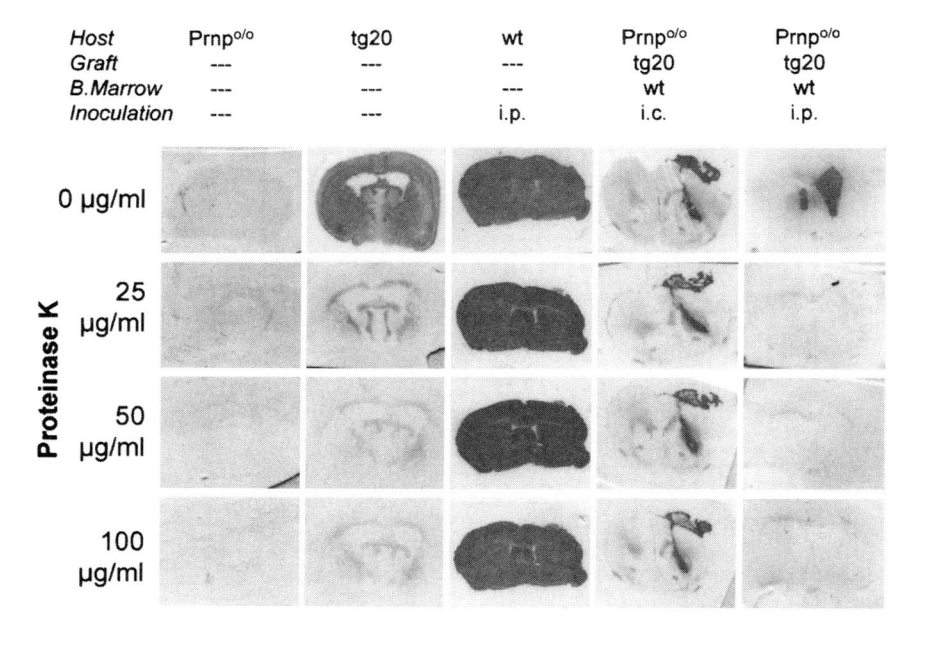

FIGURE 5. Accumulation of PrP^{Sc} in brain grafts. Histoblots showing immunoreactive PrP^c in brain sections natively (*first row*) and after digestion with increasing levels of proteinase K (*second through fourth row*). Prnp$^{o/o}$ mice (*first column*) show no immunoreactivity, while mock-inoculated *tg20* mice (which overexpress PrP^c) show proteinase K-sensitive PrP^c (*second column*), but no proteinase K-resistant PrP^c. Terminally sick scrapie-infected wild-type mice contain large amounts of both PrP^c and PrP^{Sc} (*third column*). Prnp$^{o/o}$ whose bone marrow has been reconstituted with wild-type FLCs accumulate PrP^{Sc} in their PrP^c-overexpressing grafts after i.c. (*fourth column*) but not after i.p. prion administration (*fifth column*).

The absolute necessity of PrP^c presence for the spread of scrapie from the periphery as well as within the CNS may offer a handle to interfere with this chain of events without resorting to ablation of a functional immune system such as in the case of SCID mice.

ROLE OF B LYMPHOCYTES IN NEUROINVASION

The replication of prions[40] and their transport from the periphery to the CNS[89] is dependent upon expression of PrP^c. With respect to the results described in the previous paragraph, we examined whether expression of PrP^c by B cells was necessary to support neuroinvasion. In order to study this matter we took mice with various immune defects and repopulated their LRS by adoptive transfer of hematopoietic stem cells which expressed or lacked expression of PrP^c.

Adoptive transfer of either $Prnp^{+/+}$ or $Prnp^{o/o}$ fetal liver cells (FLCs) induced formation of germinal centers in spleens of recipient mice and differentiation of FDCs as visualized by staining with antibody FDC-M1.[91] However, no FDCs were found in B- and T-cell-deficient mice reconstituted with FLCs from μMT embryos (B-cell-deficient), consistent with the notion that B cells or products thereof are required for FDC maturation.

Mice reconstituted in the fashion explained above were challenged *i.p.* with scrapie prions. All mice that received FLCs of either genotype, $Prnp^{+/+}$ or $Prnp^{o/o}$, from immunocompetent donors, succumbed to scrapie after inoculation with a high dose of prions, and most mice after a low dose. Susceptibility to disease could not be restored upon transfer of FLCs from μMT donors. Omission of the adoptive transfer procedure did not restore susceptibility to disease in any of the immune-deficient mice challenged with the low dose of prions. With the high dose inoculum, susceptibility to scrapie could be restored even in the absence of B cells and FDCs. However, reconstituted mice which received bone marrow from $TCR\alpha^{-/-}$ donors, which possess B cells and lack all T cells but those expressing $TCR\alpha^{-/-}$ receptors, regained susceptibility to scrapie, again confirming the dependency of infectibility upon the presence of B cells. Individual samples of brain and spleen from the scrapie-inoculated bone marrow chimeras were transmitted into highly susceptible indicator mice. We observed restoration of infectious titers and PrP^{Sc} deposition in spleens and brains of recipient mice either carrying $Prnp^{+/+}$ or $Prnp^{o/o}$ donor cells.[91]

B cells are clearly a cofactor in peripheral prion pathogenesis, but the identity of those cells in which prions actually replicate within lymphatic organs is uncertain. In a further step to clarify this issue, we investigated whether spleen PrP^{Sc} was associated with FDCs in repopulated mice. Double-color immunofluorescence confocal microscopy revealed deposits of PrP^{c}-immunoreactive material in germinal centers which appeared largely colocalized with the follicular dendritic network in spleens of reconstituted mice.

Taking together all the information we have gained with the above-described experiments, one can support the hypothesis that cells whose maturation depends on B cells are responsible for accumulation of prions in lymphoid tissue such as the spleen. FDCs, although their origin remains rather obscure, are a likely candidate for the site of prion replication, because their maturation correlates with the presence of B cells and their products. This hypothesis is not free of controversy; it is still possible that the follicular dendritic network serve merely as a reservoir for the accumulation of prions and that other B-cell-dependent processes are involved in the transport of the infectious agent. Prions may be transported on or within B cells directly as they cross peripheral lymphoid tissue to localize in autonomic nerve terminals. In recent studies where spleens were fractionated it was shown that prion infectivity is mainly associated with B and T lymphocytes and less with a stromal fraction containing FDCs.[92]

CONCLUSION

Peripheral pathogenesis of prion diseases is here defined as the process starting with the contact of the infectious agent with extracerebral sites, and eventually resulting in brain disease. This process occurs in distinct sequential phases. The first and very early event in disease progression is certainly accumulation of prions in the LRS. This process is dependent upon components of the host immune system. Whether prions replicate or merely accumulate in the LRS is not known with certainty. FDCs play a major role in this process, but the details are still under discussion. In order to achieve efficient neuroinvasion either B cells per se or their products are essential. One B-cell-dependent event that is of relevance is the acquisition of a functional FDC network within the germinal centers of peripheral lymphoid tissue.

The second phase of neuroinvasion appears to encompass transfer of prions from lymphoid tissue to nerve endings of the peripheral nervous system. Because lymphoid organs are predominantly innervated by nerve fibers of the sympathetic nervous system, this part of the peripheral nervous system is a prime candidate. How neuroinvasion is accomplished and how the agent is transported within the peripheral nervous system, however, is still unclear. It is worthwhile noting that the innervation of lymphoid tissue is, at least in part, controlled by lymphocytes themselves, as both T and B cells secrete nerve growth factor and, vice versa, nerve terminals secrete a variety of factors that stimulate the immune system.[93] These factors may play a critical role in the neuroinvasion process and represent a critical site for modulation of disease progression. For example, drugs which act on lymphocytes or on the sympathetic innervation of lymphoid tissue, or those that prevent cytokine release or block neurotransmission, may have a strong influence in the immune modulation and might represent useful tools for studying the cellular and molecular basis of prion neuroinvasion.

ACKNOWLEDGMENTS

We thank M. Peltola, M. König, and N. Wey for technical help, Dr. C. Weissmann for support, and Dr. K. Rajewsky for μMT mice. This work is supported by the Canton of Zürich, the Bundesämter für Gesundheit, Veterinärwesen, Bildung und Wissenschaft, and by grants from the Swiss National Research Program NFP38/ NFP38+ and from the companies Abbott and Baxter.

REFERENCES

1. WILESMITH, J.W., J.B. RYAN, W.D. HUESTON & L.J. HOINVILLE. 1992. Bovine spongiform encephalopathy: epidemiological features 1985 to 1990. Vet. Rec. **130:** 90–94.
2. ANDERSON, R.M., C.A. DONNELLY, N.M. FERGUSON *et al.* 1996. Transmission dynamics and epidemiology of BSE in British cattle. Nature **382:** 779–788.
3. WEISSMANN, C. & A. AGUZZI. 1997. Bovine spongiform encephalopathy and early onset variant Creutzfeldt-Jakob disease. Curr. Opin. Neurobiol. **7:** 695–700.
4. WILL, R., J.W. IRONSIDE, M. ZEIDLER *et al.* 1996. A new variant of Creutzfeldt-Jakob disease in the UK. Lancet **347:** 921–925.
5. CHAZOT, G., E. BROUSSOLLE, C. LAPRAS, T. BLÄTTLER, A. AGUZZI & N. KOPP. 1996. New variant of Creutzfeldt-Jakob disease in a 26-year-old French man. Lancet **347:** 1181.
6. AGUZZI, A. & C. WEISSMANN. 1996. Spongiform encephalopathies: a suspicious signature. Nature **383:** 666–667.
7. AGUZZI, A. 1996. Between cows and monkeys. Nature **381:** 734.

8. BRUCE, M.E., R.G. WILL, J.W. IRONSIDE *et al.* 1997. Transmissions to mice indicate that 'new variant' CJD is caused by the BSE agent. Nature **389:** 498–501.
9. HILL, A.F., M. DESBRUSLAIS, S. JOINER *et al.* 1997. The same prion strain causes vCJD and BSE. Nature **389:** 448–450.
10. WILL, R., S. COUSENS, C. FARRINGTON, P. SMITH, R. KNIGHT & J. IRONSIDE. 1999. Deaths from variant Creutzfeldt-Jakob disease. Lancet **353:** 9157–9158.
11. STEELMAN, V.M. 1994. Creutzfeld-Jakob disease: recommendations for infection control. Am. J. Infect. Control **22:** 312–318.
12. BROWN, P. & D.C. GAJDUSEK. 1991. Survival of scrapie virus after 3 years' interment. Lancet **337:** 269–270.
13. GRIFFITH, J.S. 1967. Self-replication and scrapie. Nature **215:** 1043–1044.
14. PRUSINER, S.B. 1982. Novel proteinaceous infectious particles cause scrapie. Science **216:** 136–144.
15. OESCH, B., D. WESTAWAY, M. WALCHLI *et al.* 1985. A cellular gene encodes scrapie PrP 27–30 protein. Cell **40:** 735–746.
16. MCKINLEY, M.P., D.C. BOLTON & S.B. PRUSINER. 1983. A protease-resistant protein is a structural component of the scrapie prion. Cell **35:** 57–62.
17. PRUSINER, S.B., M.P. MCKINLEY, K.A. BOWMAN *et al.* 1983. Scrapie prions aggregate to form amyloid-like birefringent rods. Cell **35:** 349–358.
18. STAHL, N., D.R. BORCHELT, K. HSIAO & S.B. PRUSINER. 1987. Scrapie prion protein contains a phosphatidylinositol glycolipid. Cell **51:** 229–240.
19. KRETZSCHMAR, H.A., S.B. PRUSINER, L.E. STOWRING & S.J. DEARMOND. 1986. Scrapie prion proteins are synthesized in neurons. Am. J. Pathol. **122:** 1–5.
20. MOSER, M., R.J. COLELLO, U. POTT & B. OESCH. 1995. Developmental expression of the prion protein gene in glial cells. Neuron **14:** 509–517.
21. CASHMAN, N.R., R. LOERTSCHER, J. NALBANTOGLU *et al.* 1990. Cellular isoform of the scrapie agent protein participates in lymphocyte activation. Cell **61:** 185–192.
22. MANSON, J., J.D. WEST, V. THOMSON, P. MCBRIDE, M.H. KAUFMAN & J. HOPE. 1992. The prion protein gene: a role in mouse embryogenesis? Development **115:** 117–122.
23. BENDHEIM, P.E., H.R. BROWN, R.D. RUDELLI *et al.* 1992. Nearly ubiquitous tissue distribution of the scrapie agent precursor protein. Neurology **42:** 149–156.
24. YEHIELY, F., P. BAMBOROUGH, M. DA COSTA *et al.* 1997. Identification of candidate proteins binding to prion protein. Neurobiol. Dis. **3:** 339–355.
25. RIEGER, R., F. EDENHOFER, C.I. LASMEZAS & S. WEISS. 1997. The human 37-kDa laminin receptor precursor interacts with the prion protein in eukaryotic cells. Nat. Med. **3:** 1383–1388.
26. RIEGER, R., C.I. LASMEZAS & S. WEISS. 1999. Role of the 37 kDa laminin receptor precursor in the life cycle of prions. Transfus. Clin. Biol. **6:** 7–16.
27. MARTINS, V.R., E. GRANER, J. GARCIA-ABREU *et al.* 1997. Complementary hydropathy identifies a cellular prion protein receptor. Nat. Med. **3:** 1376–1382.
28. KURSCHNER, C., J.I. MORGAN, F. YEHIELY *et al.* 1995. The cellular prion protein (PrP) selectively binds to Bcl-2 in the yeast two-hybrid system: identification of candidate proteins binding to prion protein. Brain Res. Mol. Brain Res. **30:** 165–168.
29. BÜELER, H.R., M. FISCHER, Y. LANG *et al.* 1992. Normal development and behaviour of mice lacking the neuronal cell-surface PrP protein. Nature **356:** 577–582.
30. MANSON, J.C., A.R. CLARKE, M.L. HOOPER, L. AITCHISON, I. MCCONNELL & J. HOPE. 1994. 129/Ola mice carrying a null mutation in PrP that abolishes mRNA production are developmentally normal. Mol. Neurobiol. **8:** 121–127.
31. SAKAGUCHI, S., S. KATAMINE, K. SHIGEMATSU *et al.* Accumulation of proteinase K-resistant prion protein (PrP) is restricted by the expression level of normal PrP in mice inoculated with a mouse-adapted strain of the Creutzfeldt-Jakob disease agent. J. Virol. **69:** 7586–7592.
32. BASLER, K., B. OESCH, M. SCOTT *et al.* 1986. Scrapie and cellular PrP isoforms are encoded by the same chromosomal gene. Cell **46:** 417–428.
33. COLLINGE, J., M.A. WHITTINGTON, K.C. SIDLE *et al.* 1994. Prion protein is necessary for normal synaptic function. Nature **370:** 295–297.
34. TOBLER, I., S.E. GAUS, T. DEBOER *et al.* 1996. Altered circadian activity rhythms and sleep in mice devoid of prion protein. Nature **380:** 639–642.

35. SAKAGUCHI, S., S. KATAMINE, N. NISHIDA *et al.* 1996. Loss of cerebellar Purkinje cells in aged mice homozygous for a disrupted PrP gene. Nature **380:** 528–531.
36. FISCHER, M., T. RÜLICKE, A. RAEBER *et al.* 1996. Prion protein (PrP) with amino-proximal deletions restoring susceptibility of PrP knockout mice to scrapie. EMBO J. **15:** 1255–1264.
37. NISHIDA, N., P. TREMBLAY, T. SUGIMOTO *et al.* 1999. A mouse prion protein transgene rescues mice deficient for the prion protein gene from Purkinje cell degeneration and demyelination. Lab. Invest. **79:** 689–697.
38. MOORE, R.C., I.Y. LEE, G.L. SILVERMAN *et al.* 1999. Ataxia in prion protein (PrP)-deficient mice is associated with upregulation of the novel PrP-like protein doppel. J. Mol. Biol. **292:** 797–817.
39. WEISSMANN, C. & A. AGUZZI. 1999. Perspectives: neurobiology. PrP's double causes trouble. Science **286:** 914–915.
40. BÜELER, H.R., A. AGUZZI, A. SAILER *et al.* 1993. Mice devoid of PrP are resistant to scrapie. Cell **73:** 1339–1347.
41. MANSON, J.C., A.R. CLARKE, P.A. MCBRIDE, I. MCCONNELL & J. HOPE. 1994. PrP gene dosage determines the timing but not the final intensity or distribution of lesions in scrapie pathology. Neurodegeneration **3:** 331–340.
42. BÜELER, H., A. RAEBER, A. SAILER, M. FISCHER, A. AGUZZI & C. WEISSMANN. 1994. High prion and PrPSc levels but delayed onset of disease in scrapie-inoculated mice heterozygous for a disrupted PrP gene. Mol. Med. **1:** 19–30.
43. HOPE, J., G. MULTHAUP, L.J. REEKIE, R.H. KIMBERLIN & K. BEYREUTHER. 1988. Molecular pathology of scrapie-associated fibril protein (PrP) in mouse brain affected by the ME7 strain of scrapie. Eur. J. Biochem. **172:** 271–277.
44. ROGERS, M., F. YEHIELY, M. SCOTT & S.B. PRUSINER. 1993. Conversion of truncated and elongated prion proteins into the scrapie isoform in cultured cells. Proc. Natl. Acad. Sci. USA **90:** 3182–3186.
45. SHMERLING, D., I. HEGYI, M. FISCHER *et al.* 1998. Expression of amino-terminally truncated PrP in the mouse leading to ataxia and specific cerebellar lesions. Cell **93:** 203–214.
46. GOLDFARB, L.G., P. BROWN, W.R. MCCOMBIE *et al.* 1991. Transmissible familial Creutzfeldt-Jakob disease associated with five, seven, and eight extra octapeptide coding repeats in the PRNP gene. Proc. Natl. Acad. Sci. USA **88:** 10926–10930.
47. CHIESA, R., P. PICCARDO, B. GHETTI & D.A. HARRIS. 1998. Neurological illness in transgenic mice expressing a prion protein with an insertional mutation. Neuron **21:** 1339–1351.
48. RIEK, R., S. HORNEMANN, G. WIDER, R. GLOCKSHUBER & K. WÜTHRICH. 1997. NMR characterization of the full-length recombinant murine prion protein, mPrP(23–231). FEBS Lett. **413:** 282–288.
49. DONNE, D.G., J.H. VILES, D. GROTH *et al.* 1997. Structure of the recombinant full-length hamster prion protein PrP(29– 231): the N terminus is highly flexible. Proc. Natl. Acad. Sci. USA **94:** 13452–13457.
50. SCHATZL, H.M., M. DA COSTA, L. TAYLOR, F.E. COHEN & S.B. PRUSINER. 1995. Prion protein gene variation among primates. J. Mol. Biol. **245:** 362–374.
51. PERETZ, D., R.A. WILLIAMSON, Y. MATSUNAGA *et al.* 1997. A conformational transition at the N terminus of the prion protein features in formation of the scrapie isoform. J. Mol. Biol. **273:** 614–622.
52. MURAMOTO, T., S.J. DEARMOND, M. SCOTT, G.C. TELLING, F.E. COHEN & S.B. PRUSINER. 1997. Heritable disorder resembling neuronal storage disease in mice expressing prion protein with deletion of an alpha-helix. Nat. Med. **3:** 750–755.
53. DEARMOND, S.J., H. SANCHEZ, F. YEHIELY *et al.* 1997. Selective neuronal targeting in prion disease. Neuron **19:** 1337–1348.
54. FORLONI, G., N. ANGERETTI, R. CHIESA *et al.* 1993. Neurotoxicity of a prion protein fragment. Nature **362:** 543–546.
55. ISENMANN, S., S. BRANDNER, U. SURE & A. AGUZZI. 1996. Telencephalic transplants in mice: characterization of growth and differentiation patterns. Neuropathol. Appl. Neurobiol. **21:** 108–117.

56. ISENMANN, S., S. BRANDNER, G. KUHNE, J. BONER & A. AGUZZI. 1996. Comparative *in vivo* and pathological analysis of the blood-brain barrier in mouse telencephalic transplants. Neuropathol. Appl. Neurobiol. **22:** 118–128.
57. ISENMANN, S., S. BRANDNER & A. AGUZZI. 1996. Neuroectodermal grafting: a new tool for the study of neurodegenerative diseases. Histol. Histopathol. **11:** 1063–1073.
58. BRANDNER, S., S. ISENMANN, A. RAEBER *et al.* 1996. Normal host prion protein necessary for scrapie-induced neurotoxicity. Nature **379:** 339–343.
59. AGUZZI, A. 1998. Grafting mouse brains: from neurocarcinogenesis to neurodegeneration. EMBO J. **17:** 6107–6114.
60. BRANDNER, S., S. ISENMANN, G. KUHNE & A. AGUZZI. 1998. Identification of the end stage of scrapie using infected neural grafts. Brain Pathol. **8:** 19–27.
61. CHUNG, Y.L., A. WILLIAMS, J.S. BEECH *et al.* 1995. MRI assessment of the blood-brain barrier in a hamster model of scrapie. Neurodegeneration **4:** 203–207.
62. KIMBERLIN, R.H. & J.W. WILESMITH. 1994. Bovine spongiform encephalopathy: epidemiology, low dose exposure and risks. Ann. N.Y. Acad. Sci. **724:** 210–220.
63. WELLS, G.A., A.C. SCOTT, C.T. JOHNSON *et al.* 1987. A novel progressive spongiform encephalopathy in cattle. Vet. Rec. **121:** 419–420.
64. KIMBERLIN, R.H. & C.A. WALKER. 1978. Pathogenesis of mouse scrapie: effect of route of inoculation on infectivity titres and dose-response curves. J. Comp. Pathol. **88:** 39–47.
65. SCOTT, J.R., J.D. FOSTER & H. FRASER. 1993. Conjunctival instillation of scrapie in mice can produce disease. Vet. Microbiol. **34:** 305–309.
66. DUFFY, P., J. WOLF, G. COLLINS, A.G. DEVOE, B. STREETEN & D. COWEN. 1974. Possible person-to-person transmission of Creutzfeldt-Jakob disease. N. Engl. J. Med. **290:** 692–693.
67. FRASER, H. 1982. Neuronal spread of scrapie agent and targeting of lesions within the retino-tectal pathway. Nature **295:** 149–150.
68. SAILER, A., H. BÜELER, M. FISCHER, A. AGUZZI & C. WEISSMANN. 1994. No propagation of prions in mice devoid of PrP. Cell **77:** 967–968.
69. BRANDNER, S., A. RAEBER, A. SAILER *et al.* 1996. Normal host prion protein (PrP^c) is required for scrapie spread within the central nervous system. Proc. Natl. Acad. Sci. USA **93:** 13148–13151.
70. PRUSINER, S.B., D. GROTH, A. SERBAN *et al.* 1993. Ablation of the prion protein (PrP) gene in mice prevents scrapie and facilitates production of anti-PrP antibodies. Proc. Natl. Acad. Sci. USA **90:** 10608–10612.
71. RAEBER, A.J., A. SAILER, I. HEGYI *et al.* 1999. Ectopic expression of prion protein (PrP) in T lymphocytes or hepatocytes of PrP knockout mice is insufficient to sustain prion replication. Proc. Natl. Acad. Sci. USA **96:** 3987–3992.
72. FOURNIER, J.G., F. ESCAIG HAYE, T. BILLETTE DE VILLEMEUR & O. ROBAIN. 1995. Ultrastructural localization of cellular prion protein (PrP^c) in synaptic boutons of normal hamster hippocampus. C.R. Acad. Sci. III **318:** 339–344.
73. WHITTINGTON, M.A., K.C. SIDLE, I. GOWLAND *et al.* 1995. Rescue of neurophysiological phenotype seen in PrP null mice by transgene encoding human prion protein. Nat. Genet. **9:** 197–201.
74. AGUZZI, A. 1997. Neuro-immune connection in spread of prions in the body? Lancet **349:** 742–743.
75. EKLUND, C.M., R.C. KENNEDY & W.J. HADLOW. 1967. Pathogenesis of scrapie virus infection in the mouse. J. Infect. Dis. **117:** 15–22.
76. KIMBERLIN, R.H. & C.A. WALKER. 1989. Pathogenesis of scrapie in mice after intragastric infection. Virus Res. **12:** 213–220.
77. HILL, A.F., M. ZEIDLER, J. IRONSIDE & J. COLLINGE. 1997. Diagnosis of new variant Creutzfeldt-Jakob disease by tonsil biopsy. Lancet **349:** 99.
78. FRASER, H. & C.F. FARQUHAR. 1987. Ionising radiation has no influence on scrapie incubation period in mice. Vet. Microbiol. **13:** 211–223.
79. KITAMOTO, T., T. MURAMOTO, S. MOHRI, K. DOH URA & J. TATEISHI. 1991. Abnormal isoform of prion protein accumulates in follicular dendritic cells in mice with Creutzfeldt-Jakob disease. J. Virol. **65:** 6292–6295.

80. MURAMOTO, T., T. KITAMOTO, M.Z. HOQUE, J. TATEISHI & I. GOTO. 1993. Species barrier prevents an abnormal isoform of prion protein from accumulating in follicular dendritic cells of mice with Creutzfeldt-Jakob disease. J. Virol. **67:** 6808–6810.
81. LASMEZAS, C.I., J.Y. CESBRON, J.P. DESLYS *et al.* 1996. Immune system-dependent and -independent replication of the scrapie agent. J. Virol. **70:** 1292–1295.
82. KLEIN, M.A., R. FRIGG, E. FLECHSIG & A. AGUZZI. 1997. A crucial role for B cells in neuroinvasive scrapie. Nature **390:** 687–690.
83. FRIGG, R., M.A. KLEIN, I. HEGYI, R.M. ZINKERNAGEL & A. AGUZZI. 1999. Scrapie pathogenesis in subclinically infected B-cell-deficient mice. J. Virol. **73:** 9584–9588.
84. KIMBERLIN, R.H. & C.A. WALKER. 1989 The role of the spleen in the neuroinvasion of scrapie in mice. Virus Res. **12:** 201–211.
85. GROSCHUP, M.H., F. WEILAND, O.C. STRAUB & E. PFAFF. 1996. Detection of scrapie agent in the peripheral nervous system of a diseased sheep. Neurobiol. Dis. **3:** 191–195.
86. KIMBERLIN, R.H., S.M. HALL & C.A. WALKER. 1983. Pathogenesis of mouse scrapie: evidence for direct neural spread of infection to the CNS after injection of sciatic nerve. J. Neurol. Sci. **61:** 315–325.
87. KIMBERLIN, R.H. & C.A. WALKER. 1986. Pathogenesis of scrapie (strain 263K) in hamsters infected intracerebrally, intraperitoneally or intraocularly. J. Gen. Virol. **67:** 255–263.
88. KIMBERLIN, R.H. & C.A. WALKER. 1980. Pathogenesis of mouse scrapie: evidence for neural spread of infection to the CNS. J. Gen. Virol. **51:** 183–187.
89. BLÄTTLER, T., S. BRANDNER, A.J. RAEBER *et al.* 1997. PrP-expressing tissue required for transfer of scrapie infectivity from spleen to brain. Nature **389:** 69–73.
90. BEEKES, M., E. BALDAUF & H. DIRINGER. 1996. Sequential appearance and accumulation of pathognomonic markers in the central nervous system of hamsters orally infected with scrapie. J. Gen. Virol. **77:** 1925–1934.
91. KLEIN, M.A., R. FRIGG, A.J. RAEBER *et al.* 1998. PrP expression in B lymphocytes is not required for prion neuroinvasion. Nat. Med. **4:** 1429–1433.
92. RAEBER, A.J., M.A. KLEIN, R. FRIGG, E. FLECHSIG, A. AGUZZI & C. WEISSMANN. 1999. PrP-dependent association of prions with splenic but not circulating lymphocytes of scrapie-infected mice. EMBO J. **18:** 2702–2706.
93. STRAUB, R.H., J. WESTERMANN, J. SCHOLMERICH & W. FALK. 1998. Dialogue between the CNS and the immune system in lymphoid organs. Immunol. Today **19:** 409–413.

Presenilin Function in APP Processing

WIM ANNAERT,[a] PHILIPPE CUPERS,[a] PAUL SAFTIG,[b]
AND BART DE STROOPER[a,c]

[a]Center for Human Genetics, Flanders Interuniversitary Institute for Biotechnology,
Gasthuisberg, KULeuven, Leuven, Belgium

[b]Zentrum Biochemie und Molekulare Zellbiologie, Biochemie II, Universität Göttingen,
Göttingen,Germany

ABSTRACT: Familial Alzheimer's disease (FAD) is now linked to at least three
genes encoding the amyloid precursor protein (APP) on chromosome 21, and
presenilin 1 and 2 on chromosome 14 and 1, respectively. FAD cases in whom presenilin mutations occur are more frequent than those with APP mutations.
However, altogether they only account for approximately 0.1% of all the people
suffering from Alzheimer's disease (AD),[1] and the causes of the remaining
99.9% of the sporadic form of AD or senile dementia remain unknown. Since
FAD presents with the same neuropathological features as sporadic AD, i.e.,
cognitive impairments and the amyloid plaques and tangles in the brain, our
working hypothesis is that similar molecular pathogenic mechanisms underly
both sporadic and familial AD. It follows that APP and the presenilins must be
key players in the disease. Detailed knowledge about the cell biology of these
proteins will be a rich source of insight into the pathology of AD, but will also
shed light on the fundamental neurobiology of these proteins.

WHAT THE PRESENILINS AND APP
HAVE TAUGHT US UNTIL NOW

APP is a type I transmembrane protein that becomes proteolytically cleaved by
different enzymes called secretases (reviewed in Ref. 2). Subsequent cleavage of the
ectodomain by β-secretase followed by intramembranous γ-secretase clipping generates amyloid peptides of 40 and 42 residues. It is the latter peptide $A\beta_{1-42}$ that
precipitates preferentially in amyloid plaques of Alzheimer's patients. Alternatively,
α-secretase cleaves the protein in the middle of the amyloid peptide region thereby
preventing the production of the neurotoxic peptide. It is becoming clear that these
three secretases act consecutively or even competitively, ultimately resulting in the
proteolytic breakdown of the precursor molecule through the nonamyloidogenic or
amyloidogenic pathway. The balance between both pathways is of pivotal importance in the pathogenesis of the disease. For instance in the inherited familial forms
of the disease, all clinical mutations manifestly flank the cleavage sites of APP, and
they all result in higher Aβ or more specifically $A\beta_{1-42}$ production, thereby disrupt-

[c]Address for correspondence: Bart De Strooper, M.D., Ph.D., Neuronal Cell Biology and
Gene Transfer Laboratory, Center for Human Genetics, Flanders Interuniversity Institute for
Biotechnology, Gasthuisberg, KULeuven, Herestraat 49, B-3000 Leuven, Belgium. Tel.: +32-16-
346227; fax: +32-16-347181.
e-mail: Bart.Destrooper@med.kuleuven.ac.be

ing this sensitive balance. Now that APP and the presenilins are identified, the field is focussing on the next "missing link" in the pathology, i.e., the identification of the different secretases that process APP and may be controlled by the presenilins.

α-secretase cleavage occurs at or nearby the cell surface.[3–5] Since the cleavage site is heterogeneous in nature,[6,7] it follows that probably a set of related proteases are responsible for α-secretase processing. Indeed, the protein kinase C-dependent α-cleavage of APP has been attributed to TACE,[8] while ADAM-10 and MDC9, other members of the same family of metalloproteases, are likely to perform both the regulated and constitutive cleavage of APP.[9,10] Interestingly, ADAM10 is the mammalian homologue of Kuzbanian (Kuz), a protein implied in the cleavage of Notch extracellular domain and hence Notch signaling.[11]

The β-secretase activity generates the direct substrate for the final γ-secretase cleavage, and most probably resides in the Golgi apparatus and subsequent compartments of the secretory pathway (see, for instance, Refs. 12,13). This amyloidogenic pathway is more prominently present in neuronal cultures[14] as opposed to the α-secretase pathway. Very recently, four different laboratories identified almost simultaneously the β-secretase.[15–18] BACE (β-site APP-cleaving enzyme) is a type I transmembrane protein that is, as expected, more highly expressed in brain areas and neuronal cell lines and indeed localizes to the Golgi and post-Golgi compartments.[15] The identification of a second homologue, BACE 2,[19] adds to the complexity, and further study is needed to know whether BACE 2 also contributes to the β-secretase activity. The story becomes even more complicated for γ-secretase. Cleavage by this secretase results in the generation of amyloid peptides of mainly 40 and 42 amino acid residues. The $A\beta_{1-40}$ is generally believed to be generated in the endocytic pathway while the $A\beta_{1-42}$ production site is probably in the ER, i.e., very early in the biosynthetic pathway. This implies at least two different γ-secretase activities at different locations in the cell (reviewed in Ref. 2). As β-secretase cleavage of APP precedes γ-secretase action, this implies that β-cleaved APP fragments should be transported retrogradely to reach the γ_{42} compartment. γ-secretase activity requires presenilins, and therefore they have been proposed to be identical to this enzyme (see below). Presenilin 1 and 2 are hydrophobic proteins that most likely traverse the membrane eight times. In this topology both the amino- and carboxy-terminal end and also the hydrophilic loop domain between transmembrane region six and seven are facing the cytoplasm, and are prime targets for interacting proteins.[20–23] The presenilins themselves are also proteolytically cleaved by an unknown protease called "presenilase," probably very shortly after their biosynthesis and translocation in the rough endoplasmic reticulum (ER). The resulting fragments, termed presenilin N- and C-terminal fragments, stay together as a functional heterodimer throughout their life span.[24] Clinical mutations in presenilins are scattered throughout the protein sequence, but give all rise to increased secretion of the same neurotoxic $A\beta_{1-42}$,[25–28] thereby linking presenilin function to APP processing (reviewed in Ref. 29). Last year we were able to demonstrate that presenilin 1 is critically involved in the γ_{40}- *and* γ_{42}-secretase processing. This conclusion was based on data obtained in presenilin 1 knockout mice, in whom we could demonstrate a dramatic drop in the secretion of both amyloid peptides and accumulation of β-secretase cleaved fragments.[30] A similar "knock-out" of amyloid production can be obtained when either of the aspartate residues in transmembrane region 6 or 7 of PS1 are mutated.[31] These findings tempted scientists to suggest that presenilin 1 is itself γ-secretase and a member of a new family of aspartyl proteases. There are at least two important arguments against such a hypothesis. First, no evidence is yet available that presenilins have proteolytic activity and second, there is the problem of the spatial paradox.[32] Indeed, if presenilin 1 is γ-secretase, then the enzyme (presenilin 1) should meet its substrate (β-secretase cleaved APP fragments) in the same compartment. The subcellular localization of presenilin is precisely an important matter of debate.

Many studies have used presenilin 1 overexpression, but this leads to artifacts and mislocalization of the protein in so-called "aggresomes."[33] Therefore it was important to look at the endogenous levels of presenilin 1, and preferably in cells relevant to AD, namely, neurons. Using confocal laser scanning microscopy on hippocampal neurons and subcellular fractionation experiments on brain, we could demonstrate that presenilin 1 is present in the early compartments of the secretory pathway, including the endoplasmic reticulum, the intermediate compartment and the *cis*-Golgi cisternae.[34] A clear diffusion barrier exists beyond the *cis*-Golgi as we do not detect presenilin 1 in later compartments of the secretory pathway such as lysosomes and clathrin coated vesicles. Moreover, additional functional data using the Semliki Forest Virus system to express APP in hippocampal neurons are consistent with $A\beta_{1-42}$ being mainly produced in the endoplasmic reticulum. However, these data are not easily reconciled with the $A\beta_{1-40}$ generation in the late secretory pathways. This is what we called the spatial paradox.[32] We propose therefore alternative interpretations for the "presenilin is γ-secretase" hypothesis, suggesting the possibility that presenilin 1 functions for instance by chaperoning APP to microenvironments where γ-secretases reside.

Apart from the weak homology with the *C. elegans* protein SPE-4, there is limited evidence that presenilins are mediators of protein transport. Recently, disease-causing mutations in PS1 were shown to affect the intracellular trafficking of β-catenin,[35] while weak changes were noticed in the phosphorylation and glycosylation status of TrKB in PS1 knock-out cells.[36] In this respect it is noteworthy that we and others[30,37,38] have mentioned the similarities between the processing of APP and SREBP.[39] SREBP also undergoes two cleavages, and the first cleavage by S1P is activated by SCAP, a membrane protein that structurally resembles presenilin. In the case of this SCAP-mediated SREBP-cleavage by S1P, it was now observed that a transport of the SCAP-SREBP complex to the medial-Golgi in a sterol-regulated fashion is required in order to get normal cleavage of SREBP.[40] After SREBP cleavage, SCAP returns to the ER to pick up another SREBP. On the basis of its subcellular localization it is now tempting to suggest that presenilin functions as a transport or sorting chaperone. The inhibition of γ-secretase mediated cleavage of APP can be explained as the inability of APP to reach the proper compartment or even microenvironment where the putative enzyme resides. The alternative hypothesis that presenilin is γ-secretase remains, however, likely as well.

EMERGING THERAPEUTIC STRATEGIES

Detailed molecular and cell biological studies of the disease-linked gene products has established a firm base in helping to identify specific therapeutic targets and will aid in understanding gradually the complex cascade of events ultimately resulting in AD. The general idea is to maintain the amyloid levels in the brain of AD patients below a critical level to prevent onset or progression of amyloid plaque formation. The newly identified candidate secretases and presenilins are probably the long-searched for pharmacological targets for drug development which aims at controlling the rate limiting steps in amyloid peptide generation.[41] Their precise function in the processing of APP or other yet unidentified substrates need urgently to be explored by molecular and cell biologists.

Despite the fact that the identity of γ-secretase remains a matter of debate, the recent intensive labor on presenilins by many groups clearly indicates that modulating presenilin 1 function could be an aim for the development of therapy. In this regard, one should also consider the potential side effects of such an approach and, for instance, take into account the lethal phenotype of presenilin 1 knockout mice.[42,43] In addition, presenilin 1 knockout embryos present with a neuronal migration disorder that looks very similar to the human disorder Lissencephaly Type II, indicating that presenilin 1 probably fulfills several important physiological functions during embryogenesis and development of different tissues including brain.[44] A clue to the molecular nature of these pathways came from the generation of double knockout mice.[45,46] When presenilin 2, the homologue of presenilin 1, was deleted in mice, no effects on viability or fertility were observed, suggesting that presenilin 1 can compensate for the loss of function of presenilin 2. Also, it is clear from the *in vivo* data that presenilin 1 is essential and presenilin 2 redundant for normal Notch signaling.[45,46] Notch-1 is a member of a family of large type 1 integral membrane proteins involved in complex cell fate decisions during development.[47] During its maturation, Notch-1 is proteolytically cleaved and presents as a heterodimeric receptor on the plasma membrane.[48] After ligand binding by members of the Delta-Serrate-LAG2 (DSL) family, its cytoplasmic domain becomes released by a next proteolytic cleavage step in or close to the transmembrane domain.[49] The cytoplasmic domain is a signaling factor which is transported in complex with members of the CSL (CBF1, Su(H), Lag-1) family of DNA binding proteins to the nucleus. As a consequence, genes involved in myogenesis, neuronal differentiation, and hematopoiesis are under the control of Notch.[47] Interestingly, complete deletion of both presenilin 1 and 2 genes enhanced considerably the lethal phenotype of presenilin 1 deficiency and resulted in a phenotype closely resembling that of mice deficient in Notch-1. A molecular explanation for this interference was recently provided.[37] Like APP, Notch is also proteolytically processed at an intramembranous site. Cleavage at that site, which is essential for the release of the Notch intracellular domain and the consecutive signaling to the nucleus,[49] is again dependent on presenilin 1.[37] Abolishment of cleavage in presenilin-1-deficient mice therefore interferes with the ligand-induced signaling of Notch, leading to the conclusion that presenilin 1 is a molecular switch between proteolysis and signal transduction.[32]

Our findings boil down to the point that we cannot just abolish presenilin function for the treatment of AD. Apart from its key role in embryogenesis, Notch and the Notch signaling pathway is likely to be important also in adulthood. For instance, inhibition of Notch signaling may also cause immunodeficiency and anemia because of Notch-1's role in hematopoiesis.[50] More recently, Notch-1 was demonstrated to function in postmitotic neurons of the mature mammalian CNS as it inhibits neurite outgrowth.[51] This inhibition correlates with cell to cell contact mediated Notch activation implying a role for Notch signaling in neuronal growth and maturation.[52] Furthermore, this neuritic extension becomes severely attenuated in presenilin-1-deficient neurons indicating a functional interaction between presenilin 1 and Notch-1.[53] Altogether, it is expected that complete inactivation of presenilins as a therapeutic goal in AD is unrealistic. However, such a drastic approach is probably not at all indicated. A partial inhibition of presenilin function may be already sufficient to reduce Aβ production to a level that does not drive amyloid plaques formation anymore, while maintaining high enough levels of Notch intramembranous cleavage to limit physiological consequences to an acceptable minimum. In this respect, our observations that mice bearing only one functional presenilin 1 allele (PS1$^{+/-}$PS2$^{-/-}$) develop normally and remain healthy,[45] indicate that a partial inhibition of presenilin function can be maintained without major side effects and that a therapeutic window for interference with presenilin function does exist. Without doubt, the recent identification and characterization of the secretases broadens significantly the spectrum of available drug targets for AD. The development of specific inhibitors is now a major goal of many drug companies. We at our side will provide screening assays, and use the resulting candidate drugs in our cell biological studies aimed at further understanding and elucidating the biological roles of this intriguing set of proteins.

REFERENCES

1. KIM, T.W. & R.E. TANZI. 1997. Presenilins and Alzheimer's disease. Curr. Opin. Neurobiol. **7:** 683–688.
2. SELKOE, D.J. 1998. The cell biology of beta-amyloid precursor protein and presenilin in Alzheimer's disease. Trends Cell. Biol. **8:** 447–453.
3. SISODIA, S.S. 1992. Beta-amyloid precursor protein cleavage by a membrane-bound protease. Proc. Natl. Acad. Sci. USA **89:** 6075–6079.
4. DE STROOPER, B., L. UMANS, F. VAN LEUVEN & H. VAN DEN BERGHE. 1993. Study of the synthesis and secretion of normal and artificial mutants of murine amyloid precursor protein (APP): cleavage of APP occurs in a late compartment of the default secretion pathway. J. Cell Biol. **121:** 295–304.
5. PARVATHY, S., I. HUSSAIN, E.H. KARRAN, A.J. TURNER & N.M. HOOPER. 1999. Cleavage of Alzheimer's amyloid precursor protein by alpha-secretase occurs at the surface of neuronal cells. Biochemistry **38:** 9728–9734.
6. ZHONG, Z., J. HIGAKI, K. MURAKAMI *et al.* 1994. Secretion of beta-amyloid precursor protein involves multiple cleavage sites. J. Biol. Chem. **269:** 627–632.
7. SIMONS, M., B. DE STROOPER, G. MULTHAUP, P.J. TIENARI, C.G. DOTTI & K. BEYREUTER. 1996. Amyloidogenic processing of the human amyloid precursor protein in primary cultures of rat hippocampal neurons. J. Neurosci. **16:** 899–908.
8. BUXBAUM, J.D., K.N. LIU, Y. LUO *et al.* 1998. Evidence that tumor necrosis factor alpha converting enzyme is involved in regulated alpha-secretase cleavage of the Alzheimer amyloid protein precursor. J. Biol. Chem. **273:** 27765–27767.
9. LAMMICH, S., E. KOJRO, R. POSTINA *et al.* 1999. Constitutive and regulated alpha-secretase cleavage of Alzheimer's amyloid precursor protein by a disintegrin metalloprotease. Proc. Natl. Acad. Sci. USA **96:** 3922–3927.
10. KOIKE, H., S. TOMIOKA, H. SORIMACHI *et al.* 1999. Membrane-anchored metalloprotease MDC9 has an alpha-secretase activity responsible for processing the amyloid precursor protein. Biochem. J. **343**(Pt 2): 371–375.

11. PAN, D. & G.M. RUBIN. 1997. Kuzbanian controls proteolytic processing of Notch and mediates lateral inhibition during *Drosophila* and vertebrate neurogenesis. Cell **90:** 271–280.
12. KOO, E.H. & S.L. SQUAZZO. 1994. Evidence that production and release of amyloid beta-protein involves the endocytic pathway. J. Biol. Chem. **269:** 17386–17389.
13. HAASS, C., C.A. LEMERE, A. CAPELL *et al.* 1995. The Swedish mutation causes early-onset Alzheimer's disease by beta-secretase cleavage within the secretory pathway. Nat. Med. **1:** 1291–1296.
14. ZHAO, J., L. PAGANINI, L. MUCKE *et al.* 1996. Beta-secretase processing of the beta-amyloid precursor protein in transgenic mice is efficient in neurons but inefficient in astrocytes. J. Biol. Chem. **271:** 31407–31411.
15. VASSAR, R., B.D. BENNETT, S. BABU-KHAN *et al.* 1999. Beta-secretase cleavage of Alzheimer's amyloid precursor protein by the transmembrane aspartic protease BACE. Science **286:** 735–741.
16. HUSSAIN, I., D. POWELL, D.R. HOWLETT *et al.* 1999. Identification of a novel aspartic protease (Asp 2) as beta-secretase. Mol. Cell. Neurosci. **14:** 419–427.
17. YAN, R., M.J. BIENKOWSKI, M.E. SHUCK *et al.* 1999. Membrane-anchored aspartyl protease with Alzheimer's disease. Nature **402:** 533–537.
18. SINHA, S., J.P. ANDERSON, R. BARBOUR *et al.* 1999. Purification and cloning of amyloid precursor protein beta-secretase from human brain. Nature **402:** 537–540.
19. SAUNDERS, A.J. *et al.* 1999. BACE maps to chromosome 11 and a BACE homolog, BACE2, reside in the obligate down syndrome region of chromosome 21. Science **286:** 1255a.
20. DOAN, A., G. THINAKARAN, D.R. BORCHELT *et al.* 1996. Protein topology of presenilin 1. Neuron **17:** 1023–1030.
21. LI, X. & I. GREENWALD. 1996. Membrane topology of the *C. elegans* SEL-12 presenilin. Neuron **17:** 1015–1021.
22. DE STROOPER, B., M. BEULLENS, M.B. CONTRERAS *et al.* 1997. Phosphorylation, subcellular localization, and membrane orientation of the Alzheimer's disease-associated presenilins. J. Biol. Chem. **272:** 3590–3598.
23. LI, X. & I. GREENWALD. 1998. Additional evidence for an eight-transmembrane-domain topology for *Caenorhabditis elegans* and human presenilins. Proc. Natl. Acad. Sci. USA **95:** 7109–7114.
24. CAPELL, A., J. GRUNBERG, B. PESOLD *et al.* 1998. The proteolytic fragments of the Alzheimer's disease-associated presenilin-1 form heterodimers and occur as a 100–150-kDa molecular mass complex. J. Biol. Chem. **273:** 3205–3211.
25. BORCHELT, D.R., G. THINAKARAN, C.B. ECKMAN *et al.* 1996. Familial Alzheimer's disease-linked presenilin 1 variants elevate abeta1–42/1–40 ratio *in vitro* and *in vivo*. Neuron **17:** 1005–1013.
26. DUFF, K., C. ECKMAN, C. ZEHR *et al.* 1996. Increased amyloid-beta42(43) in brains of mice expressing mutant presenilin 1. Nature **383:** 710–713.
27. SCHEUNER, D., C. ECKMAN, M. JENSEN *et al.* 1996. Secreted amyloid beta-protein similar to that in the senile plaques of Alzheimer's disease is increased *in vivo* by the presenilin 1 and 2 and APP mutations linked to familial Alzheimer's disease. Nat. Med. **2:** 864–870.
28. CITRON, M., D. WESTAWAY, W. XIA *et al.* 1997. Mutant presenilins of Alzheimer's disease increase production of 42-residue amyloid beta-protein in both transfected cells and transgenic mice. Nat. Med. **3:** 67–72.
29. HAASS, C. & B. DE STROOPER. 1999. The presenilins in Alzheimer's disease—proteolysis holds the key. Science **286:** 916–919.
30. DE STROOPER, B., P. SAFTIG, K. CRAESSAERTS *et al.* 1998. Deficiency of presenilin-1 inhibits the normal cleavage of amyloid precursor protein. Nature **391:** 387–390.
31. WOLFE, M.S., W. XIA, B.L. OSTASZEWSKI *et al.* 1999. Two transmembrane aspartates in presenilin-1 required for presenilin endoproteolysis and gamma-secretase activity. Nature **398:** 513–517.
32. ANNAERT, W. & B. DE STROOPER. 1999. Presenilins: molecular switches between proteolysis and signal transduction. Trends Neurosci. **22:** 439–443.

33. JOHNSTON, J.A., C.L. WARD & R.R. KOPITO. 1998. Aggresomes: a cellular response to misfolded proteins. J. Cell Biol. **143:** 1883–1898.
34. ANNAERT, W.G., L. LEVESQUE, K. CRAESSAERTS et al. 1999. Presenilin 1 controls gamma-secretase processing of the amyloid precursor protein in pre-Golgi compartments of hippocampal neurons. J. Cell Biol. **147:** 277–294.
35. NISHIMURA, M., G. YU, G. LEVESQUE et al. 1999. Presenilin mutations associated with Alzheimer disease cause defective intracellular trafficking of beta-catenin, a component of the presenilin protein complex. Nat. Med. **5:** 164–169.
36. NARUSE, S., G. THINAKARAN, J.J. LUO et al. 1998. Effects of PS1 deficiency on membrane protein trafficking in neurons. Neuron **21:** 1213–1221.
37. DE STROOPER, B., W. ANNAERT, P. CUPERS et al. 1999. A presenilin-1-dependent gamma-secretase-like protease mediates release of Notch intracellular domain. Nature **398:** 518–522.
38. CHAN, Y.M. & Y.N. JAN. 1998. Roles for proteolysis and trafficking in notch maturation and signal transduction. Cell **94:** 423–426.
39. BROWN, M.S. & J.L. GOLDSTEIN. 1997. The SREBP pathway: regulation of cholesterol metabolism by proteolysis of a membrane-bound transcription factor. Cell **89:** 331–340.
40. NOHTURFFT, A., R.A. DEBOSE-BOYD, S. SCHEEK, J.L. GOLDSTEIN & M.S. BROWN. 1999. Sterols regulate cycling of SREBP cleavage-activating protein (SCAP) between endoplasmic reticulum and Golgi. Proc. Natl. Acad. Sci. USA **96:** 11235–11240.
41. CUPERS, P., W.G. ANNAERT & B. DE STROOPER. 1999. The presenilins as potential drug targets in Alzheimer's disease. Emerg. Ther. Targets **3:** 413–422.
42. SHEN, J., R.T. BRONSON, D.F. CHEN, W. XIA, D.J. SELKOE & S. TONEGAWA. 1997. Skeletal and CNS defects in presenilin-1-deficient mice. Cell **89:** 629–639.
43. WONG, P.C., H. ZHENG, H. CHEN et al. 1997. Presenilin 1 is required for Notch1 and DII1 expression in the paraxial mesoderm. Nature **387:** 288–292.
44. HARTMANN, D., B.D. STROOPER & P. SAFTIG. 1999. Presenilin-1 deficiency leads to loss of Cajal-Retzius neurons and cortical dysplasia similar to human type 2 lissencephaly. Curr. Biol. **9:** 719–727.
45. HERREMAN, A., D. HARTMANN, W. ANNAERT et al. 1999. Presenilin 2 deficiency causes a mild pulmonary phenotype and no changes in amyloid precursor protein processing but enhances the embryonic lethal phenotype of presenilin 1 deficiency. Proc. Natl. Acad. Sci. USA **96:** 11872–11877.
46. DONOVIEL, D.B., A.K. HADJANTONAKIS, M. IKEDA, H. ZHENG, P.S. HYSLOP & A. BERNSTEIN. 1999. Mice lacking both presenilin genes exhibit early embryonic patterning defects. Genes Dev. **13:** 2801–2810.
47. ARTAVANIS-TSAKONAS, S., M.D. RAND & R.J. LAKE. 1999. Notch signaling: cell fate control and signal integration in development. Science **284:** 770–776.
48. BLAUMUELLER, C.M., H. QI, P. ZAGOURAS & S. ARTAVANIS-TSAKONAS. 1997. Intracellular cleavage of Notch leads to a heterodimeric receptor on the plasma membrane. Cell **90:** 281–289.
49. SCHROETER, E.H., J.A. KISSLINGER & R. KOPAN. 1998. Notch-1 signalling requires ligand-induced proteolytic release of intracellular domain. Nature **393:** 382–386.
50. VARNUM-FINNEY, B., L.E. PURTON, M. YU et al. 1998. The Notch ligand, Jagged-1, influences the development of primitive hematopoietic precursor cells. Blood **91:** 4084–4091.
51. BEREZOVSKA, O., P. MCLEAN, R. KNOWLES et al. 1999. Notch1 inhibits neurite outgrowth in postmitotic primary neurons. Neuroscience **93:** 433–439.
52. SESTAN, N., S. ARTAVANIS-TSAKONAS & P. RAKIC. 1999. Contact-dependent inhibition of cortical neurite growth mediated by Notch signaling. Science **286:** 741–746.
53. BEREZOVSKA, O., M. FORSCH, P. MCLEAN et al. 1999. The Alzheimer-related gene presenilin 1 facilitates notch 1 in primary mammalian neurons. Brain Res. Mol. Brain Res. **69:** 273–280.

Role of Presenilin-1 in Murine Neural Development

XUDONG YANG,[a] MELISSA HANDLER,[a] AND JIE SHEN[b]

Center for Neurologic Diseases, Department of Neurology, Brigham and Women's Hospital, Harvard Medical School, Boston, Massachusetts 02115, USA

ABSTRACT: Our previous studies showed that presenilin-1 (PS1) is required for murine neural and skeletal development. Here we report that the reduction in the neural progenitor cells observed in the $PS1^{-/-}$ mouse brain is due to premature differentiation of progenitor cells, rather than to increased apoptotic cell death or decreased cell proliferation. In the ventricular zone of $PS1^{-/-}$ mice, expression of the Notch1 downstream effector gene *Hes5* is reduced, and expression of the Notch1 ligand *Dll1* is elevated, indicating reduced Notch signaling. These results provide direct evidence that PS1 is involved in the regulation of neurogenesis and Notch signaling during development.

INTRODUCTION

The presenilin-1 gene (*PS1*) is a major gene responsible for familial Alzheimer's disease (FAD), and mutations in *PS1* account for approximately 50% of early-onset FAD cases.[1] Understanding the normal physiological functions of PS1 may shed light on the pathogenic mechanism of FAD-linked PS1 mutations. Studies of the *PS1* homologs in *C. elegans* and *Drosophila* provided the evidence that PS1 interacts with the LIN-12/Notch signaling pathway, which mediates cell-cell interactions that specify cell fate during development. The *PS1* homolog in *C. elegans, sel-12*, facilitates signaling mediated by LIN-12.[2] Furthermore, the wild-type human *PS1* cDNA complements the *sel-12* mutant phenotype, while PS1 containing FAD-linked mutations exhibited reduced ability to rescue *sel-12* mutations.[3,4] Fly mutants lacking both maternal and zygotic PS exhibit a neurogenic phenotype and are virtually indistinguishable from the Notch-null mutant, suggesting that PS function is required for Notch signaling in *Drosophila*.[5,6] PS is required for the proteolytic cleavage of Notch to release its intracellular domain (ICD).[5] This is further supported by studies using truncated Notch1 and primary cell cultures derived from $PS1^{-/-}$ mice.[7,8] Levels of the ICD fragment were reduced in cultured $PS1^{-/-}$ neurons and fibroblasts, indicating that PS1 facilitates proteolytic release of the ICD.

To characterize the normal physiological role of PS1 in mice, we previously generated mice with a targeted germ-line disruption of the *PS1* gene.[9] *PS1*-null mice exhibited defects in somitogenesis similar to those observed in *Notch1*-null mutant

---

[a]These authors contributed equally to the work.

[b]Address for correspondence: Jie Shen, Center for Neurologic Diseases, Department of Neurology, Brigham and Women's Hospital, Harvard Medical School, Boston, MA 02115. Tel.: (617) 525-5561; fax: (617) 525-5252.
e-mail: jshen@cnd.bwh.harvard.edu

mice,[10,11] as well as severe malformation of the axial skeleton and cerebral hemorrhage.[9,12] Furthermore, we showed that lack of PS1 results in a reduction in the neural progenitor population and a subsequent reduction in the neuronal population, indicating a critical role for PS1 in murine neurogenesis.[9] We also observed symmetric, region-specific loss of neural progenitor cells and neurons in the $PS1^{-/-}$ brain during the latter stages of neurogenesis, suggesting a neuroprotective role for PS1 during neural development.

Here, we report that the reduction in the neural progenitor population in $PS1^{-/-}$ mice is caused by premature differentiation of neural progenitor cells. To investigate the mechanism underlying this neurogenesis defect, we examined the expression of genes in the Notch signaling pathway. We find a reduction in the level of $Hes5$ transcripts as well as an increase in the level of $Dll1$ transcripts in the $PS1^{-/-}$ brain, indicating that absence of PS1 function leads to reduced Notch signaling during neural development. Taken together, our findings provide the evidence that PS1 controls the cell fate decision between neural progenitor cells and postmitotic neurons and regulates Notch signaling during neural development.

RESULTS

Beginning at embryonic day 12.5 (E12.5), it becomes evident that the ventricular zone in the $PS1^{-/-}$ brain is thinner than in the control, reflecting a reduction in the population of neural progenitor cells.[9] Three mechanisms could contribute to the reduction in the progenitor population: premature differentiation of progenitor cells, decreased proliferation, or increased apoptotic cell death. To distinguish among these possibilities, we compared the $PS1^{-/-}$ and control brains between E10.5 and E14.5 for differences in neuronal differentiation, cell proliferation, and survival.

Premature Differentiation of Neural Progenitor Cells in PS1$^{-/-}$ Mice

To assess neuronal differentiation in the $PS1^{-/-}$ and control brains, we performed immunostaining for microtubule-associated protein 2 (MAP2), a marker specific for postmitotic neurons.[14] Comparable transverse sections of the $PS1^{-/-}$ and littermate control brains were compared. In the $PS1^{-/-}$ brain at E10.5, increases in the number of MAP2-immunoreactive neurons are evident in the diencephalic neuroepithelium. At E11.5, increases in MAP2 immunoreactivity in the $PS1^{-/-}$ brain relative to the control are found in the anterior telencephalon, and more substantially in the posterior telencephalon. In the diencephalon of the $PS1^{-/-}$ brain, the MAP2-immunoreactive neurons encompass many cell layers and have largely replaced the MAP2-negative neural progenitor cells in the ventricular zone.

In summary, markedly increased numbers of postmitotic neurons accumulate in the telencephalon and diencephalon of the $PS1^{-/-}$ brain during early neural development, accompanied by a progressive reduction in size of the ventricular zone. These observations indicate that neural progenitor cells differentiate into postmitotic neurons prematurely in the absence of PS1, resulting in early depletion of the neural progenitor population.

Although premature neuronal differentiation provides an explanation for the reduction of progenitor cells in the $PS1^{-/-}$ brain, it remained possible that a decrease in cell proliferation and/or an increase in apoptotic cell death could be contributing factors as well. Cell proliferation rate was measured by the percentage of progenitor cells in S-phase during a short pulse labeling with bromodeoxyuridine (BrdU). We observed no significant differences in the BrdU-labeling patterns in the $PS1^{-/-}$ and littermate control brains at E10.5. The ratio of BrdU-labeled cells to the total number of progenitor cells in the ventricular zone of the telencephalon and diencephalon is similar in the $PS1^{-/-}$ and control brains, indicating that lack of PS1 does not lead to a reduction in the proliferation rate.

To determine whether increased apoptotic cell death might contribute to the reduction in the neural progenitor population in the $PS1^{-/-}$ brain, we assessed the number of apoptotic cells labeled by the terminal deoxynucleotidyl transferase-mediated deoxyuridine triphosphate-biotin nick end labeling (TUNEL) assay in the $PS1^{-/-}$ and control brains at E11.5 and E12.5. Quantitative comparison of the number of apoptotic cells in the $PS1^{-/-}$ and control brains revealed no significant differences, indicating that PS1 is not involved in the regulation of apoptosis during early neurogenesis.

Reduced Notch Signaling in PS1$^{-/-}$ Mice

To understand the mechanism underlying the premature neuronal differentiation observed in the $PS1^{-/-}$ brain, we examined the expression of genes in the Notch signaling pathway, which is known to be involved in cell fate determination in *Drosophila*.[15] The role of Notch receptors in murine neurogenesis is poorly understood. Mice lacking Notch1 or Notch2 function die at approximately E9 or E11, respectively, before cortical neurogenesis begins.[10,11,16] However, excess cells expressing proneural transcription factors were identified in the midbrain and hindbrain of $Notch1^{-/-}$ mice.[17] The basic helix-loop-helix transcription factors Hes1 and Hes5, which are downstream effectors of the Notch signaling pathway, have been shown to regulate murine neuronal differentiation.[18–21] We therefore first examined the levels of *Hes1* and *Hes5* transcripts to determine whether their expression is affected in $PS1^{-/-}$ mice.

In situ hybridization analysis revealed that at E11.5 the level of *Hes5* transcripts in $PS1^{-/-}$ mice is reduced in the anterior telencephalon, ganglionic eminence, and diencephalon, while expression of *Hes1* is unchanged. Consistent with previous studies,[22] *Hes5* expression is localized to the ventricular zone within each brain region. Northern analysis of poly(A)+ RNA derived from the $PS1^{-/-}$ and control brains also showed reduced levels of *Hes5* transcripts in the $PS1^{-/-}$ brain. These results indicate that lack of PS1 function leads to a reduction in *Hes5* expression, providing *in vivo* evidence for an involvement of PS1 in the Notch signaling pathway during neurogenesis and an explanation for the premature differentiation of neural progenitor cells observed in the $PS1^{-/-}$ brain.

It has been postulated in *Drosophila* that Notch and its ligand Delta are linked by a regulatory negative feedback loop under the transcriptional control of the *Enhancer-of-split* and *achaete-scute* complex gene products.[23–25] In addition, expression of *Dll1* is upregulated in the $Notch1^{-/-}$ embryo.[17] To determine whether reduced Notch signaling in $PS1^{-/-}$ mice leads to upregulation of *Dll1* expression, we examined the levels of *Dll1* transcripts by *in situ* hybridization and Northern analyses. *In situ* hybridization analysis revealed that *Dll1* expression is localized in isolated cells in the ventricular zone, consistent with previous reports.[26,27] At E11.5, the number of

Dll1-expressing cells is increased in the telencephalon and more substantially in the diencephalon of the $PS1^{-/-}$ brain. Quantitative comparison of *Dll1*-expressing cells in the telencephalon revealed a 40% increase in the density of *Dll1*-expressing cells in the $PS1^{-/-}$ neuroepithelium. Northern analysis also showed a marked increase in the level of *Dll1* transcripts, providing further support for the downregulation of Notch signaling in $PS1^{-/-}$ mice.

To determine whether PS1 regulates Notch signaling at the level of transcription, translation, and/or posttranslational maturation and activation, we examined the $PS1^{-/-}$ and control brains for differences in the levels of *Notch1* expression. *In situ* hybridization and Northern analyses of the $PS1^{-/-}$ and littermate control brains revealed no significant differences in the level of *Notch1* transcripts. Immunohistochemical analysis of comparable sections of the $PS1^{-/-}$ and control brains using a polyclonal antiserum[28] raised against the ICD of mouse Notch 1 also showed no differences in the intensity of Notch1 immunoreactivity. These results support a role for PS1 in the regulation of Notch1 posttranslational activation.

DISCUSSION

Our previous characterization of $PS1^{-/-}$ mice documented specific defects in central nervous system (CNS) development, revealing a function for PS1 in the mammalian brain.[9] Here we characterize the mechanisms underlying the progressive reduction in neural progenitor population that we observed in the $PS1^{-/-}$ brain. During early neurogenesis, very few progenitor cells in the ventricular zone exit the cell cycle to differentiate into postmitotic neurons, while the vast majority of progenitor cells remain in the cell cycle after mitosis, resulting in a steady expansion of the progenitor population. Here we have shown that lack of PS1 function leads to an increase in the number of differentiated postmitotic neurons at the expense of neural progenitor cells, indicating that PS1 regulates the cell fate decision between neural progenitor cells and postmitotic neurons in the developing brain. The premature differentiation of neural progenitor cells results in depletion of the neural progenitor population, providing an explanation for the progressive reduction in neural progenitor cells observed in the $PS1^{-/-}$ brain at E12.5, E14.5, and E16.5, particularly in the posterior portion of the brain.[9]

To understand further the mechanism by which PS1 controls cell fate decisions during neural development, we examined the expression of genes involved in the Notch signaling pathway, *Notch1*, *Dll1*, and the Notch downstream effector genes *Hes1* and *Hes5*. Previous studies have suggested a connection between Notch signaling and the regulation of neuronal differentiation. Premature neuronal differentiation has been observed at E10.5 in mutant mice lacking Hes1, Hes5, or both.[18,20] Here we have shown that expression of *Hes5* is downregulated in the $PS1^{-/-}$ brain, indicating that Notch signaling in the developing brain is reduced in the absence of PS1. Furthermore, analysis of the proteolytic processing of truncated Notch1 proteins in cultured cells derived from $PS1^{-/-}$ mice has shown that PS1 is required for efficient release of the Notch1 ICD.[7,8] The present study supports such a role for PS1 in the regulation of Notch signaling, and further provides evidence that the reduced Notch processing observed in $PS1^{-/-}$ cells is functionally significant in cell fate determination.

Lack of PS1 function was previously reported to result in reduced transcription of *Notch1* and *Dll1* in the presomitic mesoderm of the $PS1^{-/-}$ embryo, suggesting a role for PS1 in the regulation of *Notch1* and *Dll1* at the transcriptional level.[12] However, we detected unaltered levels of *Notch1* transcripts and elevated levels of *Dll1* transcripts in the embryonic brain and presomitic mesoderm of $PS1^{-/-}$ mice by Northern analysis. These results indicate that regulation of Notch signaling does not differ in the CNS and paraxial mesoderm, and that the lateral inhibition feedback mechanism first postulated in *Drosophila* is conserved in mice.

Finally, our results indicate a difference in the consequences of reduced Notch signaling during neurogenesis in *Drosophila* and mice. In *Drosophila*, loss of function mutations in Notch leads to excessive neuronal production at the expense of epidermis.[15] Our findings show that Notch1 regulates a cell fate choice between neural progenitor cells and terminally differentiated neurons early in mammalian neurogenesis, promoting regeneration of neural precursor cells at the expense of differentiation of postmitotic neurons. The early depletion of progenitor cells in the $PS1^{-/-}$ brain ultimately leads to an overall reduction in the postmitotic neuronal population.

REFERENCES

1. SELKOE, D.J. 1998. The cell biology of β-amyloid precursor protein and presenilin in Alzheimer's disease. Trends Cell Biol. **8:** 447–453.
2. LEVITAN, D. & I. GREENWALD. 1995. Facilitation of *lin-12*-mediated signalling by *sel-12*, a *Caenorhabditis elegans S182* Alzheimer's disease gene. Nature **377:** 351–354.
3. BAUMEISTER, R., U. LEIMER, I. ZWECKBRONNER, C. JAKUBEK, J. GRUNBERG & C. HAASS. 1997. Human presenilin-1, but not familial Alzheimer's disease (FAD) mutants, facilitate *Caenorhabditis elegans* Notch signalling independently of proteolytic processing. Genes Funct. **2:** 149–159.
4. LEVITAN, D., T.G. DOYLE, D. BROUSSEAU, M.K. LEE, G. THINAKARAN, H.H. SLUNT, S.S. SISODIA & I. GREENWALD. 1996. Assessment of normal and mutant human presenilin function in *Caenorhabditis elegans*. Proc. Natl. Acad. Sci. USA **93:** 14940–14944.
5. STRUHL, G. & I. GREENWALD. 1999. Presenilin is required for activity and nuclear access of Notch in *Drosophila*. Nature **398:** 522–525.
6. YE, Y., N. LUKINOVA & M.E. FORTINI. 1999. Neurogenic phenotypes and altered Notch processing in *Drosophila* presenilin mutants. Nature **398:** 525–529.
7. DE STROOPER, B., W. ANNAERT, P. CUPERS, P. SAFTIG, K. CRAESSAERTS, J.S. MUMM, E.H. SCHROETER, V. SCHRIJVERS, M.S. WOLFE, W.J. RAY, A. GOATE & R. KOPAN. 1999. A presenilin-1-dependent gamma-secretase-like protease mediates release of Notch intracellular domain. Nature **398:** 518–522.
8. SONG, W., P. NADEAU, M. YUAN, X. YANG, J. SHEN & B.A. YANKNER. 1999. Proteolytic release and nuclear translocation of Notch-1 are induced by presenilin-1 and impaired by pathogenic presenilin-1 mutations. Proc. Natl. Acad. Sci. USA **96:** 6959–6963.
9. SHEN, J., R.T. BRONSON, D.F, CHEN, W. XIA, D.J. SELKOE & S. TONEGAWA. 1997. Skeletal and CNS defects in presnilin-1 deficient mice. Cell **89:** 629–639.
10. CONLON, R.A., A.G. REAUME & J. ROSSANT. 1995. Notch 1 is required for the coordinate segmentation of somites. Development **121:** 1533–1545.
11. SWIATEK, P.J., C.E. LINDSELL, F. FRANCO DEL AMO, G. WEINMASTER & T. GRIDLEY. 1994. Notch 1 is essential for postimplantation development in mice. Genes Dev. **8:** 707–719.
12. WONG, P., H. ZHEN, H. CHEN, M.W. BECHER, D.J. SIRINATHSINGHJI, M.E. TRUMBAUER, D.L. PROCE, L.H.T. VAN DER PLOEG & S.S. SISODIA. 1997. Presenilin 1 is required for Notch 1 and D111 expression in the paraxial mesoderm. Nature **397:** 288–292.

13. SCHAEREN-WIEMERS, N. & A. GERFIN-MOSER. 1993. A single protocol to detect transcripts of various types and expression levels in neural tissue and cultured cells: *in situ* hybridization using digoxigenin-labelled cRNA probes. Histochemistry **100:** 431–440.
14. CRANDALL, J.E., M. JACOBSON & K.S. KOSIK. 1986. Ontogenesis of microtubule-associated protein 2 (MAP2) in embryonic mouse cortex. Brain Res. **393:** 127–133.
15. ARTAVANIS-TSAKONAS, S., M.D. RAND & R.J. LAKE. 1999. Notch signalling: cell fate control and signal integration in development. Science **284:** 770–776.
16. HAMADA, Y., Y. KADOKAWA, M. OKABE, M. IKAWA, J. COLEMAN & Y. TSUJIMOTO. 1999. Mutation in ankyrin repeats of the mouse *Notch2* gene induces early embryonic lethality. Development **126:** 3415–3424.
17. DE LA POMPA, J.L., A. WAKEHAM, K.M. CORREIA, E. SAMPER, S. BROWN, R.J. AGUILERA, T. NAKANO, T. HONJO, T.W. MAK, J. ROSSANT & R.A. CONLON. 1997. Conservation of the Notch signalling pathway in mammalian neurogenesis. Development **124:** 1139–1148.
18. ISHIBASHI, M., S.L. ANG, K. SHIOTA, S. NAKANISHI, R. KAGEYAMA & F. GUILLEMOT. 1995. Targeted disruption of mammalian hairy and Enhancer of split homolog-1 (HES-1) leads to up-regulation of neural helix-loop-helix factors, premature neurogenesis, and severe neural tube defects. Genes Dev. **9:** 3136–3148.
19. KAGEYAMA, R. & S. NAKANISHI. 1997. Helix-loop-helix factors in growth and differentiation of the vertebrate nervous system. Curr. Opin. Genet. Dev. **7:** 659–665.
20. OHTSUKA, T., M. ISHIBASHI, G. GRADWOHL, S. NAKANISHI, F. GUILLEMOT & R. KAGEYAMA. 1999. Hes1 and Hes5 as Notch effectors in mammalian neuronal differentiation. EMBO J. **18:** 2196–2207.
21. TOMITA, K., M. ISHIBASHI, K. NAKAHARA, S. ANG, S. NAKANISHI & R. KAGEYAMA. 1996. Mammalian hairy and Enhancer of split homolog 1 regulates differentiation of retinal neurons and is essential for eye morphogenesis. Neuron **16:** 723–734.
22. AKAZAWA, C., Y. SASAI, S. NAKANISHI & R. KAGEYAMA. 1992. Molecular characterization of a rat negative regulator with a basic helix-loop-helix structure predominantly expressed in the developing nervous system. J. Biol. Chem. **267:** 21879–21885.
23. HEITZLER, P., M. BOUROUIS, L. RUEL, C. CARTERET & P. SIMPSON. 1996. Genes of the Enhancer of split and achaete-scute complexes are required for a regulatory loop between Notch and Delta during lateral signalling in *Drosophila*. Development **122:** 161–171.
24. HEITZLER, P. & P. SIMPSON. 1993. Altered epidermal growth factor-like sequences provide evidence for a role of Notch as a receptor in cell fate decisions. Development **117:** 1113–1123.
25. HEITZLER, P. & P. SIMPSON. 1991. The choice of cell fate in the epidermis of *Drosophila*. Cell **64:** 1083–1092.
26. HENRIQUE, D., J. ADAM, A. MYAT, A. CHITNIS, J. LEWIS & D. ISH-HOROWICZ. 1995. Expression of a Delta homologue in prospective neurons in the chick. Nature **375:** 787–790.
27. BETTENHAUSEN, B., M. DE ANGELIS, D. SIMON, J. GUENET & A. GOSSLER. 1995. Transient and restricted expression during mouse embryogenesis of *Dll1*, a murine gene closely related to *Drosophila* Delta. Development **121:** 2407–2418.
28. LOGEAT, F., C. BESSIA, C. BROU, O. LEBAIL, S. JARRIAULT, N. SEIDAH & A. ISRAEL. 1998. The Notch1 receptor is cleaved constitutively by a furin-like convertase. Proc. Natl. Acad. Sci. USA **95:** 8108–8112.

Modulation of Aβ Deposition in APP Transgenic Mice by an Apolipoprotein E Null Background

M.C. IRIZARRY,[a,d] G.W. REBECK,[a] B. CHEUNG,[a] K. BALES,[b] S.M PAUL,[b] D. HOLZMAN,[c] AND B.T. HYMAN[a]

[a]*Alzheimer Disease Research Unit, Massachusetts General Hospital, Boston, Massachusetts 02114, USA*

[b]*Neuroscience Discovery Research, Lilly Research Laboratories, Indianapolis, Indiana 46202, USA*

[c]*Department of Neurology, Washington University School of Medicine, St. Louis, Missouri 63110, USA*

ABSTRACT: Several lines of evidence implicate apolipoprotein E (apoE) and its receptor—the low density lipoprotein receptor related protein (LRP)—in Alzheimer's disease (AD) pathogenesis, including increased amyloid deposition in human AD brains of people containing the apoE ε4 allele, presence of apoE and LRP in amyloid plaques, and *in vitro* uptake of amyloid precursor protein (APP) and amyloid β protein (Aβ) by LRP. Studies of crosses of apoE knockout mice with APP transgenic mice support a complex interaction between apoE and Aβ deposition. In the Tg2576 mice expressing human APP$_{K670N-M671L}$, apoE determines the amount, morphology, vascular pattern, and neuropil response to Aβ deposits. In the PDAPP mice expressing human APP$_{V717F}$, apoE also affects the anatomical localization of cerebral Aβ deposits. Thus, APP transgenic mice can serve as models to investigate genetic influences on the amount and timing of cerebral amyloidosis, the morphology of amyloid plaques, and the vulnerability of specific neuroanatomical regions to Aβ deposition.

APOLIPOPROTEIN E AND ALZHEIMER'S DISEASE

Common polymorphisms in the apolipoprotein E (apoE) gene locus have been associated with Alzheimer's disease (AD) risk. The apoE ε4 allele is consistently overrepresented in clinically and pathologically diagnosed late-onset AD (ε4 allele frequency 0.36–0.52) compared to controls (0.11–0.16), indicating that inheritance of the ε4 allele is a risk factor for developing AD; the ε2 allele is underrepresented in AD (ε2 allele frequency 0.027–0.045) compared to controls (0.086–0.126), suggesting a role as a protective genetic risk factor.[1–3] The ε4 allele is associated with an earlier age of onset of dementia in a dose-dependent manner; however, the rate of cognitive decline does not consistently vary across apoE genotypes.[4]

[d]Address for correspondence: Dr. Michael C. Irizarry, Alzheimer Disease Research Unit, Massachusetts General Hospital–East, 149 13th Street, Charlestown, MA 02129. Tel.: (617) 726-4796; fax: (617) 726-5677.
e-mail: irizarry@helix.mgh.harvard.edu

The mechanism by which apoE isoforms confer differential risk for AD is unknown. ApoE in plasma is involved in lipid transport; apoE in the central nervous system has been implicated in development, nerve growth, reinnervation, and responses to injury and repair.[5] Pathologically, apoE and the apoE receptor, the low density lipoprotein receptor related protein (LRP), are present in amyloid deposits, and the apoE ε4 allele is associated with increased amyloid deposition, but not with greater neurofibrillary tangle formation or neuronal loss when controlled for duration of illness.[4] Although apoE is present in senile plaques and amyloid angiopathy,[2,6] and amyloid β protein (Aβ)-apoE complex formation has been identified *in vitro*[7] and in human brain supernatants,[8] the effects of this interaction on Aβ fibrillogenesis and Aβ clearance are not straightforward. Depending on the experimental conditions *in vitro*, apoE can promote or inhibit Aβ polymerization.[9–13] LRP ligands—including apoE, lactoferrin, and activated α2-macroglobulin—enhance LRP-mediated clearance of Aβ by neurons in culture,[14,15] and both LRP and α2-macroglobulin polymorphisms have been linked to AD risk.[16–18] The complex interactions between apoE, APP, and Aβ suggested by these epidemiological, pathological, biochemical, and *in vitro* studies have been further corroborated by the investigation of transgenic mouse models of AD and apoE knockout mice.

APP TRANSGENIC MICE: TG2576 AND PDAPP

Amyloid precursor protein transgenic mice have been valuable model systems for assessment of the neuropathological consequences and the genetic modifiers of cerebral Aβ deposition. We evaluated the role of apoE on amyloid deposition in two different APP transgenic mice crossed onto an apoE null background.

The Tg2576 mouse expresses human APP695 with the Swedish familial AD double mutation K670N-M671L (hAPP$_{Sw}$) under the hamster PrP promoter on a C57B6/SJL mixed strain background. Amyloid deposits begin in cortical and limbic regions by 9 months of age, and are associated with dystrophic neurites, punctate phospho-tau immunoreactivity, astrocytosis, microgliosis, and vascular amyloidosis, without significant CA1 neuronal loss or neurofibrillary tangle formation.[19,20] These mice have an age-dependent behavioral and electrophysiologic phenotype, characterized by impairment in water maze and forced-choice alternation paradigms, as well as impaired induction of LTP in dentate gyrus and CA1 synapses in slice preparations, and absent potentiation of the fEPSP slope with reduced LTP of the population spike from *in vivo* recordings in the dentate gyrus.[21] There is also evidence of dysregulation of the glutamatergic system in these mice, with increased hippocampal AMPA binding in old (15 month) transgenic mice.[22]

The PDAPP mouse expresses a human APP770 minigene with the V717F familial AD mutation (hAPP$_{V717F}$) under the control of the human PDGF-b chain neuronal promoter on a mixed C57BL/6, DBA, and Swiss-Webster strain background.[23] Cortical and limbic amyloid deposition begins at 6–9 months of age in heterozygotes and 3 months of age in homozygotes, with reactive neuritic and inflammatory changes.[24] There is not significant cortical or hippocampal neuronal loss or neurofibrillary tangle formation through 18 months of age in heterozygous transgenics.[25]

A remarkable feature of both of these APP transgenic mice is the characteristic cortical and limbic localization of Aβ deposition. Amyloid plaques occur in the out-

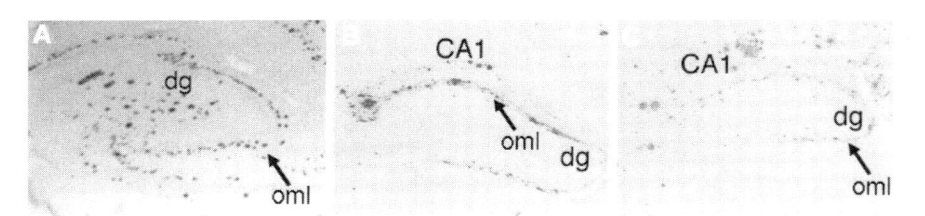

FIGURE 1. Aβ immunoreactivity. Aβ immunoreactivity in the outer molecular layer (oml) of the hippocampal dentate gyrus (dg) in human AD (**A**), 15-month Tg2576 heterozygous hAPP$_{Sw}$ transgenic mouse (**B**), and 12 month heterozygous PDAPP transgenic mouse (**C**).

er molecular layer of the dentate gyrus, in round deposits in CA1, and in mixed morphologies in neocortical areas. Diencephalon, brainstem, and cerebellum are largely spared of amyloid. The sites of amyloid deposition do not reflect the regional expression of either the hAPP$_{Sw}$ or hAPP$_{V717F}$ transgenes, which are widely expressed in neurons throughout the brain.[20,25] Instead, the anatomical pattern parallels that seen in human AD, where amyloid plaques occur in a stereotyped distribution in neocortex and hippocampus, including the outer molecular layer of the dentate gyrus (FIG. 1).[26,27] Furthermore, the morphology of amyloid plaques in aged APP transgenic mice—spanning the continuum from diffuse Aβ deposits to compact cored plaques with inflammation and neuritic dystrophy—recapitulates amyloid pathology in human AD.[24] Our studies of crosses between apoE knockout mice and APP transgenic mice indicate that apoE intimately affects the amount, morphology, and localization of Aβ deposits.

TG2576 × APOE KNOCKOUT MICE

We examined amyloid deposition in Tg2576 heterozygous APP transgenic mice on an apoE null background compared to heterozygous transgenic mice with endogenous mouse apoE at 12 months of age.[28] Mice lacking apoE had significantly reduced Aβ deposition (FIG. 2), lack of thioS deposits, absence of neuritic degeneration, and reduction of vascular amyloidosis. Aβ burden was reduced in hippocampal CA1, dentate gyrus, and cortex (FIG. 3). The anatomical pattern of Aβ deposition is similar to the Tg2576 mice containing apoE, without the redistribution of Aβ immunoreactivity in the hippocampus noted in the PDAPP apoE null mice (see below). Thus, in Tg2576 mice, apoE determines the amount and form of Aβ deposition, potentiates vascular amyloid deposition, and is required for fibrillar Aβ deposits which produce neuritic dystrophy.

PDAPP × APOE KNOCKOUT MICE

PDAPP homozygote mice on an apoE null background (PDAPP+/+ApoE0/0) analyzed at 6 months of age revealed only sparse immunoreactive Aβ deposits in the hippocampus and rarely in the cortex.[29] Aβ burden in the cortex was reduced to 11.75% of that in the PDAPP mice with endogenous mouse apoE (PDAPP+/

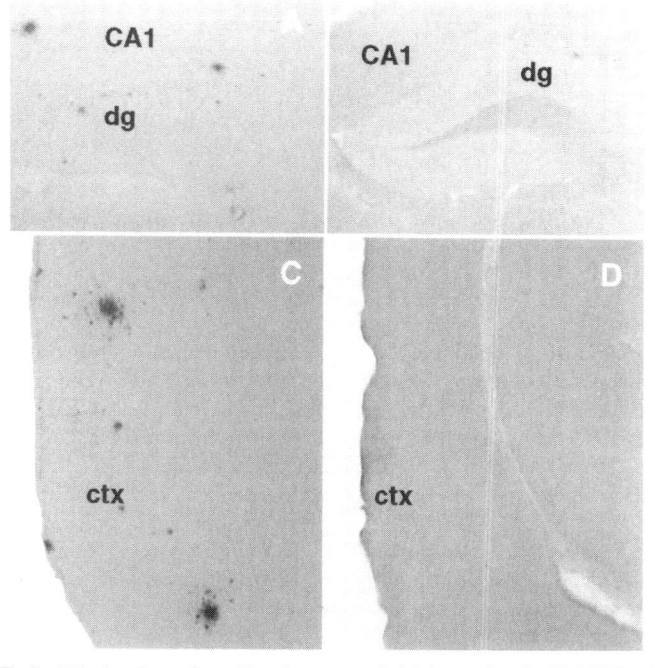

FIGURE 2. Elimination of apoE reduces amyloid depostion in Tg2576 mice. Aβ immunoreactivity in the hippocampal dentate gyrus (dg: **A**, **B**) and entorhinal cortex (ctx: **C**, **D**) of 12 month Tg2576 mice containing endogenous mouse apoE (A, C) and lacking mouse apoE (B, D).

+ApoE+/+), and reduced to 37.90% of that in the hippocampus. Furthermore, elimination of apoE in the PDAPP transgenic mouse line eliminated the formation of compact, thioS staining plaques. There were no associated differences between mice containing and lacking apoE in APP mRNA levels by RT-PCR, in APP protein levels by Western blot, or in total Aβ and Aβ$_{1-42}$ levels by ELISA in hippocampus or cortex of 2-month-old mice.[29]

We have extended these studies to characterize the regional deposition of amyloid deposits in 12 month old PDAPP+/+ApoE0/0 mice, and find a dramatic redistribution of these deposits within the cortex and the subfields of the hippocampus (FIG. 4).[30] Within the cortex, there was reduction of Aβ deposition in the mice lacking apoE. PDAPP mice with apoE had compact deposits scattered throughout the frontal cortex. PDAPP+/+ApoE0/0 mice had diffuse deposits in the deep cortical layers. Within the hippocampal subfields, the pattern of Aβ staining in the apoE null mice was altered in a very specific anatomic manner. In PDAPP+/+ApoE+/+ mice, amyloid deposits prominently in a band in the outer layer of the dentate gyrus, with focal deposits throughout the other hippocampal subfields—as in human AD. In the mice lacking apoE, the dentate gyrus is remarkably free of Aβ immunoreactivity, as is the stratum lacunosum/moleculare of CA1. The other layers of CA1 excluding the pyramidal cell layer were carpeted with Aβ. Quantitating the percent of frontal cortex, CA1, and den-

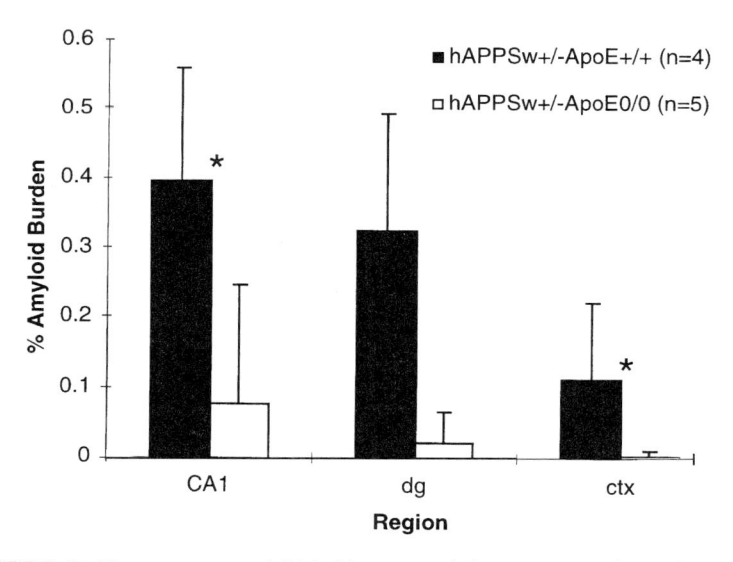

FIGURE 3. The percentage of CA1, hippocampal dentate gyrus (dg) and cortex (ctx) covered by Aβ immunoreactivity (% amyloid burden ± S.D.) over three 40-μm coronal sections spaced 960 μm apart using the antibody R1282 in 12-month Tg2576 heterozygous transgenic mice containing endogenous mouse apoE (*black*, hAPPSw+/–ApoE+/+) and lacking apoE (*white*, hAPPSw+/-ApoE0/0). Amyloid burden is significantly reduced in Tg2576 mice lacking apoE (ANOVA, p <0.0001), particularly in CA1 and cortex (*post-hoc, p <0.002).

tate gyrus covered with Aβ immunoreactivity (using R1282) in 14-μm sections shows a 78% reduction of Aβ deposition in the frontal cortex, and a virtual elimination of Aβ deposition in the dentate gyrus molecular layer in the mice lacking apoE. However, in CA1, Aβ burden increases by nearly 5-fold. Despite the prominent CA1 and CA3 hippocampal Aβ deposition in the PDAPP+/+ApoE0/0 mice, there were no thioS staining plaques in the cortex and hippocampus. There were no differences between PDAPP mice with and without apoE in the regional expression of APP by *in situ* hybridization, in total APP levels by Western blot, in soluble Aβ levels in the hippocampus or cortex by Western blot, in levels of LRP mRNA by *in situ* hybridization, or in LRP protein levels by Western blot. Thus, apoE is the first identified genetic factor involved in the specific anatomical patterning of the regional, laminar, and even sublaminar localization of Aβ deposition in the PDAPP mice. Also, as in Tg2576 mice, apoE is necessary for the development of fibrillar, thioS reactive amyloid plaques.

CONCLUSIONS

Elimination of apoE in both the PDAPP and Tg2576 transgenic mice eliminates the formation of thioS reactive plaques, implicating apoE in Aβ fibrillogenesis, stabilization of fibrillar Aβ, and/or maturation of amyloid plaques. The acceleration of diffuse amyloid deposition in CA3 and CA1 stratum radiatum/oriens of the

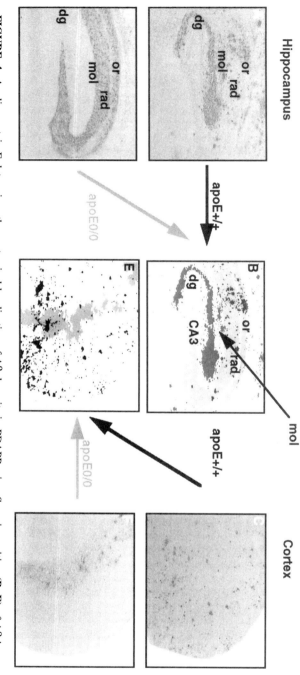

FIGURE 4. Apolipoprotein E determines the anatomical localization of Aβ deposits in PDAPP mice. Superimposition (**B, E**) of Aβ immunostaining in hippocampus (**A, B, D**) and cortex (**C, E, F**) of PDAPP+/+ApoE+/+ (**A, B** *dark*, **C, E** *dark*) and PDAPP+/+ApoE0/0 (**B** *light*, **D, E** *light*, **F**) demonstrates the specific anatomical differences in Aβ deposition. In PDAPP mice, amyloid deposits in the outer molecular layer of the dentate gyrus (dg), and all layers of CA1, CA3 (**A, B** *dark*) and cortex (**C, E** *dark*). In PDAPP mice lacking apoE, the dentate gyrus (dg) and stratum molecular of CA1 (mol) is spared, while the stratum radiatum (rad) and oreins (or) of CA1 is carpeted with diffuse Aβ (**B** *light*, **D**); in the cortex, Aβ deposition is restricted to deeper layers (**E** *light*, **F**).

PDAPP mice lacking apoE implies a competing biological function for apoE in LRP-mediated Aβ clearance. The remarkable redistribution of Aβ deposition in the PDAPP apoE null animals suggests a role for apoE in the anatomical specificity of amyloid deposition. Reintroduction of human apoE3 or apoE4 into these mouse models could test the hypothesis that these isoforms differentially shift the dynamic balance between a biophysical role for apoE in Aβ fibrillogenesis and a biological role for apoE in Aβ clearance.

ACKNOWLEDGMENTS

This work was supported by the Massachusetts ADRC and by NIH grants AG00793 and AG13956.

REFERENCES

1. SAUNDERS, A.M, W.J. STRITTMATTER, D. SCHMECHEL *et al.* 1993. Association of apolipoprotein E allele ε4 with late-onset familial and sporadic Alzheimer's disease. Neurology **43**: 1467–1472.
2. REBECK, G.W., J.S. REITER, D.K. STRICKLAND & B.T. HYMAN. 1993. Apolipoprotein E in sporadic Alzheimer's disease: allelic variation and receptor interactions. Neuron **11**: 575–580.
3. WEST, H., G.W. REBECK & B.T. HYMAN. 1994. Frequency of the apolipoprotein E ε2 allele is diminished in sporadic Alzheimer disease. Neurosci. Lett. **175**: 46–48.
4. GOMEZ-ISLA, T., H.L. WEST, G.W. REBECK *et al.* 1996. Clinical and pathological correlates of apolipoprotein E ε4 in Alzheimer's disease. Ann. Neurol. **39**: 62–70.
5. MAHLEY, R.W. 1988. Apolipoprotein E: cholesterol transport protein with expanding role in cell biology. Science **240**: 622–630.
6. GEARING, M., J.A. SCHNEIDER, R.S. ROBBINS *et al.* 1995. Regional variation in the distribution of apolipoprotein E and A-beta in Alzheimer's disease. J. Neuropathol. Exp. Neurol. **54**: 833–841.
7. LADU, M.J., M.T. FULDUTO, A.M. MANELLI, C.A. REARDON, H. MORI & D.E. FRAIL. 1994. Isoform-specific binding of apolipoprotein E to beta-amyloid. J. Biol. Chem. **269**: 23403–23406.
8. PERMANNE, B., C. PEREZ, C. SOTO, B. FRANGIONE & T. WISNIEWSKI. 1997. Detection of apolipoprotein E/dimeric soluble amyloid beta complexes in Alzheimer's disease brain supernatants. Biochem. Biophys. Res. Commun. **240**: 715–720.
9. MA, J., A. YEE, H.B. BREWER, JR., S. DAS & H. POTTER. 1994. Amyloid-associated proteins alpha 1-antichymotrypsin and apolipoprotein E promote assembly of Alzheimer beta-protein into filaments. Nature **372**: 92–94.
10. WISNIEWSKI, T., E.M. CASTANO, A. GOLABEK, T. VOGEL & B. FRANTIONE. 1994. Acceleration of Alzheimer's fibril formation by apolipoprotein E *in vitro*. Am. J. Pathol. **145**: 1030–1035.
11. EVANS, K.C., E.P. BERGER, C.G. CHO, K.H. WEISGRABER & P.T. LANSBURY, JR. 1995. Apolipoprotein E is a kinetic but not a thermodynamic inhibitor of amyloid formation: implications for the pathogenesis and treatment of Alzheimer disease. Proc. Natl. Acad. Sci. USA **92**: 763–767.
12. WOOD, S.J., W. CHAN & R. WETZEL. 1996. Seeding of A-beta fibril formation is inhibited by all three isotypes of apolipoprotein E. Biochemistry **35**: 12623–12628.
13. NAIKI, H., F. HEJYO & K. NAKAKUKI. 1997. Concentration-dependent inhibitory effects of apolipoprotein E on Alzheimer's beta-amyloid fibril formation *in vitro*. Biochemistry **36**: 6243–6250.
14. JORDAN, J., M.F. GALINDO, R.J. MILLER, C.A. REARDON, G.S. GETZ & M.J. LADU. 1998. Isoform-specific effect of apolipoprotein E on cell survival and β-amyloid-

induced toxicity in rat hippocampal pyramidal neuronal cultures. Neuroscience **18**: 195–204.

15. QIU, Z., D.K. STRICKLAND, B.T. HYMAN & G.W. REBECK. 1999. α2-Macroglobulin enhances the clearance of endogenous soluble β-amyloid peptide via low-density lipoprotein receptor-related protein in cortical neurons. Neurochemistry **73**: 1393–1398.

16. LIAO, A., R.M. NITSCH, S.M. GREENBERG et al. 1998. Genetic association of an alpha2-macroglobulin (Val1000lle) polymorphism and Alzheimer's disease. Hum. Mol. Genet. **7**: 1953–1956.

17. BLACKER, D., M.A. WILCOX, N.M. LAIRD et al. 1998. Alpha-2 macroglobulin is genetically associated with Alzheimer disease. Nat. Genet. **19**: 357–360.

18. HOLLENBACH, E., S. ACKERMANN, B.T. HYMAN & G.W. REBECK. 1998. Confirmation of an association between a polymorphism in exon 3 of the low-density lipoprotein receptor-related protein gene and Alzheimer's disease. Neurology **50**: 1905–1907.

19. HSIAO, K., P. CHAPMAN, S. NILSEN et al. 1996. Correlative memory deficits, Aβ elevation and amyloid plaques in transgenic mice. Science **274**: 99–102.

20. IRIZARRY, M.C., M. MCNAMARA, K. FEDORCHAK, K. HSIAO & B.T. HYMAN. 1997. APP-Sw transgenic mice develop age related amyloid deposits and neuropil abnormalities, but no neuronal loss in CA1. J. Neuropathol. Exp. Neurol. **56**: 965–973.

21. CHAPMAN, P.F., G.L. WHITE, M.W. JONES et al. 1999. Impaired synaptic plasticity and learning in aged amyloid precursor protein transgenic mice. Nat. Neurosci. **2**: 271–276.

22. CHA, J.-H.J., et al. 2000. Glutamate receptor dysregulation in the hippocampus of transgenic mice carrying mutated human amyloid precursor protein. Neurobiol. Dis. In press.

23. GAMES, D., D. ADAMS, R. ALLESANDRINI et al. 1995. Alzheimer-type neuropathology in transgenic mice overexpressing V717F β-amyloid precursor protein. Nature **373**: 523–527.

24. MASLIAH, E., A. SISK, M. MALLORY, L. MUCKE, D. SCHENK & D. GAMES. 1996. Comparison of neurodegenerative pathology in transgenic mice overexpressing V717F β-amyloid precursor protein and Alzheimer's disease. J. Neurosci. **16**: 5795–5811.

25. IRIZARRY, M.C., F. SORIANO, M. MCNAMARA et al. 1997. Aβ deposition is associated with neuropil changes, but not with overt neuronal loss in the PDAPP transgenic mice. J. Neurosci. **17**: 7053–7059.

26. ARNOLD, S.E., B.T. HYMAN, J. FLORY, A.R. DAMASIO & G.W. VAN HOESEN. 1991. The topographical and neuroanatomical distribution of neurofibrillary tangles and neuritic plaques in the cerebral cortex of patients with Alzheimer's disease. Cereb. Cortex **1**: 103–116.

27. HYMAN, B.T., G.W. VAN HOESEN, L.J. KROMER & A.R. DAMASIO. 1986. Perforant pathway changes and the memory impairment of Alzheimer's disease. Ann. Neurol. **20**: 473–482.

28. HOLTZMAN, D.M. et al. 2000. Apolipoprotein E facilitates neuritic and cerebrovascular plaque formation in an Alzheimer's disease model. Ann. Neurol. **47**: 739–747.

29. BALES, K., T. VERINA, R.C. DODEL et al. 1997. Lack of apolipoprotein E dramatically reduces amyloid β-protein deposition. Nat. Genet. **17**: 263–265.

30. IRIZARRY, M.C. et al. 2000. Apolipoprotein E affects the amount, form, and anatomical distribution of Aβ deposition in homozygous APPV717F transgenic mice. Acta Neuropathol. **100**: 451–458.

The Value of Transgenic Models for the Study of Neurodegenerative Diseases

DONALD L. PRICE,[a,b,c,d,g] PHILIP C. WONG,[a] ALICJA L. MARKOWSKA,[a]
MICHAEL K. LEE,[a] GOPAL THINAKAREN,[f] DONALD W. CLEVELAND,[e]
SANGRAM S. SISODIA,[f] AND DAVID R. BORCHELT[a]

*Departments of [a]Pathology, [b]Neurology, and [c]Neuroscience and
[d]Division of Neuropathology, The Johns Hopkins University School of Medicine,
Baltimore, Maryland, USA*

[e]*Ludwig Institute, University of California San Diego, La Jolla, California, USA*

[f]*Department of Pharmacological and Physiological Sciences, The University of Chicago,
Chicago, Illinois, USA*

ABSTRACT: Transgenic animal models are useful in studying the features of
APP- and PS1-linked FAD and SOD1-linked FALS. These models help to investigate the nature of the cellular/biochemical/molecular alterations in neural tissue; the character and evolution of neuronal and/or glial abnormalities; the
ways mutant proteins cause damage to neurons; and the biochemical pathways
associated with cell death. New technologies will help to define changes in a
variety of genes/gene products and the events and conformational changes in
mutant proteins that are implicated in pathogenic cascades. It is hoped such
study will result in novel treatments for testing in transgenic models that can
then be translated into new treatments for human neurodegenerative diseases.

INTRODUCTION

The neurodegenerative diseases, including Alzheimer's disease (AD) and
amyotrophic lateral sclerosis (ALS), are a heterogeneous group of age-associated,
chronic illnesses which are among the most challenging and devastating diseases in
medicine.[1-6] Many of these diseases are characterized by onset in adult life, chronic
progressive course, distinct clinical phenotypes reflecting involvement of specific
populations of neurons, and distinct cellular abnormalities often associated with the
presence of intra- or extracellular protein aggregates. For the most part, we do not
fully understand many of the factors which influence age of onset or course of disease, the basis for the vulnerabilities of subsets of neurons, or the mechanisms leading to cell dysfunction/death in these different disorders. Treatments are
symptomatic and the vast majority of patients eventually become severely disabled
and die of intercurrent illnesses.

[g]Address for correspondence: Donald L. Price, M.D., Division of Neuropathology, The Johns
Hopkins University School of Medicine, 558 Ross Research Building, 720 Rutland Avenue,
Baltimore, Maryland 21205-2196. Tel.: (410) 955-5632; fax: (410) 955-9777.
e-mail: adrc@welchlink.welch.jhu.edu

Fortunately, major clues as to pathogenesis have come from genetic studies over the past several years. Although AD and ALS usually occur as sporadic illnesses, in some instances, these disorders are caused by mutations of specific genes. For example, familial AD (FAD) and familial ALS (FALS) may show autosomal dominant inheritance: mutant genes encoding either the amyloid precursor protein (APP) or presenilins (PS1 or PS2) cause some cases of FAD; and some cases of FALS are linked to mutations in the superoxide dismutase 1 (SOD1) gene. The identification of these mutations has allowed investigators using transfection and transgenic methods to introduce mutant genes into *in vitro* and *in vivo* systems and to examine some of the molecular and biochemical events leading to cellular abnormalities associated with the presence of mutant gene products. In some of the autosomal dominant genetic neurodegenerative disorders, the mutant proteins do not necessarily lose their normal functions, but rather acquire toxic properties or participate in the formation of toxic products.[1–7] At present, many of the biochemical steps in the pathways whereby mutant gene products, directly or indirectly, damage neural cells are not fully understood. However, strategies are now available to begin to define the participants in these pathological events in *in vitro* and *in vivo* model systems. In this review we illustrate, with highly selected examples from our laboratory, how some of these issues can begin to be approached using transgenic (Tg) and gene-targeted models and by mating strategies that introduce or remove specific genes.

ALZHEIMER'S DISEASE

Mutant Genes in FAD: APP and Presenilins

In some individuals, particularly those of early onset, the illness may be inherited in an autosomal dominant manner, and mutations in three different genes (i.e., APP, PS1, and PS2) have been shown to cause this phenotype.

APP

Localized to chromosome 21, this gene is alternatively spliced to mRNA encoding several APP species, which are typical type-I integral membrane glycoproteins with an N-terminal signal peptide; a large ectodomain with sites for N-glycosylation; an alternatively spliced Kunitz-type serine protease inhibitor (KPI) domain; an Aβ region (comprised of 28 amino acids of the ectodomain and 11–14 amino acids of the adjacent transmembrane domain); a single membrane-spanning helix; and a short cytoplasmic domain.[3,5] Some APP molecules are cleaved endoproteolytically within the Aβ sequence by APP "α-secretase," an activity with unusual properties,[8] to release the ectodomain of APP (APP^{s}α),[9,10] including residues 1–16 of Aβ, into the culture medium or into the CSF.[10,11] The cleavage of APP within the Aβ domain precludes the formation of Aβ. In contrast, Aβ is generated by pathways involving the endoproteolytic cleavage of APP by activities, termed "β-" and "γ-secretase," which generate the N- and C-termini of the Aβ peptide, respectively.[2,3,5,12–15] Aβ appears to be produced in endosomes or late Golgi or, in the case of Aβ$_{42}$, possibly in the endoplasmic reticulum.

APP isoforms are present in many types of cells, including neurons and, at lower levels, astrocytes. In neurons, APP is transported within axons by the fast anterograde system;[16,17] for example, in peripheral sensory neurons of rodents, APP-695 is the predominant isoform, and full-length APP-695 and, to a lesser extent, APP-751/770 are rapidly transported anterogradely in axons.[16,17] In the entorhinal cortex, newly synthesized APP, principally APP-695, is transported via the perforant pathway to accumulate at presynaptic terminals in the hippocampal formation.[18] In the terminal fields of the perforant pathway, soluble COOH-terminally truncated APP and amyloidogenic C-terminal fragments have been identified,[18] an observation consistent with the idea that neurons and their processes are one source of the APP that give rise to $A\beta$ species. This finding is also in accord with studies of APP Tg mice, aged monkeys, and humans with AD showing that $A\beta$ deposits are often located in proximity to neurites.[19,20]

A variety of APP mutations including APPswe (a double mutation at the N-terminal of $A\beta$) and APP-717 (near the C-terminal of $A\beta$) have been reported in cases of FAD.[21,22] Cells that express mutant APP show aberrant APP processing; levels of $A\beta$ are elevated (APPswe) or a higher fraction of longer $A\beta$ peptides is secreted (APP-717) relative to cells that express wild-type APP.[3,5,23,24]

PS1 and PS2

The genes which are localized to chromosomes 14 (PS1) and 1 (PS2), respectively, are highly homologous 43- to 50-kD polytopic proteins[25,26] that contain multiple transmembrane (TM) domains as well as a hydrophilic acidic "loop" region; the N-terminus, loop, and C-terminus of PS1 are oriented towards the cytoplasm.[25] Although PS1 is synthesized as a 42- to 43-kD polypeptide, the preponderant PS1-related species that accumulates *in vitro* and *in vivo* are 27- to 28-kD N-terminal and 16- to 17-kD C-terminal derivatives[27-29] that accumulate in a 1:1 stochiometry, are tightly regulated and saturable, and are stably associated. PS genes are widely expressed at low abundance in the central nervous system.

The PS1 gene has been reported to harbor >50 different FAD mutations in >80 families, whereas only a small number of mutations have been found in PS2.[30,31] The vast majority of the genetic abnormalities are missense mutations that result in single amino acid substitutions; a mutation that deletes exon 9 from PS1 has been identified in several different FAD families.

TRANSGENIC MODELS OF $A\beta$ AMYLOIDOGENESIS

To attempt to generate animal models of amyloidogenesis and $A\beta$-associated abnormalities, many groups have created Tg mice that express wild-type APP, APP fragments, $A\beta$, or FAD-linked mutant APP or PS1 transgenes. Although early efforts were disappointing because Tg mice did not exhibit any of the cellular abnormalities characteristic of AD, more recent work has shown that multiple lines of Tg mice now exist that show $A\beta$ deposits and neuritic plaques.[3]

Using a recently engineered PrP vector,[32] Dr. Borchelt and colleagues have produced two lines of mice that express the Mo/HuAPPswe transgene product at levels which are 2- to 3-fold higher than the level of endogenous Mo-APP. Levels of $A\beta_{40}$ and $A\beta_{42}$ in brain are increased and, by 18 months of age, these Mo/HuAPPswe Tg mice develop diffuse and compact $A\beta$ immunoreactive deposits in brain.[19] Many of the amyloid deposits are surrounded by enlarged dystrophic neurites and by glial cells. Preliminary cross-sectional behavioral studies on one line of mice made congenic by backcrossing to C57BL/6J mice suggest that the mice with APPswe mutations develop memory deficits. However, the mice do not show striking evidence of tau-related pathology. Along with mutant APP mice reported by others, these mice, although they do not model the full phenotype of AD, represent excellent models of Aβ amyloidogenesis.

Using these animals, we have studied the effects of introducing other genes. For example, Tg mice that coexpress mutant A246E HuPS1 and Mo/Hu-APPswe show an acceleration of the appearance of neuritic amyloid plaques in hippocampus and cortex.[19] Moreover, when APPswe Tg mice are mated with PS1 °E9 Tg mice, double Tg progeny show an even greater acceleration of Aβ deposition in cortex and hippocampus (Drs. Lee, Price, Sisodia, Borchelt, personal observations).

These mice, as well as others, showing Aβ amyloidogenesis will be of great value in testing antiamyloidogenics strategies, whether through the use of Aβ immunization,[33,34] inhibition of β- and γ-secretase involved in production of Aβ, etc.

GENE-TARGETED MICE

Gene targeting of APP and PS1 allows examination of the consequence of ablation of specific genes. APP$^{-/-}$ mice show only a subtle phenotype.[35] However, PS1$^{-/-}$ mice fail to survive beyond the early postnatal period and exhibit severe perturbations in the development of the axial skeleton and ribs;[36,37] these abnormal developmental patterns are highly reminiscent of somite segmentation defects described in mice with functionally inactivated Notch1 and Delta Dll1 (a Notch ligand).[38,39] PS1 deficiency appears to interfere with membrane trafficking in neurons.[40] Significantly, the levels of Aβ are reduced in brains of the PS1$^{-/-}$ embryos,[40,41] providing confirmation that PS1 influences directly or indirectly APP processing with ablation of PS1 leading to decrements in levels of Aβ and mutant PS1 elevating levels of Aβ. Both wild-type and mutant PS1 rescue the developmental phenotype of PS$^{-/-}$ mice.[42,43]

AMYOTROPHIC LATERAL SCLEROSIS

ALS, the most common adult-onset motor neuron disease, manifests as weakness and muscle atrophy with occasional spastic paralysis, reflecting the selective involvement of lower, and in some cases, upper motor neurons.[44] The neuropathological features of lower motor neurons include the hyperaccumulation of phosphorylated neurofilaments, intracellular inclusions that stain with antibodies to ubiquitin, intracytoplasmic inclusions resembling Lewy bodies, fragmented Golgi, attenuated dendrites, and swellings in proximal axonal segments filled with neurofilaments. Recent evidence suggests that degrading neurons go through a series of stages culminating in apoptosis.[45]

MUTANT GENES IN FALS: SOD1

Approximately 10% of amyotrophic lateral sclerosis (ALS) cases are familial, and, in almost all cases, inheritance exhibits an autosomal dominant pattern.[46] Approximately 15–20% of patients with autosomal dominant familial ALS (FALS) have missense point mutations in the gene that encodes cytosolic Cu/Zn superoxide dismutase 1 (SOD1),[47,48] the enzyme that catalyzes the conversion of $\cdot O^-_2$ to O_2 and H_2O_2.[49,50] To date, >50 different missense mutations and more than one frame shift mutation have been identified in the SOD1 gene;[51] the phenotypes associated with different mutations may show differences, but all result in motor neuron disease.[52]

In view of the extensive studies on free radical toxicity and the role of SOD1 in scavenging superoxide, investigators initially proposed that the lesions seen in SOD1-linked FALS could result from diminished free radical scavenging activity.[47] However, multiple lines of evidence fail to support this view, but are entirely consistent with the concept that FALS-linked mutations cause SOD1 to acquire toxic properties. The following observations are consistent with this idea: 1) SOD1-linked FALS is an autosomal dominant disease and no null mutations have been identified; 2) assays of mutant SOD1 activity in transfected cells indicate that, although some FALS mutations reduce the activity of SOD1, others retain near-normal levels of enzyme activity/stability;[53–55] 3) mutant SOD1 subunits do not appear to alter the metabolism/ activities of wild-type SOD1 in a dominant negative fashion;[56] 4) most FALS mutant SOD1 rescue the growth defects of SOD1-deficient yeast,[57] which are extremely sensitive to superoxide toxicity and fail to grow in normal atmosphere if lysine or methionine is removed from culture media; 5) the mutants show chaperone facilitated copper binding;[55,58] 6) mutant enzymes appear to exhibit enhanced ability to generate free radicals;[55] 7) SOD1 null mice do not develop a FALS-like syndrome;[59] and finally, 8) multiple lines of Tg mice expressing several different FALS-linked mutant SOD1 develop many of the clinical and pathological hallmarks of motor neuron disease.[1,60–64]

The molecular mechanisms by which mutant SOD1 causes motor neuron degeneration are not well understood. Initially, two not mutually exclusive hypotheses were proposed to explain the toxic properties acquired by the mutant SOD1: 1) the improperly folded mutant SOD1 catalyzes, via −OONO and nitronium intermediates, the nitration of tyrosines on proteins critical for the proper functions and viability of motor neruons; and 2) the mutant SOD1 possesses enhanced peroxidase activities that generate H_2O_2 and elevate levels of hydroxyl radicals that oxidize targets critical for motor nerve cells. Although these hypothesis have generated many experiments, the pathogenic mechanism and molecular targets of damage are still uncertain. However, an emerging view, consistent with recent experimental results,[65–67] is that the SOD1 mutations induce conformational changes in SOD1 and allow the participation of bound copper in deleterious chemistries that generate reactive molecules which can damage, perhaps via oxidation or nitration, a variety of cell constituents required for the maintenance and survival of motor neurons. Consistent with this idea is the finding that in both sporadic and familial ALS elevations occur in free nitrotyrosine and several markers of oxidative damage.[68,69] Copper can be very toxic,[70] and free copper is virtually absent in cytoplasm. It should be stressed that there is, as of yet, little experimental proof that copper bound to mutant

SOD1 plays a key role in the generation of toxicity. However, recent work in yeast has provided information critical for designing experiments to test this hypothesis. Studies in yeast and more recently mammalian cells indicate that delivery of copper to specific proteins is mediated through distinct intracellular pathways of copper trafficking,[71–73] which involves copper carriers (or metal ion chaperones). These soluble proteins, which deliver copper ion to specific intracellular proteins, ensure the proper intracellular transport and compartmentalization of this transition metal, and thus minimizes the potential toxicity of free ionic copper. Of particular interest in this context is copper chaperone superoxide dismutase (CCS), which delivers copper to SOD1 (see below). It should be emphasized that the copper toxicity hypothesis in SOD1-linked FALS involves copper bound to the mutant enzyme, and toxicity is not related to excess or reduced levels of copper as occurs in Wilson's disease or Menke's disease, respectively.[70,74] One experiment to test this hypothesis is described below.

MUTANT SOD1 TG MICE

With regard to FALS models, transgenic mice expressing a variety of mutant SOD1 develop progressive weakness and muscle atrophy with SOD1/ubiquitin immunoreactive cytoplasmic aggregates, irregularly enlarged dendrites, abnormalities of motor axons, and, eventually, Wallerian degeneration. The G37R mutant SOD1 Tg mice accumulate the G37R SOD1 to 3–12 × levels of endogenous SOD1 in the spinal cord;[64] the mutant SOD1 retains full specific activity. Levels of the mutant transgene product determine the age of onset. At 5–7 weeks of age (~2–3 months before the appearance of clinical signs), SOD1 accumulates in irregular swollen intraparenchymal portions of motor axons, the axonal cytoskeleton is abnormal, and vacuoles are present in these axons. Radiolabeling studies have demonstrated that both endogenous SOD1 and G37R SOD1 are transported anterogradely in axons,[75] and that transport is abnormal in these mutant SOD1 mice.[76,77] Thus, toxic SOD1 is transported anterogradely, accumulates early in the disease, and is associated with early structural pathology in axons.[75] Small vacuoles are also present in dendrites,[64] and some vacuoles appear to originate in the space between the outer and inner mitochondrial membranes with prominent distention of the outer mitochondrial membrane, displacement of the inner membrane, and disruption of the cristae. The dendritic abnormalities are reminiscent of excitotoxicity. The cell bodies of some neurons showed SOD1 and ubiquitin-immunoreactive inclusions and phosphorylated NF-H immunoreactivities. Axonal and dendritic abnormalities, as well as intracellular aggregates, occur prior to the onset of clinical signs, but once Wallerian degeneration is obvious, the mice usually have clinical signs. The number of motor neurons is reduced, and astrocytes are present in ventral horns.

These SOD1 mutant mice have been used for pharmacological and "genetic" therapeutic trials.[1,78–82] In the G93A, SOD1 Tg mice have been used to test a variety of therapeutic approaches. Vitamin E and selenium modestly delay both the onset and progression of disease without affecting survival; in contrast, riluzole and gabapentin do not influence the onset/progression but do increase survival slightly.[83] Oral administration of d-penicillamine, a copper chelator, significantly delays the onset of disease.[66] Overexpression of Bcl-2 in these Tg mice extends the survival of these mice, but the presence of the gene does not change the progression of the disease.[84] In a small group of G93A SOD1 mice overexpressing a dominant negative inhibitor of interleukin-1β converting enzyme, a cell death gene, there is a modest slowing of progression of disease.[79]

To test the role of neurofilaments in motor neuron disease caused by SOD1 mutations, Tg mice expressing G37R SOD1 were crossbred to: 1) Tg mice that accumulate NF-H-β-galactosidase fusion protein (NF-H-lacZ), a multivalent protein that crosslinks neurofilaments in neuronal perikarya and limits their export to axons;[85] and 2) Tg mice expressing human NF-H subunits.[86] In G37R SOD1 mice expressing NF-H-lacZ, NF are withheld from the axonal compartment, but the disease progress is not influenced,[87] implying that neither initiation nor progression of pathology requires an axonal NF cytoskeleton and that alterations in NF biology observed in some forms of motor neuron disease may be secondary responses.[87] By contrast, the expression of wt type human NF-H transgenes in the SOD1 mutant mice increased the mean life span of the G37R SOD1 mice; the singly G37R and the compound G37R;NF-H Tg mice, respectively, had a mean life expectancy of 9.5 ± 2.8 months ($n = 20$) and 15.8 ± 1.5 months ($n = 9$).[78] In contrast to the striking axonal degeneration observed in one-year-old Tg mice expressing G37R SOD1, the compound G37R;NF-H Tg littermates showed sparing of motor neurons.[78] The reasons for this protection of G37R SOD1 mice by increased levels of human NF-H are not known.

GENE TARGETING OF SOD1 AND CCS

$SOD1^{-/-}$ mice do not develop a FALS syndrome. As mentioned above, we have hypothesized that mutant SOD1 bound copper may play a role in toxicity. Until recently, it has not been possible to reduce levels of copper in SOD1. The discovery of CCS should allow investigators to test this hypothesis. CCS, whose protein domain/crystal structure has been determined,[88,89] has been shown to interact with both wild-type and FALS-linked mutant SOD1 and copper incorporation into these molecules is CCS dependent. Thus, CCS delivers copper to SOD1. Moreover, CCS is present in the nervous system, including upper and lower motor neurons.[90] Dr. P. Wong and colleagues have gene targeted CCS, and the phenotype in the CCS null mice resembles that of the $SOD1^{-/-}$ mice.[91] The mating of $CCS^{-/-}$ mice to mutant SOD1 mice will allow testing of the hypotheses that copper plays a role in the toxicity of mutant SOD1. If mutant SOD1 Tg mice lacking CCS fail to develop disease, it would strengthen the argument that copper chemistry plays a central role in the pathogenesis of disease in mutant SOD1 Tg mice, and would encourage investigators to design approaches to intervene in the CCS-SOD1 copper trafficking pathway as therapy for individuals with SOD1-linked FALS and, potentially, for other forms of motor neuron disease.

CONCLUSIONS

Transgenic strategies have allowed investigators to produce mice that recapitulate some, if not all, of the features of APP- and PS1-linked FAD and SOD1-linked FALS[1,3,6,7] as well as aspects of other neurodegenerative diseases.[4,92-95] These models are proving to be very useful in investigations of: the nature of the cellular/ biochemical/molecular alterations in neural tissue; the character and evolution of a variety of pathologies, particularly those neuronal and/or glial abnormalities associated with protein folding/aggregation and apoptosis; the mechanisms by which the mutant proteins cause damage to specific populations of neurons; and the biochemical pathways associated with dysfunction/death of cells. The emerging view is that each of the genetic forms of these diseases results because of the presence of the mutant proteins, in some instances improperly folded or aggregated, which directly or indirectly trigger pathogenic cascades that eventually affect the structure and function of subsets of neural cells. Ultimately, some of the affected nerve cells die. Complemented by *in vitro* investigations, future studies of transgenic animals, particularly those using inducible systems,[95–97] will further define some of the *in vivo* events occurring in models of these illnesses. Moreover, new technologies, including laser capture microscopy, array technologies, and structural biophysical methods, will help to define the changes in a variety of genes/gene products and the events and conformational changes in mutant proteins that are implicated in pathogenic cascades.[88,98–101] In turn, this information will provide insight into potential therapeutic targets that can be further evaluated by designing novel treatments for testing in transgenic models. The demonstration of efficacies in these model systems should then be rapidly translated into new treatments for these devastating human neurodegenerative disorders.

ACKNOWLEDGMENTS

The authors wish to thank our many colleagues at JHMI and other institutions for their contributions to some of the original work cited in this review and for helpful discussions. Aspects of this work were supported by grants from the U.S. Public Health Service (AG05146, AG07914, AG14248, NS07435, NS37145) as well as the Metropolitan Life Foundation, American Health Assistance Foundation, Hereditary Disease Foundation, Adler Foundation, and Bristol-Myers Squibb.

REFERENCES

1. CLEVELAND, D.W. 1999. From charcot to SOD1: mechanisms of selective motor neuron death in ALS. Neuron **24:** 515–520.
2. HARDY, J. & K. GWINN-HARDY. 1998. Genetic classification of primary neurodegenerative disease. Science **282:** 1075–1079.
3. PRICE, D.L., R.E. TANZI, D.R. BORCHELT & S.S. SISODIA. 1998. Alzheimer's disease: genetic studies and transgenic models. Annu. Rev. Genet. **32:** 461–493.
4. SCHILLING, G., M.W. BECHER, A.H. SHARP *et al.* 1999. Intranuclear inclusions and neuritic pathology in transgenic mice expressing a mutant N-terminal fragment of huntingtin. Hum. Mol. Genet. **8:** 397–407.
5. SELKOE, D. 1999. Translating cell biology into therapeutic advances in Alzheimer's disease. Nature **399:** A23–A31.
6. WONG, P.C., J.D. ROTHSTEIN & D.L. PRICE. 1998. The genetic and molecular mechanisms of motor neuron disease. Curr. Opin. Neurobiol. **8:** 791–799.
7. PRICE, D.L., S.S. SISODIA & D.R. BORCHELT. 1998. Genetic neurodegenerative diseases: the human illness and transgenic models. Science **282:** 1079–1083.

8. SISODIA, S.S. 1992. β-amyloid precursor protein cleavage by a membrane-bound protease. Proc. Natl. Acad. Sci. USA **89:** 6075–6079.
9. ESCH, F.S., P.S. KEIM, E.C. BEATTIE *et al.* 1990. Cleavage of amyloid β peptide during constitutive processing of its precursor. Science **248:** 1122–1124.
10. SISODIA, S.S., E.H. KOO, K. BEYREUTHER *et al.* 1990. Evidence that β-amyloid protein in Alzheimer's disease is not derived by normal processing. Science **248:** 492–495.
11. WEIDEMANN, A., G. KÖNIG, D. BUNKE *et al.* 1989. Identification, biogenesis, and localization of precursors of Alzheimer's disease A4 amyloid protein. Cell **57:** 115–126.
12. HARDY, J. & A. ISRAËL. 1999. Alzheimer's disease: in search of γ-secretase. Nature **398:** 466–467.
13. SINHA, S., J.P. ANDERSON, R. BARBOUR *et al.* 1999. Purification and cloning of amyloid precursor protein beta-secretase from human brain. Nature **402:** 537–540.
14. VASSAR, R., B.D. BENNETT, S. BABU-KHAN *et al.* 1999. β-Secretase cleavage of Alzheimer's amyloid precusor protein by the transmembrane aspartic protease BACE. Science **286:** 735–741.
15. YAN, R., M.J. BLENKOWSKI, M.E. SHUCK *et al.* 1999. Membrane-anchored aspartyl protease with Alzheimer's disease beta-secretase activity. Nature **402:** 533–537.
16. KOO, E.H., S.S. SISODIA, D.R. ARCHER *et al.* 1990. Precursor of amyloid protein in Alzheimer disease undergoes fast anterograde axonal transport. Proc. Natl. Acad. Sci. USA **87:** 1561–1565.
17. SISODIA, S.S., E.H. KOO, P.N. HOFFMAN *et al.* 1993. Identification and transport of full-length amyloid precursor proteins in rat peripheral nervous system. J. Neurosci. **13:** 3136–3142.
18. BUXBAUM, J.D., G. THINAKARAN, V. KOLIATSOS *et al.* 1998. Alzheimer amyloid protein precursor in the rat hippocampus: transport and processing through the perforant path. J. Neurosci. **18:** 9629–9637.
19. BORCHELT, D.R., T. RATOVITSKI, J. VAN LARE *et al.* 1997. Accelerated amyloid deposition in the brains of transgenic mice co-expressing mutant presenilin 1 and amyloid precursor proteins. Neuron **19:** 939–945.
20. MARTIN, L.J., S.S. SISODIA, E.H. KOO *et al.* 1991. Amyloid precursor protein in aged nonhuman primates. Proc. Natl. Acad. Sci. USA **88:** 1461–1465.
21. GOATE, A., M.-C. CHARTIER-HARLIN, M. MULLAN *et al.* 1991. Segregation of a missense mutation in the amyloid precursor protein gene with familial Alzheimer's disease. Nature **349:** 704–706.
22. MULLAN, M., F. CRAWFORD, K. AXELMAN *et al.* 1992. A pathogenic mutation for probable Alzheimer's disease in the APP gene at the N-terminus of β-amyloid. Nat. Genet. **1:** 345–347.
23. CITRON, M., T. OLTERSDORF, C. HAASS *et al.* 1992. Mutation of the β-amyloid precursor protein in familial Alzheimer's disease increases β-protein production. Nature **360:** 672–674.
24. SUZUKI, N., T.T. CHEUNG, X.-D. CAI *et al.* 1994. An increased percentage of long amyloid β protein secreted by familial amyloid β protein precursor (βAPP$_{717}$) mutants. Science **264:** 1336–1340.
25. DOAN, A., G. THINAKARAN, D.R. BORCHELT *et al.* 1996. Protein topology of presenilin 1. Neuron **17:** 1023–1030.
26. SHERRINGTON, R., E.I. ROGAEV, Y. LIANG *et al.* 1995. Cloning of a gene bearing missense mutations in early-onset familial Alzheimer's disease. Nature **375:** 754–760.
27. LEE, M.K., H.H. SLUNT, L.J. MARTIN *et al.* 1996. Expression of presenilin 1 and 2 (PS1 and PS2) in human and murine tissues. J. Neurosci. **16:** 7513–7525.
28. PODLISNY, M.B., M. CITRON, P. AMARANTE *et al.* 1997. Presenilin proteins undergo heterogeneous endoproteolysis between Thr$_{291}$ and Ala$_{299}$ and occur as stable N- and C-terminal fragments in normal and Alzheimer brain tissue. Neurobiol. Dis. **3:** 325–337.
29. THINAKARAN, G., D.R. BORCHELT, M.K. LEE *et al.* 1996. Endoproteolysis of presenilin 1 and accumulation of processed derivatives *in vivo*. Neuron **17:** 181–190.
30. CRUTS, M. C.M. VAN DUIJN, H. BACKHOVENS *et al.* 1998. Estimation of the genetic contribution of presenilin-1 and -2 mutations in a population-based study of presenile Alzheimer disease. Hum. Mol. Genet. **71:** 43–51.

31. HARDY, J. 1997. Amyloid, the presenilins and Alzheimer's disease. Trends Neurosci. **20:** 154–159.
32. BORCHELT, D.R., J. DAVIS, M. FISCHER et al. 1997. A vector for expressing foreign genes in the brains and hearts of transgenic mice. Genet. Anal. (Biomed. Eng.) **13:** 159–163.
33. SCHENK, D., R. BARBOUR, W. DUNN et al. 1999. Immunization with amyloid-beta attenuates Alzheimer-disease-like pathology in the PDAPP mouse. Nature **400:** 173–177.
34. ST. GEORGE-HYSLOP, P.H. & D.A. WESTAWAY. 1999. Antibody clears senile plaques. Nature **400:** 116–117.
35. ZHENG, H., M.-H. JIANG, M.E. TRUMBAUER et al. 1995. β-Amyloid precursor protein-deficient mice show reactive gliosis and decreased locomotor activity. Cell **81:** 525–531.
36. SHEN, J., R.T. BRONSON, D.F. CHEN et al. 1997. Skeletal and CNS defects in *presenilin-1*-deficient mice. Cell **89:** 629–639.
37. WONG, P.C., H. ZHENG, H. CHEN et al. 1997. Presenilin 1 is required for *Notch1* and *Dll1* expression in the paraxial mesoderm. Nature **387:** 288–292.
38. CONLON, R.A., A.G. REAUME & J. ROSSANT. 1995. *Notch 1* is required for the coordinate segmentation of somites. Development **121:** 1533–1545.
39. HRABE DE ANGELIS, M., J. MCINTYRE & A. GOSSLER. 1997. Maintenance of somite borders in mice requires the *Delta* homologue *Dll1*. Nature **386:** 717–721.
40. NARUSE, S., G. THINAKARAN, J.-J. LUO et al. 1998. Effects of PS1 deficiency on membrane protein trafficking in neurons. Neuron **21:** 1213–1221.
41. DE STROOPER, B., P. SAFTIG, K. CRAESSAERTS et al. 1998. Deficiency of presenilin-1 inhibits the normal cleavage of amyloid precursor protein. Nature **391:** 387–390.
42. DAVIS, J.A., S. NARUSE, H. CHEN et al. 1998. An Alzheimer's disease-linked PS1 variant rescues the developmental abnormalities of *PS1*-deficient embryos. Neuron **20:** 603–609.
43. QIAN, S., P. JIANG, X. GUAN et al. 1998. Mutant human presenilin 1 protects presenilin 1 null mouse against embryonic lethality and elevates $A\beta_{1-42/43}$ expression. Neuron **20:** 611–617.
44. ROWLAND, L.P. 1994. Natural history and clinical features of amyotrophic lateral sclerosis and related motor neuron diseases. *In* Neurodegenerative Diseases. D.B. Calne, Ed.: 507–521. W.B. Saunders. Philadelphia.
45. MARTIN, L.J. 1999. Neuronal death in amyotrophic lateral sclerosis is apoptosis: possible contribution of a programmed cell death mechanism. J. Neuropathol. Exp. Neurol. **58:** 459–471.
46. BROWN, R.H., JR. 1997. Amyotrophic lateral sclerosis: insights from genetics. Arch. Neurol. **4:** 1246–1250.
47. DENG, H.-X., A. HENTATI, J.A. TAINER et al. 1993. Amyotrophic lateral sclerosis and structural defects in Cu,Zn superoxide dismutase. Science **261:** 1047–1051.
48. ROSEN, D.R., T. SIDDIQUE, D. PATTERSON et al. 1993. Mutations in Cu/Zn superoxide dismutase gene are associated with familial amyotrophic lateral sclerosis. Nature **362:** 59–62.
49. FRIDOVICH, I. 1986. Superoxide dismutases. Adv. Enzymol. Relat. Areas Mol. Biol. **58:** 61–97.
50. STADTMAN, E.R. 1992. Protein oxidation and aging. Science **257:** 1220–1224.
51. WONG, P.C. & D.R. BORCHELT. 1995. Motor neuron disease caused by mutations in superoxide dismutase 1. Curr. Opin. Neurol. **8:** 294–301.
52. CUDKOWICZ, M.E., D. MCKENNA-YASEK, C. CHEN et al. 1998. Limited corticospinal tract involvement in amyotrophic lateral sclerosis subjects with the A4V mutation in the copper/zinc superoxide dismutase gene. Ann. Neurol. **43:** 703–710.
53. BORCHELT, D.R. M.K. LEE, H.H. SLUNT et al. 1994. Superoxide dismutase 1 with mutations linked to familial amyotrophic lateral sclerosis possesses significant activity. Proc. Natl. Acad. Sci. USA **91:** 8292–8296.
54. BOWLING, A.C., J.B. SCHULZ, R.H. BROWN, JR. & M.F. BEAL. 1993. Superoxide dismutase activity, oxidative damage, and mitochondrial energy metabolism in familial and sporadic amyotrophic lateral sclerosis. J. Neurochem. **61:** 2322–2325.
55. YIM, M.B., J.H. KANG, H.S. YIM et al. 1996. A gain-of-function of an amyotrophic lateral sclerosis-associated Cu,Zn-superoxide dismutase mutant: an enhancement of

free radical formation due to a decrease in K_m for hydrogen peroxide. Proc. Natl. Acad. Sci. USA **93:** 5709–5714.

56. BORCHELT, D.R., M. GUARNIERI, P.C. WONG *et al.* 1995. Superoxide dismutase 1 subunits with mutations linked to familial amyotrophic lateral sclerosis do not affect wild-type subunit function. J. Biol. Chem. **270:** 3234–3238.

57. RABIZADEH, S., E.B. GRALLA, D.R. BORCHELT *et al.* 1995. Mutations associated with amyotrophic lateral sclerosis convert superoxide dismutase from an antiapoptotic gene to a proapoptotic gene: studies in yeast and neural cells. Proc. Natl. Acad. Sci. USA **92:** 3024–3028.

58. CORSON, L.B., V.C. CULOTTA & D.W. CLEVELAND. 1998. Chaperone-facilitated copper binding is a property common to several classes of familial amyotrophic lateral sclerosis-linked superoxide dismutase mutants. Proc. Natl. Acad. Sci. USA **95:** 6361–6366.

59. REAUME, A.G., J.L. ELLIOTT, E.K. HOFFMAN *et al.* 1996. Motor neurons in Cu/Zn superoxide dismutase-deficient mice develop normally but exhibit enhanced cell death after axonal injury. Nat. Genet. **13:** 43–47.

60. BRUIJN, L.I., M.W. BECHER, M.K. LEE *et al.* 1997. ALS-linked SOD1 mutant G85R mediates damage to astrocytes and promotes rapidly progressive disease with SOD1-containing inclusions. Neuron **18:** 327–338.

61. DAL CANTO, M.C. & M.E. GURNEY. 1994. Development of central nervous system pathology in a murine transgenic model of human amyotrophic lateral sclerosis. Am. J. Pathol. **145:** 1271–1280.

62. GURNEY, M.E., H. PU, A.Y. CHIU *et al.* 1994. Motor neuron degeneration in mice that express a human Cu,Zn superoxide dismutase mutation. Science **264:** 1772–1775.

63. RIPPS, M.E., G.W. HUNTLEY, P.R. HOF *et al.* 1995. Transgenic mice expressing an altered murine superoxide dismutase gene provide an animal model of amyotrophic lateral sclerosis. Proc. Natl. Acad. Sci. USA **92:** 689–693.

64. WONG, P.C., C.A. PARDO, D.R. BORCHELT *et al.* 1995. An adverse property of a familial ALS-linked SOD1 mutation causes motor neuron disease characterized by vacuolar degeneration of mitochondria. Neuron **14:** 1105–1116.

65. BRUIJN, L.I., M.F. BEAL, M.W. BECHER *et al.* 1997. Elevated free nitrotyrosine levels, but not protein-bound nitrotyrosine or hydroxyl radicals, throughout amyotrophic lateral sclerosis (ALS)-like disease implicate tyrosine nitration as an aberrant *in vivo* property of one familial ALS-linked superoxide dismutase 1 mutant. Proc. Natl. Acad. Sci. USA **94:** 7606–7611.

66. HOTTINGER, A.F., E.G. FINE, M.E. GURNEY *et al.* 1997. The copper chelator *d*-penicillamine delays onset of disease and extends survival in a transgenic mouse model of familial amyotrophic lateral sclerosis. Eur. J. Neurosci. **9:** 1548–1551.

67. WIEDAU-PAZOS, M., J.J. GOTO, S. RABIZADEH *et al.* 1996. Altered reactivity of superoxide dismutase in familial amyotrophic lateral sclerosis. Science **271:** 515–518.

68. BEAL, M.F., R.J. FERRANTE, S.E. BROWNE *et al.* 1997. Increased 3-nitrotyrosine in both sporadic and familial amyotrophic lateral sclerosis. Ann. Neurol **42:** 646–654.

69. FERRANTE, R.J., S.E. BROWNE, L.A. SHINOBU *et al.* 1997. Evidence of increased oxidative damage in both sporadic and familial amyotrophic lateral sclerosis. J. Neurochem. **69:** 2064–2074.

70. WAGGONER, D.J., T.B. BARTNIKAS & J.D. GITLIN. 1999. The role of copper in neurodegenerative disease. Neurobiol. Dis. **6:** 221–230.

71. CULOTTA, V.C., L.W.J. KLOMP, J. STRAIN *et al.* 1997. The copper chaperone for superoxide dismutase. J. Biol. Chem. **272:** 23469–23472.

72. PUFAHL, R.A., C.P. SINGER, K.L. PEARISO *et al.* 1997. Metal ion chaperone function of the soluble Cu(I) receptor Atx1. Science **278:** 853–856.

73. VALENTINE, J.S. & E.B. GRALLA. 1997. Delivering copper inside yeast and human cells. Science **278:** 817–818.

74. HARRIS, Z.L. & J.D. GITLIN. 1996. Genetic and molecular basis for copper toxicity. Am. J. Clin. Nutr. **63:** 836S–341S.

75. BORCHELT, D.R., P.C. WONG, M.W. BECHER *et al.* 1998. Axonal transport of mutant superoxide dismutase 1 and focal axonal abnormalities in the proximal axons of transgenic mice. Neurobiol. Dis. **5:** 27–35.

76. WILLIAMSON, T.L. & D.W. CLEVELAND. 1999. Slowing of axonal transport is a very early event in the toxicity of ALS-linked SOD1 mutants to motor neurons. Nat. Neurosci. **2**: 50–56.
77. ZHANG, B., P.-H. TU, F. ABTAHIAN *et al.* 1997. Neurofilaments and orthograde transport are reduced in ventral root axons of transgenic mice that express human SOD1 with a G93A mutation. J. Cell Biol. **139**: 1307–1315.
78. COUILLARD-DESPRÉS, S., Q. ZHU, P.C. WONG *et al.* 1998. Protective effect of neurofilament NF-H overexpression in motor neuron disease induced by mutant superoxide dismutase. Proc. Natl. Acad. Sci. USA **95**: 9626–9630.
79. FRIEDLANDER, R.M., R.H. BROWN, V. GAGLIARDINI *et al.* 1997. Inhibition of ICE slows ALS in mice. Nature **388**: 31.
80. JULIEN, J.-P. 1999. Neurofilament functions in health and disease. Curr. Opin. Neurobiol. **9**: 554–560.
81. KLIVENYI, P., R.J. FERRANTE, R.T. MATTHEWS *et al.* 1999. Neuroprotective effects of creatine in a transgenic animal model of amyotrophic lateral sclerosis. Nat. Med. **5**: 347–350.
82. PASINELLI, P., D.R. BORCHELT, M.K. HOUSEWEART *et al.* 1998. Caspase-1 is activated in neural cells and tissue with amyotrophic lateral sclerosis-associated mutations in copper-zinc superoxide dismutase. Neurobiology **95**: 15763–15768.
83. GURNEY, M.E., F.B. CUTTINGS, P. ZHAI *et al.* 1996. Benefit of vitamin E, riluzole, and gabapentin in a transgenic model of familial amyotrophic lateral sclerosis. Ann. Neurol. **39**: 147–157.
84. KOSTIC, V., V. JACKSON-LEWIS, F. DE BILBAO *et al.* 1997. Bcl-2: prolonging life in a transgenic mouse model of familial amyotrophic lateral sclerosis. Science **277**: 559–562.
85. EYER, J. & A. PETERSON. 1994. Neurofilament-deficient axons and perikaryal aggregates in viable transgenic mice expressing a neurofilament-β-galactosidase fusion protein. Neuron **12**: 389–405.
86. CÔTÉ, F., J.-F. COLLARD & J.-P. JULIEN. 1993. Progressive neuronopathy in transgenic mice expressing the human neurofilament heavy gene: a mouse model of amyotrophic lateral sclerosis. Cell **73**: 35-46.
87. EYER, J., D.W. CLEVELAND, P.C. WONG & A.C. PETERSON. 1998. Pathogenesis of two axonopathies does not require axonal neurofilaments. Nature **391**: 584–587.
88. LAMB, A.L., A.K. WERNIMONT, R.A. PUFAHL *et al.* 1999. Crystal structure of the copper chaperone for superoxide dismutase. Nat. Struct. Biol. **6**: 724–729.
89. SCHMIDT, P.J., T.D. RAE, R.A. PUFAHL *et al.* 1999. Multiple protein domains contribute to the action of the copper chaperone for superoxide dismutase. J. Biol. Chem. **274**: 23719–23725.
90. ROTHSTEIN, J.D., M. DYKES-HOBERG, L.B. CORSON *et al.* 1999. The copper chaperone CCS is abundant in neurons and astrocytes in human and rodent brain. J. Neurochem. **72**: 422–429.
91. WONG, P.C., D. WAGGONER, J. SUBRAMANIAM *et al.* 2000. Copper chaperone for superoxide dismutase is essential to activate mammalian Cu/Zn superoxide dismutase. Proc. Natl. Acad. Sci. USA **97**: 2886–2891.
92. ISHIHARA, Y., M. HONG, B. ZHANG *et al.* 1999. Age-dependent emergence and progression of a taupathy in transgenic mice overexpressing the shortest human tau isoform. Neuron **24**: 751–762.
93. LEE, V.M.-Y. & J.Q. TROJANOWSKI. 1999. Neurodegenerative taupathies: human disease and transgenic mouse models. Neuron **24**: 507–510.
94. LIN, X., C.J. CUMMINGS & H.Y. ZOGHBI. 1999. Expanding our understanding of polyglutamine diseases through mouse models. Neuron **24**: 499–502.
95. TREMBLAY, P., Z. MEINER, M. GALOU *et al.* 2000. Doxycycline control of prion protein transgene expression modulates prion disease in mice. Proc. Natl. Acad. Sci. USA **95**: 12580–12585.
96. GINGRICH, J.R. & J. RODER. 1998. Inducible gene expression in the nervous system of transgenic mice. Annu. Rev. Neurosci. **21**: 377–405.
97. MANSUY, I.M., D.G. WINDER, T.M. MOALLEM *et al.* 1998. Inducible and reversible gene expression with the rtTA system for the study of memory. Neuron **21**: 257–265.

98. FEND, F., M.R. EMMERT-BUCK, R. CHUAQUI *et al.* 1999. Immuno-LCM: laser capture microdissection of immunostained frozen sections for mRNA analysis. Am. J. Pathol. **154:** 61–66.

99. FINK, L., W. SEEGER, L. ERMERT *et al.* 1998. Real-time quantitative RT-PCR after laser-assisted cell picking. Nat. Med. **4:** 1329–1333.

100. LUO, L., R.C. SALUNGA, H. GUO *et al.* 1999. Gene expression profiles of laser-capture adjacent neuronal subtypes. Nat. Med. **5:** 117–122.

101. SIMONE, N.L., R.F. BONNER, J.W. GILLESPIE *et al.* 1998. Laser-capture microdissection: opening the microscopic frontier to molecular anaysis. Trends Genet. **14:** 272–276.

Identifying Proteases That Cleave APP

MARTIN CITRON[a]

Department of Neuroscience, Amgen Inc., Thousand Oaks, California 91320, USA

BACKGROUND

When the sequence of the amyloid precursor protein was published more than 12 years ago,[1] it became immediately clear that the amyloid β-peptide (Aβ), the main constituent of the amyloid plaques in Alzheimer's disease, is part of a large precursor protein. Theoretically, the N-terminus of Aβ could be derived from the APP gene by two mechanisms: by internal translation from the methionine immediately before the first amino acid of the Aβ-peptide,[2] or by proteolytic cleavage by enzyme(s) termed β-secretase. While no evidence for the internal translation hypothesis has been found,[3] numerous lines of evidence demonstrate that β-secretase cleavage of APP is required for Aβ generation, for example, the aminoterminal soluble form of APP (APPsβ) predicted to arise from β-secretase cleavage of the APP has been detected,[4] and protease inhibitor-like compounds have been shown to affect β-secretase cleavage products. Generation of the N-terminus is followed by C-terminal cleavage by enzyme(s) termed γ-secretase to release the final Aβ-product from the β-secretase cleavage fragment C99 (FIG. 1). In addition to this amyloidogenic pathway, APP can also undergo nonamyloidogenic processing by α-secretase, which cleaves APP within the Aβ domain to generate APPsα (the ectodomain of APP ending at the α-secretase cleavage site) and C83 (the C-terminal tail of APP). C83 can then undergo γ-secretase cleavage leading to the release of p3, a shortened form of Aβ (FIG. 1). Finally, it is important to keep in mind that only a minority of APP molecules enters the α- or β-secretase cleavage pathway, but the majority is degraded in the endoplasmic reticulum.[5]

THE PROBLEM

As evidence for a seminal role of Aβ in Alzheimer's disease pathogenesis has accumulated, it has become clear that blocking Aβ production promises therapeutic benefit for Alzheimer's disease. Proteases are considered good drug targets, and therefore the development of inhibitors of Aβ generating proteases is one of the top priorities in the development of Alzheimer's disease modifying agents. Obviously, the more information about a protease is available, the better inhibitors can be generated. Ideally, one would like to have the pure active enzyme available for rapid screening and high resolution structural information data to rationally design inhibitors. This approach has been successfully used for the HIV protease inhibitors

[a]Address for correspondence: Martin Citron, Department of Neuroscience, Amgen Inc., One Amgen Center Drive, Thousand Oaks, CA 91320. Tel.: (805) 447-4520; fax: (805) 480-1347. e-mail: mcitron@amgen.com

that have been launched as AIDS drugs. However, the complex proteolytic machinery that processes APP is not completely understood. It is not even known how many enzymes are involved. First, there are the three broad classes of activities, α-, β- and γ-secretases, and one would focus on inhibiting β- and/or γ-secretases while leaving the nonamyloidogenic α-secretase untouched. But even within one category there may be multiple different enzymes which cleave either at the exact same site or within a few amino acids distance. For example, it has been proposed, but not proven, that the two γ-secretase cleavages at amino acid 40 and amino acid 42 are made by different enzymes[6,7] and that even for just the 42 cleavage multiple activities are involved.[8] How would one isolate a secretase candidate enzyme? How would one know which enzymes are really important?

SOURCES OF CANDIDATE ENZYMES

Proposing Candidates from the Literature

A number of human proteases are known from the biochemical literature and are already available in pure form. Some of these candidates can under the right conditions cleave APP or synthetic fragments thereof close to or at the α-, β- and γ-secretase cleavage sites *in vitro*. This method of identifying candidates does not require much work and thus can beat all other experimental approaches in terms of speed. The obvious limitation is that only already known proteins are promoted to further analysis.

Biochemical Purification

Because proteases within the brain cleave APP to produce Aβ, one should be able to purify the relevant enzymes from brain extracts using APP or fragments thereof as test substrates. This method should cover unknown enzymes, but has some major intrinsic disadvantages. The necessary tissue homogenization destroys the subcellular compartmentalization leading to the release of various proteases that may be capable of cleaving APP *in vitro*, but not in intact cells. Furthermore, an *in vitro* assay that is simple but reflects the structure of the cleavage site within the large APP protein must be developed or the effort is doomed from the start. Finally, major work may be involved in cloning the candidate genes from enriched preparations of enzymatic activity. These first two methods have dominated the secretase field until very recently.

Expression Cloning

This method is based on the idea that transient overexpression of a secretase should increase proteolytic processing of APP by the overexpressed enzyme, leading to the release of APP metabolites that can be monitored to track the overexpressed secretase. This method covers unknown enzymes and tracks activity in intact cells on the native substrate, thus avoiding the artifacts of the biochemical purification method. In addition, the separate cloning effort is not necessary. However, the approach is technically demanding, laborious, and based on the assumption that overexpression of a secretase—in the presence of the normal cellular APP processing

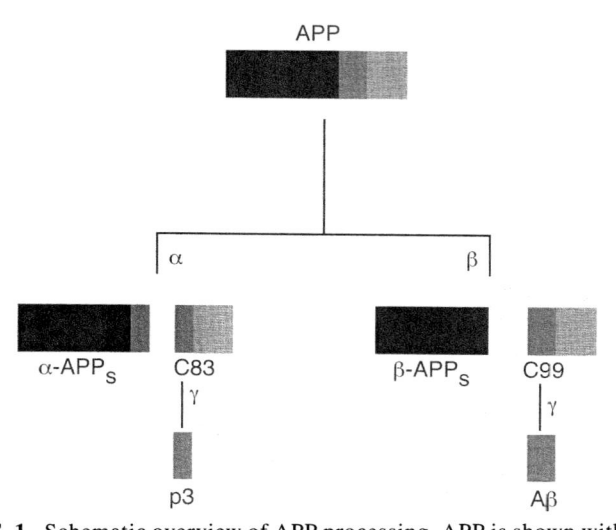

FIGURE 1. Schematic overview of APP processing. APP is shown with the large N-terminal ectodomain in *black*, the Aβ region in *gray*, and the C-terminus in *light gray* (not drawn to scale). APP can be processed by α-secretase to yield secreted α-APPs and the membrane bound C83 fragment or by β-secretase to yield β-APPs and the membrane bound C99 fragment. These membrane bound fragments can each undergo γ-secretase cleavage to give rise to the secreted fragments Aβ and p3.

machinery including the candidate—will impact APP processing. The method has not been widely used to identify secretases.

Genomic Approach

With the advent of large scale sequencing of human genes comes the possibility of just testing all new human proteases for secretase activity. Because the sequence of the proteases is available from the start, the cloning is easier than in the biochemical purification method, but the genomic method fails if the desired secretase does not look like a typical protease, or if its gene has not been sequenced yet. This method will play an increasingly important role as more and more sequence information becomes available.

VALIDATION OF CANDIDATE ENZYMES

All the methods listed above may lead to candidate proteases that have at least some properties expected of a secretase enzyme. A complete validation of the candidate enzymes then becomes critical and rate limiting. One should not stop the validation process once a candidate has fullfilled just one or two liberal criteria, e.g., *in vitro* cleavage around the expected site, but rather go all the way and match as many properties of the enzyme as possible. Some criteria are less important than others, for example, the exact subcellular localization of a secretase activity may be hard to predict, so one should not exclude a candidate just because it is found in more sub-cellular compartments than predicted; however, candidate enzymes that are exclusively cytoplasmic can be ruled out for α-, β-, and γ-secretase. Another criterion holding for all three enzyme classes is that they should be widely expressed and constitutively active. For β-secretase high neuronal expression was predicted, but for γ-secretase it is not known whether activity in neurons would be necessarily higher than expression in other cell types.

When we validated our β-secretase candidate BACE,[9] we used a validation "funnel" that allows to rapidly narrow down the number of candidate genes. A similar set of criteria could be proposed for γ-secretase candidate testing. Candidates are sequentially put through the various tests. The tests are not necessarily sorted by increasing rigor, but by throughput such that easy assays with high throughput weed out most of the candidates and only very few enzymes make it to the low throughput validation steps that require a lot of work. The inclusion of high throughput assays is critical for genomic or expression cloning approaches which start out with a huge number of candidate genes.

We began by expressing 860,000 clones in pools of 100 and searched for those genes that caused increased $A\beta_{42}$ or $A\beta_{42}/A\beta_{40}$ upon transient transfection. Next we excluded genes that also increased APPsα production, arguing that such genes would not be specific for the amyloidogenic pathway. Obviously, β-secretase candidates should lead to increased APPsβ production. At this point we had to move to a low throughput mode in which nonautomated bench type experiments with a turn-around time of several days to a few months were used to make the case that BACE is β-secretase. These experiments included: demonstration that BACE overexpression leads to increased C99 levels, while full-length APP is unaffected; proof that overexpressed BACE causes cleavage exactly and only at the known sites of β-secretase cleavage; and demonstration that BACE has the same P1 specificity as β-secretase. To directly demonstrate the right protease activity, one needs to prove that the purified enzyme cleaves a pure substrate at the right position, a criterion that BACE fulfilled. A similar *in vitro* experiment would be required to conclude that a candidate gene is γ-secretase. Finally, we had to show that BACE is not just capable of but required for β-secretase cleavage. The most complete demonstration would require gene targeting in an animal model of Aβ formation, but because this ultimate validation experiment would take more than a year, we used as an approximation an antisense transfection study which convincingly demonstrated that at least in the 293 cell line model BACE is required for β-secretase cleavage.

The identification of BACE as the major β-secretase will now allow more rapid β-secretase inhibitor development. Moreover, a paradigm for secretase validation has been established that could be easily adapted for γ-secretase candidates.

REFERENCES

1. KANG, J., H.-G. LEMAIRE, A. UNTERBECK *et al*. 1987. The precursor of Alzheimer's disease amyloid A4 protein resembles a cell-surface receptor. Nature **325:** 733–736.
2. BREIMER, L.H., & P. DENNY. 1987. Alzheimer amyloid aspects. Nature **326:** 749–750.
3. CITRON, M., C. HAASS & D. SELKOE. 1993. Production of amyloid β-peptide by cultured cells: no evidence for internal initiation of translation at Met_{596}. Neurobiol. Aging **14:** 571–573.

4. SEUBERT, P., T. OLTERSDORF, M.G. LEE et al. 1993. Secretion of β-amyloid precursor protein cleaved at the amino-terminus of the β-amyloid peptide. Nature **361:** 260–263.
5 KUENTZEL, S.L., S.M. ALI, R.A. ALTMAN et al. 1993. The Alzheimer β-amyloid protein precursor/protease nexin-II is cleaved by secretase in a trans-Golgi secretory compartment in human neuroglioma cells. Biochem. J. **295:** 367–378.
6. CITRON, M., T.S. DIEHL, T. GORDON et al. 1996. Evidence that $A\beta_{42}$ and $A\beta_{40}$ are generated from the β-amyloid precursor protein by different protease activities. Proc. Natl. Acad. Sci. USA **93:** 13170–13175.
7. KLAFKI, H.W., D. ABRAMOWSKI, R. SWOBODA et al. 1996. The carboxyl termini of β-amyloid peptides 1–40 and 1–42 are generated by distinct γ-secretase activities. J. Biol. Chem. **271** 28655–28659.
8. MURPHY, M.P., L.J. HICKMAN, C.B. ECKMAN et al. 1999. γ-Secretase: evidence for multiple proteolytic activities and influence of membrane positioning of substrate on generation of amyloid β-peptides of varying length. J. Biol. Chem. **274:** 11914–11923.
9. VASSAR, R., B.D. BENNETT, S. BABU-KHAN et al. 1999. β-Secretase cleavage of Alzheimer's amyloid precursor protein by the transmembrane aspartic protease BACE. Science **286:** 735–741.

Toward the Characterization and Identification of γ-Secretases Using Transition-state Analogue Inhibitors

CHAD L. MOORE,[a] THEKLA S. DIEHL,[b] DENNIS J. SELKOE,[b] AND MICHAEL S. WOLFE[b,c]

[a]Department of Pharmaceutical Sciences, University of Tennessee, Memphis, Tennessee 38163, USA

[b]Center for Neurologic Diseases, Brigham and Women's Hospital and Harvard Medical School, Boston, Massachusetts 02115, USA

ABSTRACT: The amyloid-β protein (Aβ), strongly implicated in the etiology of Alzheimer's disease (AD), is formed from the amyloid-β precursor protein (APP) through sequential proteolysis by β- and γ-secretases. Cleavage by γ-secretase takes place within the middle of the single transmembrane region of APP and results primarily in 40- and 42-amino acid Aβ C-terminal variants, $A\beta_{40}$ and $A\beta_{42}$. The latter form of Aβ is highly fibrillogenic, is invariably elevated in autosomal-dominant forms of AD, and is the major Aβ component found presymptomatically in cerebral deposits. Thus, blocking production of Aβ in general and $A\beta_{42}$ in particular is considered an important therapeutic goal. We have developed transition-state analogue inhibitors of γ-secretase as molecular probes for characterizing the active site of this enzyme, as pharmacological tools for understanding its role in biology, and as affinity labels toward its definitive identification. Specifically, we found that: (1) difluoro ketone and difluoro alcohol peptidomimetics are effective inhibitors of γ-secretase activity in APP-transfected cells, strongly suggesting an aspartyl protease mechanism; (2) γ-secretases that form $A\beta_{40}$ and $A\beta_{42}$ are pharmacologically distinct but are nevertheless closely similar; (3) large hydrophobic P1 substituents increase the inhibitory potency of these peptidomimetics, suggesting a large complementary S1 pocket for γ-secretases; (4) $A\beta_{42}$ production is increased several fold over control by these γ-secretase inhibitors after replacement with inhibitor-free media; (5) a bromoacetamide derivative of one of these analogues continues to inhibit total Aβ and $A\beta_{42}$ production hours after replacement with compound-free media and should help identify the target(s) of these protease transition-state mimics.

INTRODUCTION

Postmortem analysis invariably reveals that the Alzheimer's disease (AD) brain is littered with neuritic plaques.[1] The principle protein component of these plaques is the 4-kDa amyloid-β protein (Aβ), derived from the amyloid-β precursor protein

[c]Address for correspondence: Michael S. Wolfe, Center for Neurologic Diseases, Brigham and Women's Hospital, Harvard Medical School, Boston, MA 02115. Tel.: (617) 525-5511; fax: (617) 525-5252.
e-mail: wolfe@cnd.bwh.harvard.edu

(APP) via sequential proteolysis by β- and γ-secretases. Cleavage by β-secretase occurs just outside the single transmembrane domain of APP to release the large ectodomain, and subsequent processing of the membrane-associated C-terminal fragment by γ-secretase takes place in the middle of the transmembrane region to produce 40- and 42-amino acid C-terminal Aβ variants, $A\beta_{40}$ and $A\beta_{42}$. While Aβ is prone to self-association into fibrils that are neurotoxic,[2] the longer and more hydrophobic $A\beta_{42}$ is particularly fibrillogenic.[3] Moreover, mutations in APP and in the polytopic presenilins that cause autosomal-dominant familial Alzheimer's disease (FAD) all increase $A\beta_{42}$ production,[4] and $A\beta_{42}$ is the principal Aβ isoform found presymptomatically in early, diffuse plaques.[5] Thus, $A\beta_{42}$ is particularly implicated in the pathogenesis of AD.

Both β- and γ-secretases are considered important targets for the development of new therapeutic agents to treat AD. β-Secretase has recently been identified as a new membrane-tethered aspartyl protease,[6–9] a major step toward developing effective inhibitors as drug candidates. γ-Secretase, however, has not been definitively identified. We have shown through inhibitor studies that γ-secretases have properties of aspartyl proteases,[10] and modeling and mutagenesis support a helical conformation of the APP transmembrane region for its initial interaction with γ-secretase.[10,11] Based on these results, we found that two conserved transmembrane aspartates in presenilin-1 are each required for two separate proteolytic events: γ-secretase cleavage of APP and presenilin endoproteolysis.[12] Similar results have been obtained with presenilin-2.[13] These findings are consistent with the hypothesis that presenilins are γ-secretases, novel intramembrane-cleaving aspartyl proteases activated through autoproteolysis.[14] While β-secretase has clear sequence homology with other known aspartyl proteases, the eight-transmembrane presenilins bear no obvious resemblance to them. Moreover, presenilins apparently do not facilitate γ-secretase proteolysis by themselves but require other limiting cofactors.[15] Thus, the issue of whether presenilins are γ-secretases is unsettled.

We have taken a pharmacological approach to this problem, designing transition-state analogue inhibitors of γ-secretases as a means of probing the characteristics of these mysterious enzymes, determining their role in biology, and developing affinity labels toward their identification. Using these inhibitors, we provide evidence that γ-secretases possess a large S1 pocket and that the γ-secretase that forms $A\beta_{42}$ has a lower affinity for substrate than does the protease that leads to $A\beta_{40}$. Moreover, N-terminal modification of one of these inhibitors to a bromoacetamide derivative resulted in a compound that continued to block Aβ production in cell culture after replacement with inhibitor-free media, consistent with the formation of a covalent complex between the inhibitor and its target protein(s). Such irreversible inhibitors may be useful molecular tools for identifying γ-secretases and specifically testing whether presenilins are the targets of these protease transition-state analogues.

EXPERIMENTAL METHODS

General Procedures for the Synthesis of Peptide Analogues

The various difluoro ketone peptidomimetic transition-state analogues were synthesized as previously described.[10,16] N-Boc-protected L-amino aldehydes were obtained from the *N*-Boc-protected L-amino acids via their *N,O*-dimethylhydroxamide (Weinreb amides). The aldehyde was added to activated zinc and ethyl bromodifluoroacetate in dry tetrahydrofuran under reflux for 30 min to provide the pseudopeptide difluoro alcohol intermediates. These were hydrolyzed with 1 eq NaOH or LiOH in 1:1 acetonitrile:water, and the carboxylic acid product was coupled to Val-Ile-OMe overnight with 1.1 eq HATU and 3 eq diisopropylethylamine in DMF. After TFA-mediated removal of the Boc group, the N-terminus was extended with Boc-L-valine. Bromoacetylation was accomplished by Boc deprotection followed by EDC-mediated coupling with bromoacetic acid. Difluoro alcohols were oxidized to ketones using 7 eq Dess-Martin periodinane reagent for 3 h as previously described.

Cell lines, Compound Treatments, and ELISAs

Chinese hamster ovary (CHO) cells stably transfected with the 751 amino-acid splice variant of human APP and the *neo* gene[17] were grown to confluence in Dulbecco's modified Eagle's medium containing 200 µg/mL G418 (Gibco BRL). Stock concentrations of the peptide analogues in DMSO were added to media to reach the final concentrations with 1% DMSO. Positive controls contained 1% DMSO alone. After 4 h, the media were either replaced or removed and then centrifuged at 3000 *g* for 5 min. The supernatant fluids were stored at −80°C until the assays were carried out. Sandwich ELISAs for total Aβ and $A\beta_{42}$ were performed as previously described.[18,19] Capture antibodies were 266 (to residues 13–28) for total Aβ and 21F12 (to residues 33–42) for $A\beta_{42}$. Reporter antibody was biotinylated 3D6 (to residues 1–5) in each assay.

Immunoprecipitation and Western Blotting

Cell lysates were precleared with protein A-sepharose at 4°C for 30 min, and proteins were precipitated with primary antibody C7 directed against the APP C-terminus for 2 h.[12] Beads were washed twice with 0.2% NP-40 buffer, and heated to 100°C for 5 min in reducing SDS-sample buffer. The precipitated proteins were separated by SDS-PAGE on 4–20% Tris-glycine gels. Immunoblotting using polyvinylidene difluoride membranes was done by probing the membranes overnight with antibody 13G8 (directed against the APP C-terminus), and by developing with peroxidase-conjugated secondary antibodies and enhanced chemiluminescence (ECL, Amersham).

RESULTS AND DISCUSSION

We previously reported that substrate-based difluoro ketone peptidomimetic transition-state analogues inhibit both $A\beta_{40}$ and $A\beta_{42}$ production at the level of γ-secretase. Levels of the soluble ectodomains, α- and β-APP$_s$, were not reduced, demonstrating that α- and β-secretase activities were not inhibited.[16] We found that a number of changes in the flanking residues of the analogue still allowed γ-secretase inhibition.[10] Such loose sequence specificity in the inhibitors mirrored similar observations with substrates.[11,20–22] Moreover, we have observed that difluoro alcohol analogues, while less effective, also block Aβ production.[10] Difluoro ketones are readily hydrated to closely mimic the transition state of aspartyl protease catalysis,

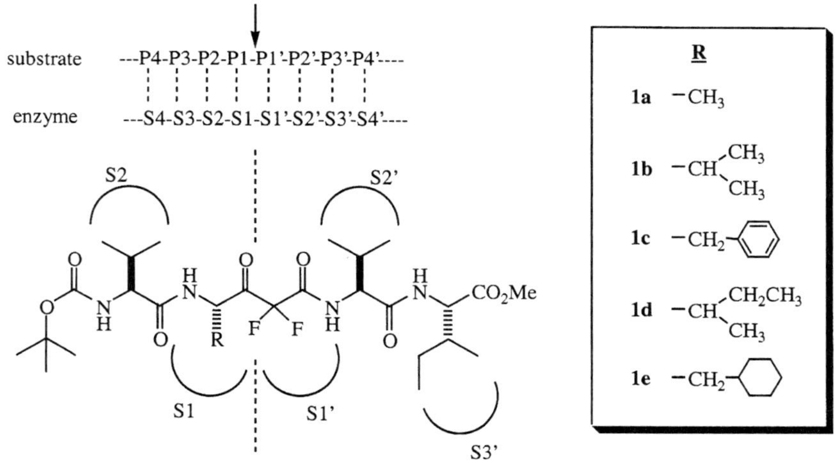

FIGURE 1. Structure of difluoro ketone transition-state analogue inhibitors with alterations in the P1 position. P sites on the protease substrates and the complementary S pockets in the enzyme are defined as shown.

but certain analogues of this type can also inhibit serine and cysteine proteases.[23,24] In contrast, difluoro alcohols are only known to inhibit aspartyl proteases.[25,26] These results therefore suggest that γ-secretases are aspartyl proteases.

To further explore the issue of loose sequence specificity, we synthesized a series of difluoro ketone transition-state mimics with alterations in the P1 position (FIG. 1). All of the compounds (**1a–e**) effectively blocked total Aβ and Aβ_{42} production at 25 and 50 μM. Although the potencies of the compounds were somewhat variable between experiments, the rank order of potency within a given experiment consistently showed **1e**>**1d**>**1c**>**1b**>**1a** (FIG. 2). Thus, the preference for P1 substituent was cyclohexylmethyl>*sec*-butyl>benzyl$\geq$*iso*-propyl>methyl, suggesting a relatively large S1 pocket for γ-secretases. These findings are consistent with other observations, noted above, showing that γ-secretases have loose sequence specificity.

Compound **6e** was further tested for effects on other APP metabolites. γ-Secretase substrates C99 and C83 increased dramatically (FIG. 3) and with a similar dose-response effect as seen for inhibition of Aβ production, indicating that **6e** inhibits Aβ production at the level of γ-secretase. Similar analysis of C99 and C83 levels 4 h after replacement with media alone showed that the inhibition of γ-secretase by this compound is reversible. We also found that α- and β-APP$_s$ levels were not lowered by this compound, indicating that α- and β-secretase activities were not inhibited (data not shown). Thus, despite the recent cloning and identification of β-secretase as a membrane-tethered aspartyl protease,[6–9] the difluoro ketone analogues reported here are apparently selective for γ-secretase. Installation of the cyclohexylmethyl group in P1 also led to the identification of a difluoro alcohol (the immediate synthetic precursor to **1e**) equipotent to its difluoro ketone counterpart toward inhibiting total Aβ production (IC$_{50}$ ~ 5 μM; data not shown). This difluoro alcohol was an order of magnitude more potent than other difluoro alcohols we have previously reported,[10] providing strong additional evidence that γ-secretase is an aspartyl protease.

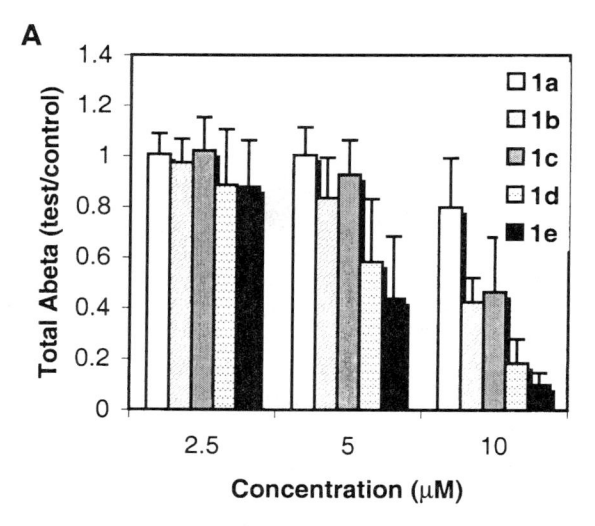

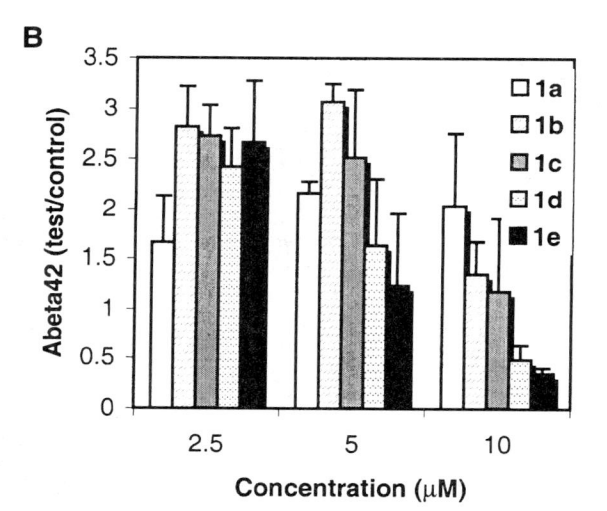

FIGURE 2. Effect of transition-state analogues **1a–1e** (**A**) on total Aβ and (**B**) on Aβ$_{42}$ production in CHO cells stably transfected with human APP.

As we have observed before with related peptidomimetics,[10] the rank order of potencies for inhibition of Aβ$_{40}$ and Aβ$_{42}$ production was essentially the same (compare FIGS. 2A and 2B, especially at 10 μM), suggesting that the active site topologies for γ$_{40}$- and γ$_{42}$-secretases are closely similar. Nevertheless, these related γ-secretase activities are apparently distinct, since Aβ$_{40}$ production is more sensitive to γ-secretase inhibitors than is Aβ$_{42}$ production, as demonstrated in FIG. 2 and reported by others and us.[10,16,27,28] Moreover, subinhibitory concentrations of γ-secretase inhib-

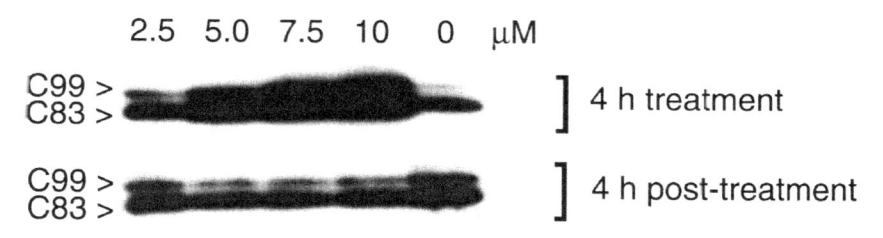

2.5 5.0 7.5 10   0   μM

C99 >
C83 >   ] 4 h treatment

C99 >
C83 >   ] 4 h post-treatment

FIGURE 3. Levels of γ-secretase substrates C83 and C99 in APP-transfected CHO cells (**A**) after 4 h treatment with peptidomimetic **1e**, and (**B**) after a subsequent 4-h recovery phase with inhibitor-free media.

itors elicit profound increases in $A\beta_{42}$ production; all γ-secretase inhibitors reported to date show this effect.[10,16,27–30]

Because the ability of compounds to increase $A\beta_{42}$ production closely correlates with their inhibitory potency against γ-secretase activity, we hypothesize that partial inhibition of $A\beta_{40}$ production increases the availability of substrate C99 for $A\beta_{42}$ production. That is, γ_{42}-secretase has a higher K_m for substrate than γ_{40}-secretase, a conclusion supported by a recent study with peptide aldehyde γ-secretase inhibitors.[31] In support of this hypothesis, we found that after effective inhibition of γ-secretase activity with difluoro ketone analogues, replacement with inhibitor-free medium resulted in substantial elevations in $A\beta_{42}$ production, while $A\beta_{40}$ levels simply returned to that of control (FIG. 4). Apparently, γ_{40}-secretase is at or close to saturation in this cell line, while γ_{42}-secretase is not. Substrate levels are increased by the presence of inhibitor (e.g., FIG. 3). After removal of the inhibitor, γ_{40}-secretase activity returns to control levels. In contrast, γ_{42}-secretase can now bind more substrate. These findings have implications for therapy: γ-secretase inhibitors with poor pharmacokinetic profiles may have the unintended consequence of elevating $A\beta_{42}$.

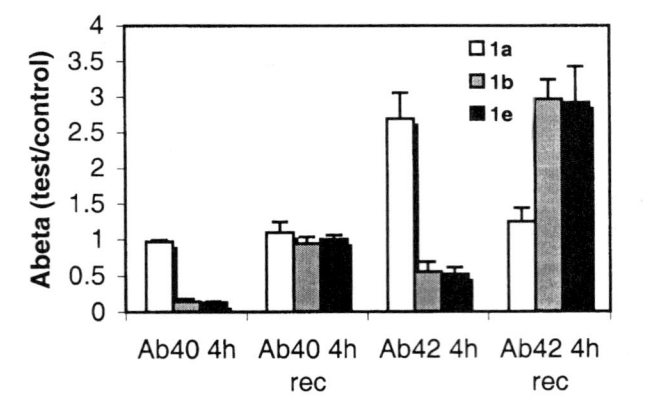

FIGURE 4. Levels of $A\beta_{40}$ and $A\beta_{42}$ secreted from APP-transfected CHO cells after 4-h treatment with 10 μM **1a**, **1b**, or **1e** and after a subsequent 4-h recovery phase with inhibitor-free media.

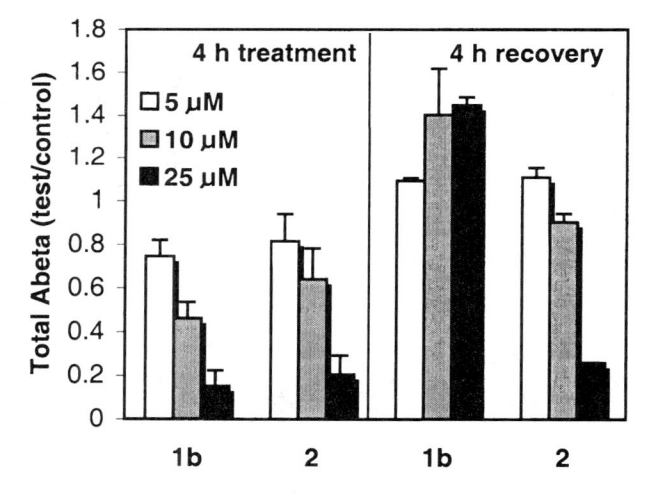

FIGURE 5. Levels of total Aβ production secreted from APP-transfected CHO cells after 4-h treatment with 5–25 μM of N-terminal Boc-containing **1b** or its *N*-bromoacetyl counterpart **2** and after a subsequent recovery phase with inhibitor-free media.

To identify the target of these γ-secretase inhibitors, we have designed derivatives of these peptide analogues that may bind covalently and irreversibly. The N-terminal Boc group of **1b** was replaced with a bromoacetyl group, a functionality susceptible to nucleophilic attack that has been extensively employed as a means of creating affinity labels.[32–37] Thus, the difluoro ketone transition-state mimic should interact with the two active site aspartates of γ-secretase,[38] while the bromoacetamide should react with any proximal nucleophilic residues (e.g., Ser, Cys, Thr) to form a stable covalent bond and irreversibly inactivate the enzyme. As expected, we found that the Boc-containing **1b** reversibly inhibits γ-secretase: Upon replacement with inhibitor-free media, Aβ production returned to control levels (FIG. 5). In comparison, the bromoacetamide **2** is not quite as potent during the initial 4-h treatment; however, upon removal of the compound, Aβ production was still inhibited. Irreversible protease transition-state analogue inhibitors of this type may be important biochemical tools for identifying γ-secretases and specifically testing the hypothesis that presenilins are these proteases.

[NOTE ADDED IN PROOF: Since the submission of this manuscript, we have determined that bromoacetamide derivatives of these transition-state analogue inhibitors of γ-secretase bind directly and specifically to heterodimeric presenilins.[39]]

ACKNOWLEDGMENTS

This work was supported by NIH grants NS 37537 to MSW and AG 12749 to DJS. We thank Talat Rahmati for expert technical help with the ELISAs.

REFERENCES

1. SELKOE, D.J. 1999. Translating cell biology into therapeutic advances in Alzheimer's disease. Nature **399**: A23–A31.
2. LORENZO, A. & B.A. YANKNER. 1994. Beta-amyloid neurotoxicity requires fibril formation and is inhibited by congo red. Proc. Natl. Acad. Sci. USA **91**: 12243–12247.
3. JARRETT, J.T., E.P. BERGER & P.T. LANSBURY, JR. 1993. The carboxy terminus of the beta amyloid protein is critical for the seeding of amyloid formation: implications for the pathogenesis of Alzheimer's disease. Biochemistry **32**: 4693–4697.
4. HARDY, J. 1997. The Alzheimer family of diseases: many etiologies, one pathogenesis? Proc. Natl. Acad. Sci. USA **94**: 2095–2097.
5. IWATSUBO, T., D.M. MANN, A. ODAKA et al. 1995. Amyloid beta protein (A beta) deposition: A beta 42(43) precedes A beta 40 in Down syndrome. Ann. Neurol. **37**: 294–299.
6. VASSAR, R., B.D. BENNETT, S. BABU-KHAN et al. 1999. Beta-secretase cleavage of Alzheimer's amyloid precursor protein by the transmembrane aspartic protease BACE. Science **286**: 735–741.
7. SINHA, S., J.P. ANDERSON, R. BARBOUR et al. 1999. Purification and cloning of amyloid precursor protein beta-secretase from human brain [in process citation]. Nature **402**: 537–540.
8. YAN, R., M.J. BIENKOWSKI, M.E. SHUCK et al. 1999. Membrane-anchored aspartyl protease with Alzheimer's disease beta- secretase activity [in process citation]. Nature **402**: 533–537.
9. HUSSAIN, I., D. POWELL, D.R. HOWLETT et al. 1999. Identification of a novel aspartic protease (Asp 2) as beta-secretase. Mol. Cell. Neurosci. **14**: 419–427.
10. WOLFE, M.S., W. XIA, C.L. MOORE et al. 1999. Peptidomimetic probes and molecular modeling suggest Alzheimer's γ-secretases are intramembrane-cleaving aspartyl proteases. Biochemistry **38**: 4720–4727.
11. LICHTENTHALER, S.F., R. WANG, H. GRIMM et al. 1999. Mechanism of the cleavage specificity of Alzheimer's disease gamma-secretase identified by phenylalanine-scanning mutagenesis of the transmembrane domain of the amyloid precursor protein. Proc. Natl. Acad. Sci. USA **96**: 3053–3058.
12. WOLFE, M.S., W. XIA, B.L. OSTASZEWSKI et al. 1999. Two transmembrane aspartates in presenilin-1 required for presenilin endoproteolysis and γ-secretase activity. Nature **398**: 513–517.
13. STEINER, H., K. DUFF, A. CAPELL et al. 1999. A loss of function mutation of presenilin-2 interferes with amyloid beta-peptide production and notch signaling. J. Biol. Chem. **274**: 28669–28673.
14. WOLFE, M.S., J. DE LOS ANGELES, D.D. MILLER et al. 1999. Are presenilins intramembrane-cleaving proteases? Implications for the molecular mechanism of Alzheimer's disease. Biochemistry **38**: 11223–11230.
15. THINAKARAN, G., C.L. HARRIS, T. RATOVITSKI et al. 1997. Evidence that levels of presenilins (PS1 and PS2) are coordinately regulated by competition for limiting cellular factors. J. Biol. Chem. **272**: 28415–28422.
16. WOLFE, M.S., M. CITRON, T.S. DIEHL et al. 1998. A substrate-based difluoro ketone selectively inhibits Alzheimer's gamma-secretase activity. J. Med. Chem. **41**: 6–9.
17. XIA, W., J. ZHANG, D. KHOLODENKO et al. 1997. Enhanced production and oligomerization of the 42-residue amyloid beta-protein by Chinese hamster ovary cells stably expressing mutant presenilins. J. Biol. Chem. **272**: 7977–7982.
18. JOHNSON-WOOD, K., M. LEE, R. MOTTER et al. 1997. Amyloid precursor protein processing and A beta 42 deposition in a transgenic mouse model of Alzheimer disease. Proc. Natl. Acad. Sci. USA **94**: 1550–1555.
19. SEUBERT, P., C. VIGO-PELFREY, F. ESCH et al. 1992. Isolation and quantification of soluble Alzheimer's beta-peptide from biological fluids. Nature **359**: 325–327.
20. MARUYAMA, K., T. TOMITA, K. SHINOZAKI et al. 1996. Familial Alzheimer's disease-linked mutations at Val717 of amyloid precursor protein are specific for the increased secretion of A beta 42(43). Biochem. Biophys. Res. Commun. **227**: 730–735.

21. TISCHER, E. & B. CORDELL. 1996. Beta-amyloid precursor protein: location of trans-membrane domain and specificity of gamma-secretase cleavage. J. Biol. Chem. **271:** 21914–21919.

22. LICHTENTHALER, S.F., N. IDA, G. MULTHAUP *et al.* 1997. Mutations in the transmembrane domain of APP altering gamma-secretase specificity. Biochemistry **36:** 15396–15403.

23. PARISI, M.F. & R.H. ABELES. 1992. Inhibition of chymotrypsin by fluorinated alpha-keto acid derivatives. Biochemistry **31:** 9429–9435.

24. ANGLIKER, H., J. ANAGLI & E. SHAW. 1992. Inactivation of calpain by peptidyl fluoro-methyl ketones. J. Med. Chem. **35:** 216–220.

25. THAISRIVONGS, S., D.T. PALS, W.M. KATI *et al.* 1986. Design and synthesis of potent and specific renin inhibitors containing difluorostatine, difluorostatone, and related analogues. J. Med. Chem. **29:** 2080–2087.

26. DOHERTY, A.M., I. SIRCAR, B.E. KORNBERG *et al.* 1992. Design and synthesis of potent, selective, and orally active fluorine-containing renin inhibitors. J. Med. Chem. **35:** 2–14.

27. CITRON, M., T.S. DIEHL, G. GORDON *et al.* 1996. Evidence that the 42- and 40-amino acid forms of amyloid beta protein are generated from the beta-amyloid precursor protein by different protease activities. Proc. Natl. Acad. Sci. USA **93:** 13170–13175.

28. KLAFKI, H., D. ABRAMOWSKI, R. SWOBODA *et al.* 1996. The carboxyl termini of beta-amyloid peptides 1–40 and 1–42 are generated by distinct gamma-secretase activities. J. Biol. Chem. **271:** 28655–28659.

29. HIGAKI, J., D. QUON, Z. ZHONG & B. CORDELL. 1995. Inhibition of beta-amyloid for-mation identifies proteolytic precursors and subcellular site of catabolism. Neuron **14:** 651–659.

30. HIGAKI, J.N., S. CHAKRAVARTY, C.M. BRYANT *et al.* 1999. A combinatorial approach to the identification of dipeptide aldehyde inhibitors of beta-amyloid production. J. Med. Chem. **42:** 3889–3898.

31. ZHANG, L., L. SONG & E.M. PARKER. 1999. Calpain inhibitor I increases beta-amyloid peptide production by inhibiting the degradation of the substrate of gamma-secretase: evidence that substrate availability limits beta-amyloid peptide production. J. Biol. Chem. **274:** 8966–8972.

32. PONGS, O. & E. LANKA. 1975. Affinity labeling of the ribosomal decoding site with an AUG-substrate analog. Proc. Natl. Acad. Sci. USA **72:** 1505–1509.

33. CHANG, C.H., T.J. LOBL, D.R. ROWLEY & D.J. TINDALL. 1984. Affinity labeling of the androgen receptor in rat prostate cytosol with 17 beta-[(bromoacetyl)oxy]-5 alpha-androstan-3-one. Biochemistry **23:** 2527–2533.

34. BATEMAN, R.C., JR., Y.A. KIM, C. SLAUGHTER & L.B. HERSH. 1990. *N*-Bromoacetyl-D-leucylglycine: an affinity label for neutral endopeptidase 24.11. J. Biol. Chem. **265:** 8365–8368.

35. SMAR, M.W., J.J. ARES, T. NAKAYAMA *et al.* 1992. Selective irreversible inhibitors of aldose reductase. J. Med. Chem. **35:** 1117–1120.

36. SAFRAN, M., A.P. FARWELL, H. ROKOS & J.L. LEONARD. 1993. Structural requirements of iodothyronines for the rapid inactivation and internalization of type II iodothyro-nine 5'-deiodinase in glial cells. J. Biol. Chem. **268:** 14224–14229.

37. KULIOPULOS, A., N.P. NELSON, M. YAMADA *et al.* 1994. Localization of the affinity peptide-substrate inactivator site on recombinant vitamin K-dependent carboxylase. J. Biol. Chem. **269:** 21364–21370.

38. JAMES, M.N., A.R. SIELECKI, K. HAYAKAWA & M.H. GELB. 1992. Crystallographic analysis of transition state mimics bound to penicillopepsin: difluorostatine- and difluorostatone-containing peptides. Biochemistry **31:** 3872–3886.

39. ESLER, W.P., W.T. KIMBERLY, B.L. OSTASZEWSKI *et al.* 2000. Transition-state analogue inhibitors of γ-secretase bind directly to presenilin-1. Nat. Cell Biol. **2:** 428–434.

Recent Advances in the Understanding of the Processing of APP to Beta Amyloid Peptide

S. SINHA,[a] J. ANDERSON, V. JOHN, L. McCONLOGUE, G. BASI,
E. THORSETT, AND D. SCHENK

Elan Pharmaceuticals, South San Francisco, California 94080, USA

INTRODUCTION

Numerous lines of evidence suggest that the 42 amino-acid long form of beta amyloid peptide ($A\beta_{42}$) plays a key role in the pathogenesis of Alzheimer's disease (AD). This evidence includes the observations that multiple missense mutations in the amyloid precursor protein (APP), presenilin-1 (PS-1) or presenilin-2 (PS-2) all result in the overproduction of $A\beta_{42}$.[1,2] $A\beta$ is produced from the APP through sequential proteolytic processing events, carried out by two independent enzyme activities termed beta- and gamma-secretase.[3] Once the peptide is produced it can, under some conditions, go on to form amyloid deposits (senile plaques) in the brain parenchyma, which are a hallmark of AD. Efforts to block the production of $A\beta$ have been pursued over the past several years, towards the goal of therapeutic treatment for AD. This effort has resulted in compounds that are effective in inhibiting gamma secretase-like cleavage of APP into $A\beta$[4,5] and, very recently, have resulted in the independent identification of beta-secretase by several groups including our own.[6–8] The identification of this novel, membrane bound aspartyl proteinase has increased therapeutic opportunities for Alzheimer's disease aimed at the inhibition of $A\beta$ peptide production.

METHODS

A maltose-binding protein (MBP) fusion protein with the C-terminal 125 amino acids of APP attached to it (MBP-C125) was expressed in *E. coli* and used as a substrate to assess beta-secretase activity. Beta secretase activity was determined using MBP-C125 (10 μg/ml) in a buffered solution of 20 mM sodium acetate pH 4.8, and 0.06% Triton X-100. Specific cleavage products were determined using biotinylated antibody 192[9] as described previously.[10] Purification of the β-secretase enzyme activity from human brain was achieved by a sequential four-step procedure, incorporating an affinity purification step with immobilized P_{10}-P_4·StatVal inhibitor peptide.

[a]Address for correspondence: Sukanto Sinha, Ph.D., Elan Pharmaceuticals, 800 Gateway Blvd., So. San Francisco, CA 94080. Tel.: (650) 877-7635; fax: (650) 553-7196.
e-mail: ssinha@elanpharma.com

RESULTS

Initial studies using total membranes isolated from human brain detected a membrane-bound activity with properties similar to that expected for beta-secretase. The partially purified enzyme activity cleaved APP between aa 596–597 (APP695 numbering), thus generating the free N-terminus of Aβ. This was determined using the 192 antibody, which specifically reacts with β-cleaved APP that ends at exactly aa 596, and hence is diagnostic for beta-secretase-like activity. Various tissues and cell lines were surveyed for β-cleavage activity, by extracting P2 membranes from each source with 0.2% Triton X-100, and assaying for β-cleavage. Human and mouse brain and brain regions had uniformly high levels of enzyme activity, whereas little activity was detected in other tissues. Amongst cell lines, neurons had the highest level of enzyme activity, while 293, Cos, and CHO cells exhibited lower levels. Thus the enzyme activity is highest in cells of CNS lineage, and present in cell lines commonly used for analysis of APP metabolism, in line with the observation that β-sAPP (soluble APP, cleaved by beta-secretase) production is enhanced in CNS-derived cells, such as fetal neurons in culture.[1]

A number of synthetic peptide substrates, based on the beta-secretase cleavage site in APP, were designed to further understand the specificity of the beta-secretase activity and to identify potential inhibitors. Of the various peptides made, the tetradecapeptide P10-P4' was also made replacing the P1 Leu residue with the amino-acid Statine (Sta) and this was shown to be inhibitory to the enzyme activity with an IC_{50} ~40 μM. Further improvement in the inhibitory properties were achieved by replacement of the P1' Asp with Val, which resulted in strongly inhibitory peptide, IC_{50} ~30 nM, that was then used to develop an inhibitor affinity matrix for beta-secretase purification.

The enzyme activity is purified ~300,000-fold using this procedure, yielding a ~70 kDa protein, homogenous by silver-stained SDS-PAGE analysis. N-terminal sequence was used for isolation of cDNA clones encoding full length beta-secretase by a combination of PCR and conventional cDNA library screening. A full-length clone predicted to encode a polypeptide comprising 501 amino acids, p501, was obtained from a human fetal neuronal cell library.

The p501 clone shows sequence homology with both cathepsin D and pepsin, two other well-characterized aspartyl proteinases. It is unusual in that it has a consensus sequence for a transmembrane domain, consistent with its biochemical properties.

Transfection of cells with the p501 beta-secretase clone with wild type APP in 293 cells resulted in a very marked elevation in secreted Aβ peptide and β-sAPP (soluble APP, cleaved by beta-secretase). Little, if any decrease was seen in the levels of α-sAPP (soluble APP, cleaved by alpha-secretase), supporting the notion that cleavage of APP at the beta- and alpha- sites occur by distinct enzymes.

CONCLUSIONS

We and others[6–8] have now identified the putative enzyme involved in the rate-limiting cleavage of APP to the Aβ peptide. The identification of this enzyme has been sought throughtout the last decade, in the pursuit of potential inhibitors that might be useful for reducing Aβ peptide levels and hence might be of therapeutic benefit for Alzheimer's disease. The proteinase encoded by p501 fits all the criteria expected and predicted for beta-secretase. Much work is now required to develop orally active compounds effective in inhibiting this enzyme *in vivo* to test their potential utility for treatment of AD.

REFERENCES

1. SUZUKI, N., T.T. CHEUNG, X.D. CAI *et al.* 1994. An increased percentage of long amyloid beta protein secreted by familial amyloid beta protein precursor (beta APP717) mutants. Science **264:** 1336–1340.
2. CITRON, M., D. WESTAWAY, W. XIA *et al.* 1997. Mutant presenilins of Alzheimer's disease increase production of 42-residue amyloid beta-protein in both transfected cells and transgenic mice [see comments]. Nat. Med. **3:** 67–72.
3. SELKOE, D.J. 1998. The cell biology of beta-amyloid precursor protein and presenilin in Alzheimer's disease [in process citation]. Trends Cell Biol. **8:** 447–453.
4. HIGAKI, J., D. QUON, Z. ZHONG & B. CORDELL. 1995. Inhibition of beta-amyloid formation identifies proteolytic precursors and subcellular site of catabolism. Neuron **14:** 651–659.
5. WOLFE, M.S., W. XIA, C.L. MOORE *et al.* 1999. Peptidomimetic probes and molecular modeling suggest that Alzheimer's gamma-secretase is an intramembrane-cleaving aspartyl protease. Biochemistry **38:** 4720–4727.
6. SINHA, S., J.P. ANDERSON, R. BARBOUR *et al.* 1999. Purification and cloning of amyloid precursor protein β secretase from human brain. Nature **402:** 537–540.
7. VASSAR, R., B.D. BENNETT *et al.* 1999. Beta-secretase cleavage of Alzheimer's amyloid precursor protein by the transmembrane aspartic protease BACE. Science **286:** 735–741.
8. YAN, R., M.J. BIENKOWSKI, M.E. SHUCK *et al.* 1999. Membrane-anchored aspartyl protease with Alzheimer's disease β-secretase activity. Nature **402:** 533–537.
9. SEUBERT, P., T. OLTERSDORF, M.G. LEE *et al.* 1993. Secretion of beta-amyloid precursor protein cleaved at the amino terminus of the beta-amyloid peptide. Nature **361:** 260–263.
10. Assays for Detecting Beta-Secretase. 1999. US Patent #5,942,400.

Presenilin-1: A Component of Synaptic and Endothelial Adherens Junctions

ANASTASIOS GEORGAKOPOULOS,[a] PHILIPPE MARAMBAUD,[a]
VICTOR L. FRIEDRICH, JR.,[b] JUNICHI SHIOI,[a]
SPIROS EFTHIMIOPOULOS,[a] AND NIKOLAOS K. ROBAKIS[a,c]

[a]Department of Psychiatry and Fishberg Research Center for Neurobiology, and
[b]Departments of Biochemistry and Molecular Biology, Mount Sinai School of Medicine,
New York, New York 10029, USA

Presenilin-1 (PS1) is an integral membrane protein involved in the development of familial Alzheimer disease (FAD). Cadherin-based cell-cell interactions control critical events in cell-cell adhesion and recognition. We obtained evidence that PS1 accumulates at cell-cell contact sites where it colocalizes with components of the cadherin-based adherens junctions. At these sites, PS1 is linked to the cortical cytoskeleton and is found at intercellular junctions. PS1 fragments form detergent-stable complexes with E-cadherin, β-catenin, and α-catenin, all components of adherens junctions. PS1 overexpression in human kidney cells enhances cell-cell adhesion. Together, our data show that PS1 incorporates into the cadherin/catenin adhesion system and modulates cell-cell adhesion. PS1 concentrates at synaptic contacts and forms complexes with brain E- and N-cadherin, known synaptic components. The PS1 incorporation into the cadherin/catenin complex makes it a potential target for PS1 FAD mutations.[1]

Presenilin-1 (PS1) mutations are responsible for most cases of early-onset autosomal dominant familial Alzheimer disease (FAD). PS1 protein is a polytopic transmembrane peptide expressed in many tissues including brain where it is enriched in neurons. Structural studies suggest that PS1 crosses the membrane six or eight times with the N- and C-termini and the large hydrophilic loop all located in the cytoplasm. PS1 has been mainly localized in the endoplasmic reticulum (ER)/Golgi system and in vesicular structures. Most cellular full-length PS1 is cleaved within the large cytoplasmic loop to yield N-terminal fragments of approximately 30 kDa and C-terminal fragments of approximately 20 kDa. Following cleavage of the full-length protein, PS1 fragments stay together as a stable 1:1 heterodimer. Recently it was shown that PS1 binds members of the armadillo family of proteins including δ- and β-catenin and promotes processing and signaling of Notch1 receptor. Other studies suggest that PS1 functions in protein trafficking, neuroprotection, chromosome segregation, and processing of selected proteins including APP (for a comprehensive review and reference list of the cellular biology of PS1, see Ref. 3). Theories proposed to explain the mechanism by which PS1 mutations induce FAD include increased production

[c]Address for correspondence: Dr. Nikolaos K. Robakis, Dept. of Psychiatry and Fishberg Research Center for Neurobiology, Mount Sinai School of Medicine, Box 1229, One Gustave Levy Place, New York, NY 10029-6547. Tel.: (212) 241-9380; fax: (212) 831-1947.
e-mail: nikolaos.robakis@mssm.edu

of Aβ, destabilization of β-catenin, inhibition of PS1 proteolysis, and increased apoptosis (for review, see Ref. 3).

Classical cadherins, including E(epithelial)- and N(neural)-cadherin, are a family of cell surface single-pass transmembrane proteins that control critical events in cell-cell adhesion, recognition, and tissue development and maintenance. These functions are mediated by the extracellular domain of cadherins, which in the dimeric state promotes Ca^{++}-dependent homophilic interactions between same-class cadherins on opposing cell surfaces (for review, see Ref. 4). Cadherin-based adherens junctions (AJ) are specialized forms of cellular adhesive organelles where plasmalemmal cadherins form complexes with cytosolic catenins. According to this model, the conserved cytoplasmic sequence of cadherins binds to either β- or γ-catenin which in turn binds to α-catenin. The latter protein binds to α-actinin and F-actin, thus linking the cadherin/catenin system to the cortical actin cytoskeleton. Homophilic interactions of the extracellular sequence of specific cadherins with same-class cadherins on the surface of neighboring cells regulate cell-cell adhesion and communication in tissues and organs. In addition, cell surface cadherins mediate the intracellular transduction of extracellular signals.[4]

Recently, we obtained evidence that PS1 forms complexes with the cadherin/catenin cell-cell adhesion system and is recruited to intercellular and synaptic contacts.[1] Confocal microscopy showed that in confluent epithelial cells, PS1 localizes at cell-cell adhesion sites in close association with E-cadherin, β-catenin, and α-catenin, all of which are components of the cadherin-based AJ. In cells not forming cell-cell contacts, PS1 was mostly found in the ER/Golgi network. Immunogold electron microscopy also localized PS1 at intercellular junctions along the lateral plasma membrane. That PS1 concentrates at cell-cell contact sites in close association with E-cadherin and catenins suggests PS1 may be a part of the cadherin/catenin adhesion system. Indeed, we found PS1 fragments in detergent-stable complexes with E-cadherin, β-catenin, and α-catenin. Furthermore, quantitative immunoprecipitations and velocity gradient centrifugation revealed single complexes containing both PS1 fragments, E-cadherin, β-catenin, and α-catenin. Thus, detection of complexes containing PS1 and the basic structural components of the cadherin/catenin cell adhesion system indicates that PS1 is a component of this system. In support of this conclusion, we found that PS1 is recruited to Ca^{++}-induced cell-cell contact sites where PS1 fragments form complexes with cell surface E-cadherin. Interestingly, removal of extracellular Ca^{++} resulted in a specific decrease of the cellular PS1/E-cadherin complexes. These data suggest the presence of signal transduction mechanisms that regulate the stability of PS1/cadherin complexes in response to changes in extracellular Ca^{++}. *In vivo* experiments showed that in epithelial tissue PS1 concentrates at cell-cell contact sites suggesting a PS1 function in cell-cell adhesion. In support of this suggestion, over-expression of PS1 stimulated cell-cell aggregation.[1] The localization of PS1 at intercellular sites is consistent with the detection of PS1 fragments in clathrin-coated vesicle membranes,[5] suggesting a PS1 trafficking to the cell surface.

Recent reports suggest that PS1 mediates processing of Notch1, a surface receptor involved in cell-cell interactions during development.[6] This suggestion however, is inconsistent with the intracellular localization of PS1.[7] Our data showing that PS1 is recruited to intercellular contact sites suggests that PS1 processes Notch1 at the plasma membrane at sites of cell-cell contact, and could therefore constitute part of the Notch signaling system.

Cadherins and associated catenins are expressed in highly dynamic and specific patterns throughout embryonic development and adult life of the vertebrate nervous system.[8] At least fifteen different classic cadherins have been detected in various developmental stages of the central nervous system (CNS). In early development, various cadherins are regionally expressed in the brain thus defining specific neuromeric subdivisions. This expression pattern suggests that cadherin-mediated adhesion plays a role in establishing the cytoarchitecture of the CNS.[9] Later in development, cadherins are expressed in the elongating neurites, and may be involved in target recognition and synapse formation as the targets of cadherin-expressing neurites usually express the same type of cadherin. Thus, homophillic cadherin binding at axo-dendritic interfaces generates synaptic specificity.[9] Several cadherins, including N- and R (retinal)-cadherin have been shown to promote neurite outgrowth by functioning as homophilic guidance molecules for the navigation of neuronal processes (for review, see Ref. 8). Cadherins are expressed in the mature CNS, and the cadherin/catenin adhesion system has been localized at the synapse where it functions to link pre- and postsynaptic membranes (for review, see Ref. 9), and to regulate synaptic plasticity including long term potentiation.[10]

Immunocytochemical experiments showed that in brain, PS1 is mainly expressed in neuronal dendrites and cell bodies, whilst it is mostly absent from axons. Nonneuronal cells contain low levels of PS1.[11] We used a stereological methodology to quantitate both the total number of neurons in AD and normal brain tissue, and the number of neurons expressing PS1.[12] Our results show that although there is a significant decrease in the number of neurons that do not express PS1, neuronal population that contain PS1 are preserved in AD. These data suggest that presenilins may have neuroprotective properties, and similar suggestions have been made by several other groups.[13–15]

In brain tissue, we detected PS1 in complexes with E-cadherin, N-cadherin, and β-catenin, suggesting that PS1 is an integral component of the brain cadherin/catenin complex. Furthermore, electron microscopy showed that brain PS1 concentrates at synaptic junctions,[1] whereas confocal microscopy colocalized PS1 with synaptic markers (FIG. 1). Together, our results suggest that PS1 is a component of the synaptic cadherin/catenin AJ complex, and that PS1 has a synaptic function. Synapses are specialized contact sites between neurons in the brain. These contacts are vital for the interneuronal communication required for the processing, integration, storage, and retrieval of information. Efficient function of the synapse and the synaptic signal transduction mechanisms are critical for the proper functioning and information processing in the CNS. That PS1 is a component of the synaptic cadherin/catenin complex makes that complex a potential target for PS1 FAD mutations, as they could affect any of the steps required for the interaction of PS1 with other components of the complex. Such perturbations of protein-protein interactions within multimeric complexes is a mechanism for dominant "gain of aberrant function or loss of function" effects of disease-associated mutations.[16,17] Furthermore, the incorporation of a defective (mutant) PS1 within the synaptic structure may influence the transmission of signals from the pre- to postsynaptic terminals or may otherwise interfere with synaptic plasticity and function. In this context, it is interesting to note that

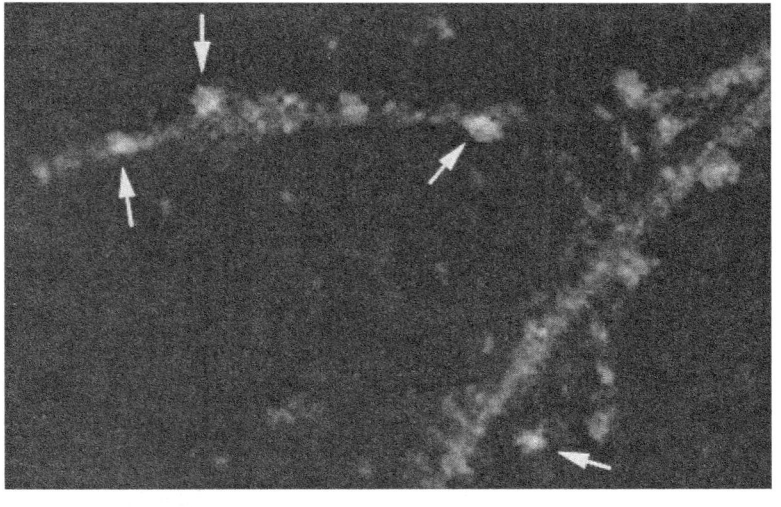

FIGURE 1. Synaptic localization of PS1 using confocal microscopy. PS1 and synapto-physin colocalize at synaptic boutons indicated by *arrows*.

among the neuropathological phenotypes of AD, synapse abnormalities show the best correlation with the degree of dementia.[18] In addition, synapses also contain APP,[19,20] and although a function for APP has not yet been clearly established, several lines of evidence suggest that APP may actually promote cell adhesion.[21,22] In any event, the synaptic colocalization of both proteins makes this brain structure a candidate locus for the interaction of these two peptides, an interaction that may be of critical importance for the development of AD. This is particularly important in the face of recent evidence that PS1 plays a role in the processing of APP and pro-duction of Aβ.[23,24]

Our observation, that PS1 is a component of the cadherin/catenin adherens junc-tions has important implications for the role of this protein in tissue development and maintenance. Continued expression and function of adherens junctions is required for the dynamic cellular rearrangements that take place in neuronal and nonneuronal tissues during development and for the maintenance of tissues in adult organisms. The crucial role E-cadherin plays in normal development is indicated by the lethal phenotype displayed by E-cadherin-null mice fetuses, which is probably due to the abnormal tissue adhesion and organogenesis.[25] It was recently shown that PS1 null mice die at birth and display severe organogenesis abnormalities including skeletal deformities and impaired neurogenesis.[13] Together with our data, these observations raise the possibility that the lethal phenotype of PS1 null mice might be due to a mal-function of the cadherin-based cell-cell adhesion system.

We obtained evidence that PS1 forms complexes with the endothelial adherens junctions (Serban *et al.*, in preparation). The endothelium forms and regulates the main barrier to the passage of macromolecules and circulating cells from blood to tissues including brain tissue. This endothelial permeability is regulated by intercellular junctions with adherens junctions playing a prominent role. Incorporation of defective (i.e., FAD mutant) PS1 in the endothelial adherens junctions could change the permeability of the blood-brain barrier, and this change may adversely affect neuronal survival.

REFERENCES

1. GEORGAKOPOULOS, A., P. MARAMBAUD, S. EFTHIMIOPOULOS *et al.* 1999. Presenilin-1 forms complexes with the cadherin/catenin cell-cell adhesion system and is recruited to intercellular and synaptic contacts. Mol. Cell **4:** 893–902.
2. ANNAERT, W. & B. DE STROOPER. 1999. Presenilins: molecular switches between proteolysis and signal transduction. Trends Neurosci. **22:** 439–443.
3. SELKOE, D.J. 1999. Translation cell biology into therapeutic advances in Alzheimer's disease. Nature **399:** 23–31.
4. YAP, A.S., W.M. BRIEHER & B.M. GUMBINER. 1997. Molecular and functional analysis of cadherin-based adherens junctions. Annu. Rev. Cell Dev. Biol. **13:** 119–146.
5. EFTHIMIOPOULOS, S., E. FLOOR, A. GEORGAKOPOULOS *et al.* 1998. Enrichment of presenilin 1 peptides in neuronal large dense-core and somatodendritic clathrin-coated vesicles. J. Neurochem. **71:** 2365–2372.
6. DE STROOPER, B., W. ANNAERT, P. CUPERS *et al.* 1999. A presenilin-1-dependent gamma-secretase-like protease mediates release of Notch intracellular domain. Nature **398:** 518–522.
7. HARDY, J. & A. ISRAEL. 1999. In search of gamma secretase. Nature **398:** 466–467.
8. REDIES, C. & M. TAKEICHI. 1996. Cadherins in the developing central nervous system: an adhesive code for segmental and functional subdivisions. Dev. Biol. **180:** 413–423.
9. UEMURA, T. 1998. The cadherin superfamily at the synapse more members, more missions. Cell **93:** 1095–1098.
10. TANG, L., C.P. HUNG & E.M. SCHUMAN. 1998. A role for the cadherin family of cell adhesion molecules in hippocampal long-term potentiation. Neuron **6:** 1165–1175.
11. ELDER, G.A., N. TEZAPSIDIS, J. CARTER *et al.* 1996. Identification and neuron specific expression of the S182/presenilin 1 protein in human and rodent brains. J. Neurosci. Res. **45:** 308–320.
12. GIANNAKOPOULOS, P., C. BOURAS, E. KOVARI *et al.* 1997. Presenilin-1-immunoreactive neurons are preserved in late-onset Alzheimer's disease. Am. J. Pathol. **150:** 429–436.
13. SHEN, J., R.T. BRONSON, D.F. CHEN *et al.* 1997. Skeletal and CNS defects in presenilin-1-deficient mice. Cell **89:** 629–639.
14. ROPERCH, J.P., V. ALVARO, S. PRIEUR *et al.* 1998. Inhibition of presenilin 1 expression is promoted by p53 and p21WAF-1 and results in apoptosis and tumor suppression. Nat. Med. **4:** 835–838.
15. BURSZTAJN, S., R. DESOUZA, D.L. MCPHIE *et al.* 1998 Overexpression in neurons of human presenilin-1 or a presenilin-1 familial Alzheimer disease mutant does not enhance apoptosis. J. Neurosci. **18:** 9790–9799.
16. KAUSHAL, S. & H.G. KHORANA. 1994. Structure and function in rhodopsin. 7. Point mutations associated with autosomal dominant retinitis pigmentosa. Biochemistry **33:** 6121–6128.
17. NISHIMURA, M., G. YU, G. LEVESQUE *et al.* 1999. Presenilin mutations associated with Alzheimer disease cause defective intracellular trafficking of beta-catenin, a component of the presenilin protein complex. Nat. Med. **5:** 164–169.
18. TERRY, R.D., E. MASLIAH & L.A. HANSEN. 1994. Structural basis of the cognitive alterations in Alzheimer disease. *In* Alzheimer Disease. R.D. Terry, R. Katzman & K.L. Bick, Eds. Raven Press, Ltd. New York.
19. SIMONS, M., E. IKONEN, P.J. TIENARI *et al.* 1995. Intracellular routing of human amyloid protein precursor: axonal delivery followed by transport to dendrites. J. Neurosci. Res. **41:** 121–128.

20. SISODIA, S.S., E.H. KOO, P.N. HOFFMAN *et al.* 1993. Identification and transport of full-length amyloid precursor proteins in rat peripheral nervous system. J. Neurosci. **13:** 3136–3142.
21. BREEN, K.C., M. BRUCE & B.H. ANDERTON. 1991. Beta amyloid precursor protein mediates neuronal cell-cell and cell-surface adhesion. J. Neurosci. Res. **28:** 90–100.
22. SCHUBERT, D., L.W. JIN, T. SAITOH & G. COLE. 1989. The regulation of amyloid beta protein precursor secretion and its modulatory role in cell adhesion. Neuron **3:** 689–694.
23. DE STROOPER, B., P. SAFTIG, K. CRAESSAERTS *et al.* 1998. Deficiency of presenilin-1 inhibits the normal cleavage of amyloid precursor protein. Nature **39:** 387–390.
24. WOLFE, M.S., W. XIA, B.L. OSTASZEWSKI *et al.* 1999. Two transmembrane aspartates in presenilin-1 required for presenilin endoproteolysis and gamma-secretase activity. Nature **398:** 513–517.
25. LARUE, L., M. OHSUGI, J. HIRCHENHAIN & R. KEMLER. 1994. E-cadherin null mutant embryos fail to form a trophectoderm epithelium. Proc. Natl. Acad. Sci. USA **91:** 8263–8267.

α-Secretase Activity of the Disintegrin Metalloprotease ADAM 10

Influences of Domain Structure

FALK FAHRENHOLZ,[a] SANDRA GILBERT, ELZBIETA KOJRO, SVEN LAMMICH, AND ROLF POSTINA

Institut für Biochemie, Johannes Gutenberg-Universität, Mainz, Germany

ABSTRACT: Disintegrin metalloproteases from different organisms form the ADAM (a disintegrin and metalloprotease) family. All members display a common domain organization and possess four potential functions: proteolysis, cell adhesion, cell fusion, and cell signaling. Members of the ADAM family are responsible for the proteolytic cleavage of transmembrane proteins and release of their extracellular domain. The proteolytic process is referred to as ectodomain shedding, which is activated by phorbol esters and inhibited by hydroxamic acid-based inhibitors. We have shown that the disintegrin metalloprotease ADAM 10 has both constitutive and regulated α-secretase activity. Expression of a dominant negative mutant of ADAM 10 in HEK cells decreases the secretion of APPsα. In order to investigate the influence of distinct protein domains of ADAM 10 on α-secretase activity, several deletion mutants of ADAM 10 were constructed. Our findings demonstrate that the deletion of the disintegrin domain results in a mutant ADAM 10 with remaining α-secretase activity, whereas the deletion of the prodomain destroys the proteolytic activity of ADAM 10.

INTRODUCTION

Both during and after its transport through the secretory pathway to the cell surface, a fraction of the amyloid precursor protein molecules (APP) undergoes endoproteolytic cleavage within the sequence of the amyloid β-peptides (Aβ). This principal secretory cleavage is effected by the protease(s) designated as α-secretase(s). Soluble N-terminal APP (APPsα) fragments of 105–125 kDa are released into vesicle lumens and from the cell surface. The α-secretase activity can be significantly enhanced by events that involve the activation by second messengers, as recently reviewed.[1] Protein kinase C was the first signal transduction-related molecule to be implicated in this mechanism.[2]

The stimulation of α-secretase activity and an increase of secreted APPsα might be beneficial for the treatment of Alzheimer's disease for several reasons: In principle, proteolytic cleavage of APP within the Aβ sequence precludes the formation of the amyloidogenic peptides. Furthermore, APPsα has a trophic effect on cerebral

[a]Address for correspondence: Falk Fahrenholz, Institut für Biochemie, Johannes Gutenberg-Universität, Becherweg 30, D-55128 Mainz, Germany. Tel.: +6131-3925833; fax: +6131-3925348.

e-mail: ibc1950@mail.uni-mainz.de

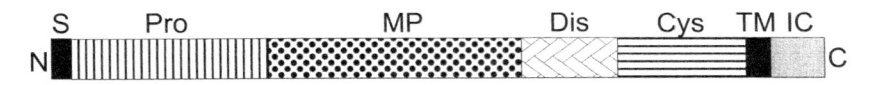

FIGURE 1. Domain organization of ADAMs. The extracellular region of these class I membrane domain proteins are composed of multiple domains. Potential functions are given in brackets. S, signal sequence; Pro, prodomain; MP, metalloprotease domain (proteolysis); Dis, disintegrin domain (adhesion); Cys, cysteine-rich domain (fusion); TM, transmembrane domain; IC, intracellular domain (signaling). The length of the domains reflects the number of amino acids in the domains of ADAM 10.

neurons in culture and has neuroprotective properties.[3] Meziane *et al.* reported that in behavioral paradigms, APPsα has memory-enhancing effects in normal and amnestic mice.[4]

DISINTEGRIN METALLOPROTEASES

Recently it has been demonstrated that the disintegrin metalloprotease ADAM 10 has both constitutive and regulated α-secretase activity and many properties expected for the proteolytic processing of APP.[5] At present, 30 disintegrin metalloproteases from different organisms like *Drosophila melanogaster, Caenorhabditis elegans,* and *Xenopus laevis,* as well as from several mammals, are known and form the ADAM (a disintegrin and metalloprotease) family.[6] All ADAMs display a common domain organization (FIG. 1) and possess four potential functions: proteolysis, cell adhesion, cell fusion, and cell signaling. About one-half of the known ADAMs contain in their metalloprotease domain a catalytic site sequence with three histidine residues (HEXXHXXGXXH) that chelate a zinc ion and one glutamic residue involved in the acid-catalyzed cleavage of peptide bonds. This extended zinc binding site is typical for a superfamily of metalloproteases, the metzincins. Their name is derived from the highly conserved methionine close to the zinc binding site, which is involved in the formation of the active conformation.

Members of the ADAM family are responsible for the proteolytic cleavage of transmembrane proteins and release of their extracellular domain. This proteolytic process is referred to as ectodomain shedding, which is activated by phorbol esters and inhibited by hydroxamic acid-based inhibitors. ADAM 17 specifically cleaves the precursor of tumor necrosis factor-α (TNFα).[7,8] This enzyme, also called TNFα-converting enzyme or TACE, shows the highest homology to ADAM 10 (21% amino acid identity). The latter has also been shown to cleave pro-TNFα *in vitro.*[9] ADAM 9 converts the membrane localized form of the heparin-binding EGF-like growth factor (pro-HB-EGF) to its soluble form.[10] In *Drosophila melanogaster* neurogenesis, the metalloprotease disintegrin protein Kuzbanian (Kuz) is required in the early embryo for neural inhibition.[11] There is evidence that this process mediated by Kuz involves a specific cleavage in the extracellular domain of the transmembrane receptor Notch and/or of the membrane bound Notch Ligand Delta.[12,13] Kuz and mammalian ADAM 10 share a high level of sequence similarity throughout the molecule (41% amino acid identity).

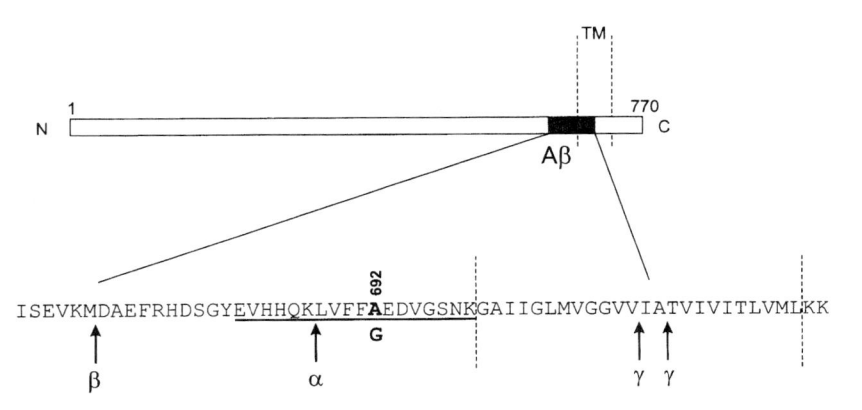

FIGURE 2. Sites of APP cleavage by secretases. The cleavage sites of the largest APP alternative splice form, comprising 770 amino acids, are shown by arrows; the mutation A692G close to the α-secretase site leading to a mixed phenotype of AD and cerebral hemorrhage with amyloidosis (CHWA) is indicated by a bold typed letter. The position of octadecapeptides corresponding to residues 11–28 in Aβ used for *in vitro* assays of α-secretase activity of purified ADAM 10 is underlined.

CONSTITUTIVE AND REGULATED α-SECRETASE ACTIVITY OF ADAM 10

Studies in various cell types confirmed that the major α-secretory cleavage site is after Lys[16] in the Aβ domain, but multiple minor cleavages around this site have been observed.[14,15] Principal determinants of APP cleavage by α-secretase appear to be the distance of the hydrolyzed bond from the membrane (12–13 residues) and a local helical conformation.[16]

We have shown that ADAM 10 purified from bovine kidney proteolytically cleaves an octadecapeptide amino acid sequence of APP (FIG. 2; residues 11–28 in Aβ) between Lys[16] and Leu[17] as expected for an enzyme with α-secretase activity. The activity of ADAM 10 was dependent on the conformation of its substrate: replacement of Ala[21] in Aβ$_{11-28}$ by glycine reduced both the α-helical conformation and the velocity of cleavage by ADAM 10.[5] This position corresponds to a naturally occurring Ala→Gly mutation at position 692 of APP$_{770}$,[17] which was identified in patients with cerebral hemorrhages due to amyloid angiopathy.

Overexpression of bovine ADAM 10 in HEK cells led to a severalfold increase of APPsα (FIG. 3; lanes 1 and 2) and of the C-terminal p10 fragment (not shown). This enhanced α-secretase activity due to overexpression of ADAM 10 could be further increased by stimulation of protein kinase C with phorbol esters (FIG. 3; lanes 6 and 7), a characteristic feature of the α-secretase.[2,18]

Cell-surface biotinylation experiments demonstrated that the proteolytically activated form of ADAM 10 is localized mainly in the plasma membrane of HEK cells.[5] This result supported the view that cleavage of the transmembrane protein APP occurs by a membrane-bound endoprotease at the cell surface.[16,19–21] On the other

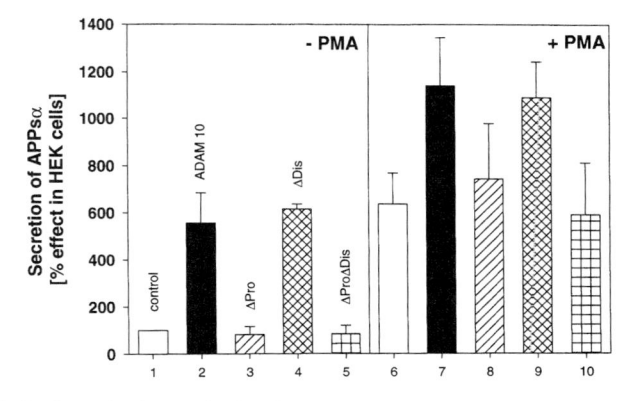

FIGURE 3. Quantitative analysis of secreted APPsα from HEK cells and HEK cells stably expressing either ADAM 10 or three different deletion mutants of ADAM 10. Cells were incubated for 4.5 h in the absence or presence of PMA. Then the proteins of the culture medium were precipitated, separated by SDS-PAGE and subsequently transferred to a PVDF membrane. The membrane was probed with the antibody 6E10 (Senetek), followed by alkaline phosphatase-coupled anti-mouse IgG (Tropix, Bedford, MA). For detection of bands corresponding to APPsα, the chemiluminescence substrate CDPstar (Tropix) was used. The emitted light was detected using a digital camera and quantified. (Software: Aida, version 2.0 provided by Raytest, Straubenhardt, Germany).

hand, several reports provided evidence that APP is cleaved by the α-secretase in a trans-Golgi compartment of the secretory pathway.[22–25] ADAM 10 was predominantly found as proenzyme intracellularly in the Golgi, presumably in an inactive form.[5]

INFLUENCE OF THE PRODOMAIN AND THE DISINTEGRIN DOMAIN ON THE α-SECRETASE ACTIVITY OF ADAM 10

The proteolytic activity of several members of the metzincin family is regulated by a cysteine residue in the prodomain. According to the "cysteine-switch" mechanism,[26] the conserved cysteine in the prodomain complexes at the fourth coordination site of the zinc ion in the catalytic center and inhibits the entrance of the water molecule which is responsible for hydrolysis. Only after proteolytic removal of the prodomain, the latent inhibition is released. Several ADAMs, including ADAM 10, contain the recognition site RX(K/R)R for furin-like pro-protein convertases between their prodomain and their metalloprotease domain. For both ADAM 9 and ADAM 12, it has been shown that the post-translational proteolytic removal of the prodomain within the trans-Golgi network is an important step for their conversion from a latent pro-form to an active enzyme.[27,28]

To examine the effect of the prodomain on the α-secretase activity of ADAM 10, a deletion mutant was constructed lacking the prodomain (ΔPro). After stable overexpression of the ΔPro mutant in HEK cells, the same α-secretase activity was found as in control HEK cells (FIG. 3; lanes 1 and 3). Stimulation of HEK cells and cells overexpressing the ΔPro mutant with the phorbol ester PMA resulted in a sixfold increase of α-secretase activity due to stimulation of endogenous ADAM 10 in HEK cells, with no significant further increase in cells overexpressing the ΔPro mutant (FIG. 3; lanes 3 and 8). Therefore, the expression of ADAM 10 as a proenzyme seems to be a prerequisite for the proteolytic activity of ADAM 10. The prodomain obviously plays an important role for the correct folding of the latent proenzyme in the endoplasmatic reticulum and/or the further transport in the secretory pathway.[29] Our finding is supported by the hypothesis that the prodomain acts as an intramolecular or steric chaperone for the folding and activity of several proteases containing prosequences.[30,31]

For ADAM 2 and ADAM 15, it has been shown that they interact via their disintegrin domain with integrin receptors on neighboring cells.[32,33] To investigate whether the disintegrin domain has any supporting function for the proteolytic activity of ADAM 10, a deletion mutant of ADAM 10 lacking the disintegrin domain (ΔDis) was constructed. The overexpression of the mutant protein ΔDis in HEK cells led to an enhanced α-secretase activity as compared to control cells (FIG. 3; lanes 1 and 4). This activity could further be increased by stimulation with PMA (FIG. 3; lanes 6 and 9). Obviously, the disintegrin domain is not a prerequisite for α-secretase activity of ADAM 10. Further removal of the prodomain from the proteolytically active deletion mutant ΔDis led to a catalytically inactive mutant ΔProDis (FIG. 3; lanes 5 and 10). This observation confirms the hypothesis that the prodomain is important for the α-secretase activity of ADAM 10. Nevertheless, the role of the disintegrin domain in α-secretase acivity and substrate specificity has to be further examined.

EFFECT OF A DOMINANT NEGATIVE ADAM 10 MUTANT ON α-SECRETASE ACTIVITY

To inhibit the endogenous α-secretase activity in HEK cells, the point mutation E384A was introduced into the zinc binding site of the bovine ADAM 10 protease. A mutant Kuz-protein with a mutation at the same site acted as a dominant negative form in *Drosophila melanogaster*.[12] HEK cells stably expressing mutant ADAM 10 E384A (HEK/DN) showed a substantially decreased secretion of APPsα without effecting the expression of APP. The inhibitory effect was most apparent in PMA-treated cells: only about 25% of enzymatic activity was observed (FIG. 4; lanes 3 and 4). Thus, this point mutation resulted in a dominant negative form of the protease, and significantly decreased constitutive and stimulated endogenous α-secretase activity.

CONCLUSIONS

The disintegrin metalloprotease ADAM 10 has many properties expected for a physiologically relevant APP processing enzyme with constitutive and regulated α-secretase activity. Evidence was provided that also TACE (ADAM 17) may be involved in the regulated α-secretase cleavage of APP.[34] ADAM 9 has been shown to cleave peptides derived from APP. However, it does not target the major α-secretase site *in vitro*.[27] Two yeast aspartyl proteases have recently been described which cleave APP in yeast at the expected α-secretase cleavage site.[35] Thus, with the observation of heterogeneity of cleavages in this site,[14,15] this could indicate that apart from ADAM 10 other enzymes may act as α-secretases.

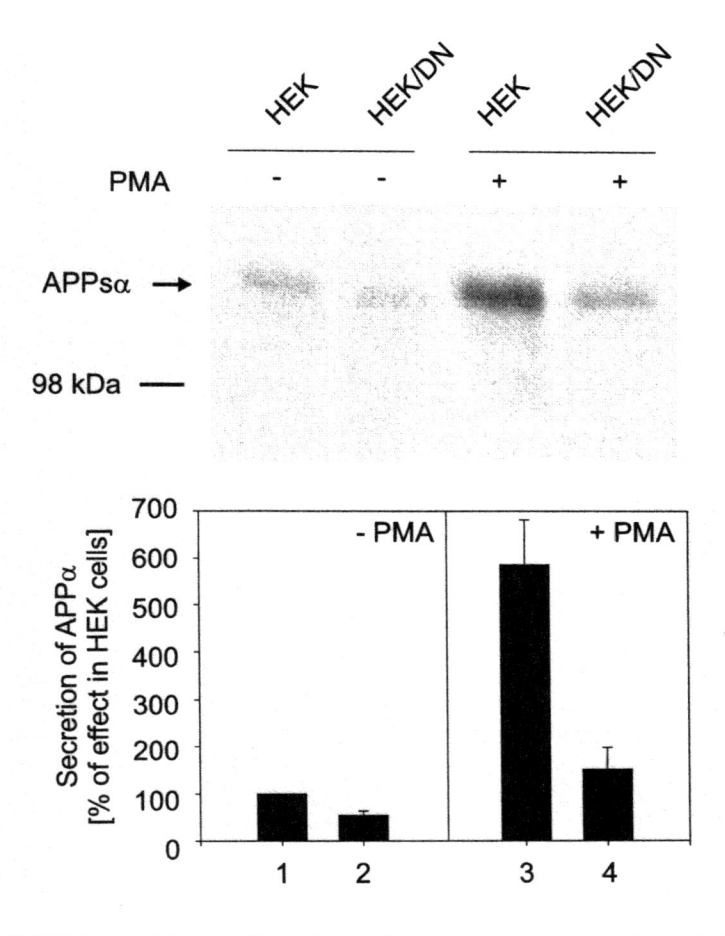

FIGURE 4. Inhibition effect of a dominant negative ADAM 10 form (DN) of the endogenous α-secretase activity on HEK cells. The basal and PMA-stimulated α-secretase activity of HEK cells stably expressing the dominant negative ADAM 10 form (DN) was compared with the effect in control HEK cells. *Upper part*: Cells were incubated in the absence or presence of 1 μM PMA. After 4 h, the medium was collected and the proteins were precipitated and subjected to immunoelectrophoretic blot analysis with antibody 6E10 (Senetek, St. Louis) followed by a secondary [^{35}S]-labeled anti-mouse IgG antibody (Amersham). *Lower part*: Quantitative analysis of secreted APPsα after immunoblot analysis. The results are expressed as percentage of secreted APPsα in control HEK cells and are the averages ± SD of at least three experiments.

REFERENCES

1. MILLS, J. & P.B. REINER. 1999. Regulation of amyloid precursor protein cleavage. J. Neurochem. **72:** 443–460.
2. HUNG, A.Y., C. HAASS, R.M. NITSCH, *et al.* 1993. Activation of protein kinase C inhibits cellular production of the amyloid beta-protein. J. Biol. Chem. **268:** 22959–22962.
3. ARAKI, W., N. KITAGUCHI, Y. TOKUSHIMA, *et al.* 1991. Trophic effect of beta-amyloid precursor protein on cerebral cortical neurons in culture. Biochem. Biophys. Res. Commun. **181:** 265–271.
4. MEZIANE, H., J.-C. DODART, C. MATHIS, *et al.* 1998. Memory enhancing effects of secreted forms of the β-amyloid precursor protein in normal and amnestic mice. Proc. Natl. Acad. Sci. USA **95:** 12683–12688.
5. LAMMICH, S., E. KOJRO, R. POSTINA, *et al.* 1999. Constitutive and regulated α-secretase cleavage of Alzheimer's amyloid precursor protein by a disintegrin metalloprotease. Proc. Natl. Acad. Sci. USA **96:** 3922–3927.
6. BLACK, R.A. & J.M. WHITE. 1998. ADAMs: focus on the protease domain. Curr. Opin. Cell Biol. **10:** 654–659.
7. BLACK, R.A., C.T. RAUCH, C.J. KOZLOSKY, *et al.* 1997. A metalloproteinase disintegrin that releases tumour-necrosis factor-α. Nature **385:** 729–733.
8. MOSS, M.L., S.-L.C. JIN, M.E. MILLA, *et al.* 1997. Cloning of a disintegrin metalloproteinase that processes precursor tumour-necrosis factor-α. Nature **385:** 733–736.
9. ROSENDAHL, M.S., S.C. KO, D.L. LONG, *et al.* 1997. Identification and characterization of a pro-tumor necrosis factor-α-processing enzyme from the ADAM family of zinc metalloproteases. J. Biol. Chem. **272:** 24588–24593.
10. IZUMI, Y., M. HIRATA, H. HASUWA, *et al.* 1998. A metalloprotease-disintegrin, MDC9/meltrin-γ/ADAM9 and PKCδ are involved in TPA-induced ectodomain shedding of membrane-anchored heparin-binding EGF-like growth factor. EMBO J. **17:** 7260–7272.
11. ROOKE, J., D. PAN, T. XU & G.M. RUBIN. 1996. KUZ, a conserved metalloprotease-disintegrin protein with two roles in *Drosophila* neurogenesis. Science **273:** 1227–1231.
12. PAN, D. & G.M. RUBIN. 1997. Kuzbanian controls proteolytic processing of Notch and mediates lateral inhibition during Drosophila and vertebrate neurogenesis. Cell **90:** 271–280.
13. QI, H., M.D. RAND, X. WU, *et al.* 1999. Processing of the Notch Ligand Delta by the metalloprotease Kuzbanian. Science **283:** 91–94.
14. ZHONG, Z., J. HIGAKI, K. MURAKAMI, *et al.* 1994. Secretion of β-amyloid precursor protein involves multiple cleavage sites. J. Biol. Chem. **269:** 627–632.
15. SIMONS, M., B. DE STROOPER, G. MULTHAUP, P.J. TIENARI, C.G. DOTTI & K. BEYREUTHER. 1996. Amyloidogenic processing of the human amyloid precursor protein in primary cultures of rat hippocampal neurons. J. Neurosci. **16:** 899–908.
16. SISODIA, S.S. 1992. β-Amyloid precursor protein cleavage by a membrane-bound protease. Proc. Natl. Acad. Sci. USA **89:** 6075–6079.
17. HENDRIKS, L., C.M. VAN DUIJN, P. CRAS, *et al.* 1992. Presenile dementia and cerebral hemorrhage linked to a mutation at codon 692 of the β-amyloid precursor protein gene. Nature Genet. **1:** 218–221.
18. BUXBAUM, J.D., E.H. KOO & P. GREENGARD. 1993. Protein phosphorylation inhibits production of Alzheimer amyloid/A4 peptide. Proc. Natl. Acad. Sci. USA **90:** 9195–9198.
19. HAASS, C., E.H. KOO, A. MELLON, A.Y. HUNG & D.J. SELKOE. 1992. Targeting of cell-surface β-amyloid precursor protein to lysosomes: alternative processing into amyloid-bearing fragments. Nature **357:** 500–503.
20. IKEZU, T., B.D. TRAPP, K.S. SONG, A. SCHLEGEL, M.P. LISANTI & T. OKAMOTO. 1998. Caveolae, plasma membrane microdomains for α-secretase-mediated processing of the amyloid precursor protein. J. Biol. Chem. **273:** 10485–10495.
21. PARVATHY, S., I. HUSSEIN, E.H. KARRAN, A.J. TURNER & N.M. HOOPER. 1999. Cleavage of Alzheimer's amyloid precursor protein by α-secretase occurs at the surface of neuronal cells. Biochemistry **38:** 9728–9734.

22. KUENTZEL, S.L., S.M. ALI, R.A. ALTMAN, B.D. GREENBERG & T.J. RAUB. 1993. The Alzheimer beta-amyloid protein precursor/protease nexin-II is cleaved by secretase in a trans-Golgi secretory compartment in human neuroglioma cells. Biochem. J. 295: 367–378.

23. DE STROOPER, B., L. UMANS, F. VAN LEUVEN & H. VAN DEN BERGHE. 1993. Study of the synthesis and secretion of normal and artificial mutants of murine amyloid precursor protein (APP): cleavage of APP occurs in a late compartment of the default secretion pathway. J. Cell Biol. 121: 295–304.

24. SAMBAMURTI, K., J. SHIOI, J.P. ANDERSON, M.A. PAPPOLLA & N.K. ROBAKIS. 1992. Evidence for intracellular cleavage of the Alzheimer's amyloid precursor in PC12 cells. J. Neurosci. Res. 33: 319–329.

25. TOMITA, S., K. YUTAKA & T. SUZUKI. 1998. Cleavage of Alzheimer's amyloid precursor protein (APP) by secretases occurs after O-glycosylation of APP in the protein secretory pathway. J. Biol. Chem. 273: 6277–6284.

26. GRAMS, F., R. HUBER, L.F. KRESS, L. MORODER & W. BODE. 1993. Activation of snake venom metalloproteinases by a cysteine switch-like mechanism. FEBS Lett. 335: 76–80.

27. ROGHANI, M., J.D. BECHERER, M.L. MOSS, et al. 1999. Metalloprotease-disintegrin MDC9: intracellular maturation and catalytic activity. J. Biol. Chem. 274: 3531–3540.

28. LOECHEL, F., B.J. GILPIN, E. ENGVALL, R. ALBRECHTSEN & U.M. WEWER. 1998. Human ADAM 12 (meltrin α) is an active metalloprotease. J. Biol. Chem. 273: 16993–16997.

29. LOECHEL, F., M.T. OVERGAARD, C. OXVIG, R. ALBRECHTSEN & U.M. WEWER. 1999. Regulation of human ADAM 12 protease by the prodomain. J. Biol. Chem. 274: 13427–13433.

30. SHINDE, U.P., J.J. LIU & M. INOUYE. 1997. Protein memory through altered folding mediated by intramolecular chaperones. Nature 389: 520–522.

31. PETERS, R.J., A.K. SHIAU, J.L. SOHL, et al. 1998. Pro region C-terminus: protease active site interactions are critical in catalyzing the folding of α-lytic protease. Biochemistry 37: 12058–12067.

32. ALMEIDA, E.A.C., A.-P. J. HUOVILA, A.E. SUTHERLAND, et al. 1995. Mouse egg integrin α6β1 functions as a sperm receptor. Cell 81: 1095–1104.

33. ZHANG, XI-P., T. KAMATA, K. YOKOYAMA, W. PUZON-MCLAUGHLIN & Y. TAKADA. 1998. Specific interaction of the rRecombinant disintegrin-like domain of MDC-15 (metargidin, ADAM 15) with integrin αvβ3. J. Biol. Chem. 273: 7345–7350.

34. BUXBAUM, J.D., K.-N. LIU, Y. LUO, et al. 1998. Evidence that tumor necrosis factor-α converting enzyme is involved in regulated α-secretase cleavage of the Alzheimer amyloid protein precursor. J. Biol. Chem. 273: 27765–27767.

35. KOMANO, H., M. SEEGER, S. GANDY, G.T. WANG, G.A. KRAFFT & R.S. FULLER. 1998. Involvement of cell surface glycosyl-phosohatidylinositol-linked aspartyl proteases in alpha-secretase-type cleavage and ectodomain solubilization of human Alzheimer beta-amyloid precursor protein in yeast. J. Biol. Chem. 273: 31648–31651.

Rapid Notch1 Nuclear Translocation after Ligand Binding Depends on Presenilin-associated γ-Secretase Activity

OKSANA BEREZOVSKA,[a,e] CHRISTINE JACK,[a] PAMELA McLEAN,[a]
JON C. ASTER,[b] CAROL HICKS,[c] WEIMING XIA,[d] MICHAEL S. WOLFE,[d]
GERRY WEINMASTER,[c] DENNIS J. SELKOE,[d] AND BRADLEY T. HYMAN[a]

[a]*Alzheimer's Disease Research Laboratory, Massachusetts General Hospital,
Charlestown, Massachusetts 02129, USA*

[b]*Department of Pathology, Brigham and Women's Hospital,
Boston, Massachusetts 02115, USA*

[c]*Department of Biological Chemistry, UCLA School of Medicine,
Los Angeles, California 90024, USA*

[d]*Center for Neurologic Diseases, Brigham and Women's Hospital,
Boston, Massachusetts 02115, USA*

ABSTRACT: Recent data suggest an intimate relationship between the familial
Alzheimer disease gene presenilin 1 (PS1) and proteolytic processing of both
the amyloid precursor protein (APP) and the important cell signaling molecule, Notch1. We now show, using mammalian cells transfected with full-length
Notch1, that the C terminal domain of Notch1 rapidly translocates to the nucleus upon stimulation with the physiologic ligand Delta and initiates a CBF1-
dependent signal transduction cascade. Using this assay, we demonstrate that
the same aspartate mutations in PS1 that block APP processing also prevent
Notch1 cleavage and translocation to the nucleus. Moreover, we show that two
APP γ-secretase inhibitors also diminish Notch1 nuclear translocation in a
dose-dependent fashion. However, Notch1 signaling, assessed by measuring the
activity of CBF1, a downstream gene, was reduced but not completely abolished in the presence of either aspartate mutations or γ-secretase inhibitors.
Our results support the hypothesis that similar PS1-related enzymatic activity
is necessary for both APP and Notch1 processing, yet suggest that Notch signaling may remain relatively preserved with moderate levels of γ-secretase
inhibition.

INTRODUCTION

Mutations in presenilin genes (PS1 and PS2) are associated with the majority of
early onset familial Alzheimer's disease (AD). PS mutations alter proteolytic processing of a large single transmembrane domain protein, β-amyloid precursor protein (APP), by enzymatic activity of β- and γ-secretases, which results in markedly

[e]Address for correspondence: Dr. Oksana Berezovska, Alzheimer's Disease Research Laboratory, Massachusetts General Hospital, 149-13th Street, Charlestown, MA 02129. Tel.: (617) 724-
8330; fax: (617) 726-5677.
e-mail: berezovskaja@helix.mgh.harvard.edu

elevated levels of amyloid β-protein (Aβ) deposition in the brains of AD patients.[1,2] Recently, PS1 has been suggested as a candidate for the enzyme that cleaves both APP and Notch1.[3–7]

RESULTS AND DISCUSSION

Chinese hamster ovary (CHO) cells were transfected with full- length Notch1 tagged with EGFP on its C-terminus [N1(FL)-EGFP] and then treated with conditioned medium (CM) containing soluble Fc-conjugated Delta (Dl-Fc), or with control media without Dl-Fc.[8] The cells were fixed at different time points of ligand treatment and immunostained for GFP. The fluorescent signal in the nucleus corresponding to the accumulation of Notch's EGFP-labeled C-terminus was quantified using confocal microscopy. We observed the presence of Notch-EGFP in the nucleus as early as 3–5 min after adding preclustered Dl-Fc. To determine whether the nuclear translocation resulted in activation of Notch signaling pathway, we assessed transactivation of a CBF1-luciferase reporter construct co-transfected with Notch1 into CHO cells.[9] We found that CBF1-luciferase activity in WT PS1 CHO cells transfected with N1(FL) and treated with Dl-Fc showed 4–6 times activation in comparison to an empty vector transfected cells.

Next we used a nuclear translocation assay to examine the role of PS1 in Notch1 nuclear translocation/signaling. We transfected CHO cells stably expressing either wild-type PS1 (WT PS1), or mutated PS1 (D257A, or D385A), which have previously been shown to lead to a significant diminution of APP γ-secretase activity,[3] with N1(FL) and then treated them with Dl-Fc. There was no fluorescent signal in the nucleus of either D257A or D385A PS1 expressing cells even 24 h after exposure of the cells to the ligand (FIG. 1). This suggests that both aspartate mutations in PS1 abolish, and not simply delay, ligand-induced Notch1-EGFP nuclear translocation. In addition,

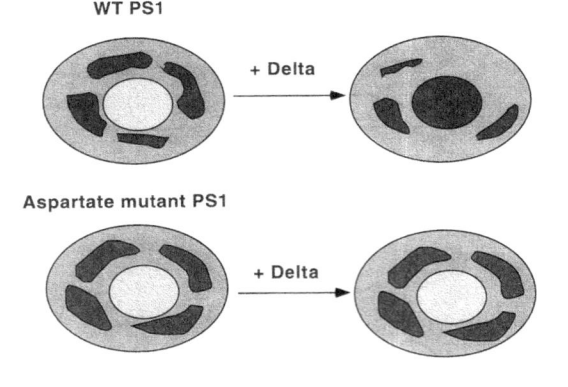

FIGURE 1. Schematic representation of Notch1 nuclear translocation after ligand binding in N1(FL)-EGFP transfected CHO cells. A marked accumulation of the green fluorescence was found in the nucleus of WT PS1, but not in D257A or D385A aspartate mutant CHO cells 24 h after treatment with Delta, Notch's ligand.

Western blot analysis showed significant reduction in NICD generation in PS1 aspartate mutant cells in comparison to WT PS1 cells. This agrees with the findings by Ray *et al.*[6] that the same aspartate mutations inhibited Notch γ-secretase-like proteolysis.

In addition to the experiments in which we introduced specific PS1 mutations, we used pharmacological agents, γ-secretase inhibitors MW115 and MW167, which have been shown to inhibit γ-secretase cleavage of APP,[3,10] to test the hypothesis that APP γ-secretase-like activity is important for ligand-induced Notch1 cleavage/nuclear translocation. We demostrated that ligand-induced Notch1 cleavage/nuclear translocation also was effectively inhibited by these two γ-secretase inhibitors in a dose-dependent manner. This is consistent with DeStrooper's data showing inhibition of cleavage of constitutively active truncated Notch1 (mNotchΔEC) by the APP γ-secretase inhibitor MW167.[4]

An alternative hypothesis explaning the lack of response of Notch1 to the ligand in D257A and D385A PS1 cells would be if PS1 mutations affected trafficking of Notch1 or protease to the site of cleavage, the cell-surface membrane.[11–14] To test this hypothesis we transfected WT PS1, D257A PS1, and D385A PS1 CHO cells with a N1(FL) construct, bearing an extracellular-domain HA tag, which has previously been shown to be biologically active.[15] Immunostaining for HA without addition of permeabilizing agents showed an identical pattern of staining in all three cell lines. This suggests that the D257A and D385A mutations do not affect Notch1 access to the plasma membrane and supports the idea that these mutations impact Notch1 signaling by interfering with Notch1 proteolysis and/or nuclear translocation. A similar conclusion was reached by Ray *et al.*[6] who showed that PS1 aspartate mutations affect neither the ability of PS1 to bind Notch in ER/Golgi, nor traffic to the plasma membrane.

SUMMARY

C-terminal domain of Notch1 rapidly translocates to the nucleus (3–5 min) upon stimulation with the physiologic ligand Delta, and results in transcriptional activation of CBF1, a downstream component of Notch signaling pathway. Two PS1 transmembrane aspartate mutations (D257A and D385A) do not affect Notch1 trafficking to the cell surface. The two PS1 aspartate mutations and γ-secretase inhibitors impair Notch1 proteolytic processing and nuclear translocation. We conclude that identical PS1-dependent γ-secretase enzymatic activity is necessary for both Notch1 and APP processing.

ACKNOWLEDGMENTS

This work was supported by grants PO AG 15379 and AG 14744.

REFERENCES

1. LEMERE, C.A., F. LOPERA, K.S. KOSIK, *et al.* 1996. The E280A presenilin 1 Alzheimer mutation produces increased Aβ$_{42}$ deposition and severe cerebellar pathology. Nature Med. **2:** 1146–1150.

  2. GÓMEZ-ISLA, T., W.B. GROWDON, M.J. MCNAMARA, *et al.* 1999. The impact of different presenilin 1 and presenilin 2 mutations on amyloid deposition, neurofibrillary changes and neuronal loss in the familial Alzheimer's disease (AD) brain: evidence for other phenotype modifying factors. Brain **122:** 1709–1719.
  3. WOLFE, M.S., W. XIA, B.L. OSTASZEWSKI, *et al.* 1999. Two transmembrane aspartates in presenilin-1 required for presenilin endoproteolysis and γ-secretase activity. Nature **398:** 513–517.
  4. DE STROOPER, B., W. ANNAERT, P. CUPER, *et al.* 1999. A presenilin-1-dependent γ-secretase-like protease mediates release of Notch intracellular domain. Nature **398:** 518–521.
  5. SONG, W., P. NADEAU, M. YUAN, *et al.* 1999. Proteolytic release and nuclear translocation of Notch-1 are induced by presenilin-1 and impaired by pathogenic presenilin-1 mutations. Proc. Natl. Acad. Sci. USA **96:** 6959–6063.
  6. RAY, W., M. YAO, J. MUMM, *et al.* 1999. Cell surface presenilin-1 participates in the gamma-secretase-like proteolysis of Notch. J. Biol. Chem. **274:** 36801–36807.
  7. STEINER, H., K. DUFF, A. CAPELL, *et al.* 1999. A loss of function mutation of presenilin-2 interferes with amyloid-peptide production and Notch signaling. J. Biol. Chem. **274:** 28669–28673.
  8. WANG, S., A.D. SDRULLA, G. DISIBIO, *et al.* 1998. Notch receptor activation inhibits oligodendrocyte differentiation. Neuron **21:** 63–75.
  9. BEREZOVSKA, O., P. MCLEAN, R. KNOWLES, *et al.* 1999. Notch1 inhibits neurite outgrowth in postmitotic primary neurons. Neuroscience **93:** 433–439.
 10. WOLFE, M., M. CITRON, T.S. DIEHL, *et al.* 1998. A substrate-based difluoro ketone selectively inhibits Alzheimer's gamma-secretase activity. J. Med. Chem. **41:** 6–9.
 11. NARUSE, S., G. THINAKARAN, J.J. LUO, *et al.* 1998. Effect of PS1 deficiency on membrane protein trafficking in neurons. Neuron **21:** 1213–1221.
 12. LEVITAN, D. & I. GREENWALD. 1998. Effect of Sel-12 presenilin on Lin-12 localization and function in *Caenorhabditis elegans.* Development **125:** 3599–3606.
 13. GUO, Y., I. LIVNE-BAR, L. ZHOU & B.L. GOULIANNE. 1999. Drosophila presenilin is required for neuronal differentiation and affects Notch subcellular localization and signaling. J. Neurosci. **19:** 8435–8442.
 14. YE, Y., N. LUKINOVA & M.E. FORTINI. 1999. Neurogenic phenotypes and altered Notch processing in Drosophila presenilin mutants. Nature **398:** 525–529.
 15. RAND, M., L.M. GRIMM, S. ARTAVANIS-TSAKONAS, *et al.* 2000. Calcium depletion dissociates and activates heterodimeric Notch receptors. Mol. Cell. Biol. **20:** 1825–1835.

GSK3β Forms a Tetrameric Complex with Endogenous PS1-CTF/NTF and β-Catenin

Effects of the D257/D385A and FAD-linked Mutations

G. TESCO AND R.E. TANZI[a]

Genetics and Aging Unit, Massachusetts General Hospital and Harvard Medical School, Charlestown, Massachusetts 02129, USA

ABSTRACT: We have previously shown that the endogenous C-terminal fragment of presenilin 1 co-immunoprecipitates with endogenous β-catenin. Since PS1 has been suggested to be involved in β-catenin stabilization, we further investigated whether GSK3β, responsible for β-catenin phosphorylation and degradation, is part of the PS1/β-catenin complex. In naïve H4 and CHO cells, PS1 co-immunoprecipitated with both endogenous β-catenin and GSK3β. In addition, GSK3β endogenously binds to the PS1-CTF/NTF complex and β-catenin in naïve CHO cells. GSK3β also co-immunoprecipitated with PS1 full length in CHO cell lines overexpressing PS1 wild type. Given that it has been recently shown that PS1 mutations of aspartate 257 or 385 result in prevention of PS1 endoproteolysis and inhibition of γ-secretase activity, we also tested whether PS1 endoproteolysis is required for β-catenin/GSK3β/PS1 binding and whether PS1 FAD-linked mutations affect GSK3β recruitment in the PS1/β-catenin complex. GSK3β was detected in PS1 immunoprecipitates from H4 cell lines overexpressing PS1 wild type, ΔE10, A286E, L246V and in CHO cell lines overexpressing aspartate or M146L mutations. The latter data show that the absence of PS1 endoproteolysis (D257A/D385A and ΔE10) or the presence of PS1-FAD mutations does not interfere with β-catenin/GSK3β/PS1 complex formation.

INTRODUCTION

Missense mutations in presenilin 1 (PS1) and presenilin 2 (PS2) are responsible for roughly 40% of early-onset familial Alzheimer's disease. To date, over 70 different PS1 mutations have been described, and five FAD mutations have been identified in PS2.[1] In naïve cell lines and brain, full-length PS1 is not easily detectable because the protein constitutively undergoes endoproteolytic cleavage resulting in the production of a fragment of ~20 kDa (C-terminal fragment or CTF) and a fragment of ~30 kDa (N-terminal fragment or NTF), which then associate in a heterodimeric complex. FAD-linked mutations in these proteins are associated with an increase in $A\beta_{1-42}$ both *in vivo* and *in vitro*.[2] In neuronal cultures derived from PS1-deficient mouse embryos, γ-secretase cleavage of APP is dramatically decreased, resulting in

[a]Address for correspondence: Rudolph E. Tanzi, Ph.D., Genetics and Aging Unit, Massachusetts General Hospital, 149-13th Street, Charlestown, MA 02129. Tel.: (617) 726-6845; fax (617) 726-5677.

e-mail: tanzi@helix.mgh.harvard.edu

attenuated production of Aβ.[3] More recently, it has been shown that two transmembrane aspartates in PS1 are required for presenilin endoproteolysis and γ-secretase activity,[4] suggesting that PS1 is an essential cofactor for γ-secretase or is itself γ-secretase.

The identification of presenilin-interacting proteins can provide a better understanding of presenilin functions. Strong evidence exists for an interaction between PS1 and β-catenin.[5–11] β-Catenin is a multifunctional protein which plays a key role in the Wingless pathway during axis development and in the regulation of cell-cell adhesion.[12] The cytoplasmic level of β-catenin is highly regulated by phosphorylation and then subsequent degradation by the proteasome. In the steady state, glycogen synthase kinase3β (GSK3β) phosphorylates β-catenin at its N-terminus. When the Wingless pathway is activated, GSK3β is inhibited producing an increase in the cytoplasmic level of β-catenin and making the protein available for transportation to the nucleus where it can bind the TCF/LEF1 family of transcription factors and regulate gene transcription.

Regarding the role of β-catenin/PS1 complex and the effect of PS1 FAD-linked mutations, different studies have reported opposite effects of PS1 in the regulation of β-catenin. Zhang et al.[8] reported that PS1 FAD-linked mutations destabilize β-catenin increasing its degradation and that decreased amounts of β-catenin make neurons more susceptible to apoptotic stimuli. More recently, Kang et al.[11] reported that PS1 FAD-linked mutations increased the half-life of β-catenin because of a defect in GSK3β recruitment into the β-catenin/PS1 complex. The latter finding is in contrast with that of Takashima et al.[13] who reported that the FAD-linked mutations increase the amount of GKS3β co-immunoprecipitated with PS1.

The aim of this study was to test the effect of different PS1 FAD-linked mutations (PS1L286V, PS1A246E, PS1Δ10, and PS1M146L) and PS1 mutations of aspartate

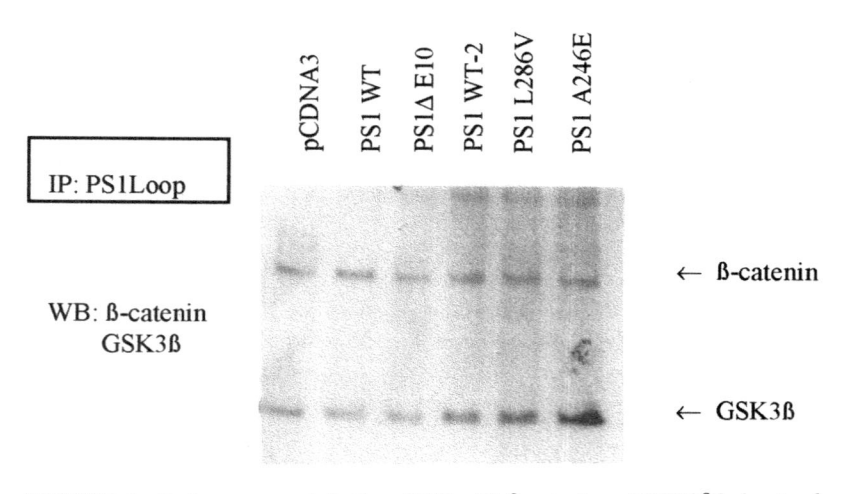

FIGURE 1. Co-immunoprecipitation of PS1 with β-catenin and GSK3β in lysates from H4 human neuroglioma PS1 stably transfected cell lines. Immunoprecipitation with αPS1 Loop antibody and Western blot with anti-β-catenin antibody and anti-GSK3β antibody.

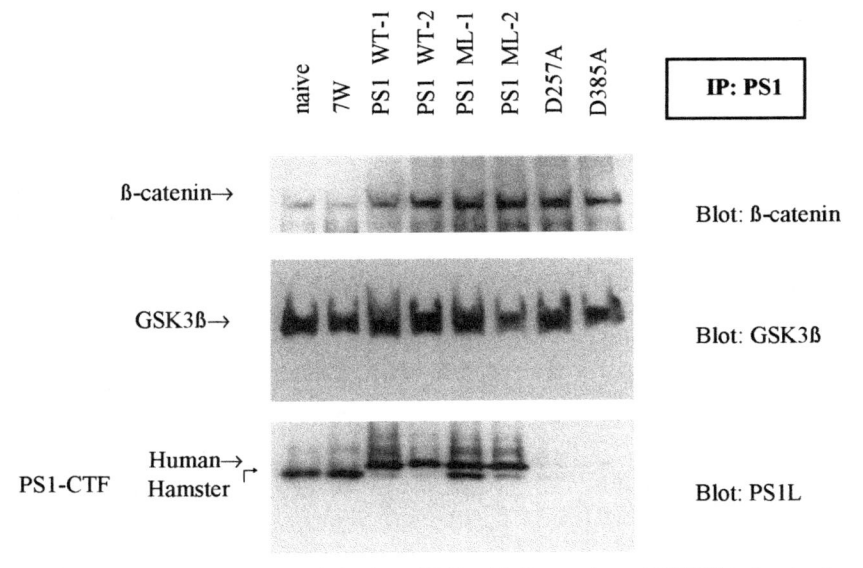

FIGURE 2. Co-immunoprecipitation of PS1 with β-catenin and GSK3β in lysates from CHO naïve and stably transfected cell lines. Cell line 7W was stably transfected with APP751 alone. All other cell lines were stably transfected with both APP751 and PS1 wild-type or mutant. Immunoprecipation with αPS1 Loop antibody and Western blot with anti-β-catenin antibody, anti-GSK3β antibody and αPS1 Loop antibody.

257 or 385 on β-catenin/GSK3β/PS1 complex using two different cell lines (CHO and H4 human neuroglioma).

RESULTS

H4 stable cell lines expressing vector alone (pCDNA3), PS1 wild-type, PS1L286V, PS1A246E, and PS1ΔE10-pCDNA3 construct[14] were lysed and subjected to immunoprecipitation with αPS1 Loop antibody as previously described[6] (FIG. 1). PS1 co-immunoprecipitated with both endogenous β-catenin and endogenous GSK3β in control (vector alone) H4 cells. Accordingly, both β-catenin and GSK3β were detected in PS1 immunoprecipitates from cell lines overexpressing PS1 WT, PS1L286V, PS1A246E, or PS1ΔE10. PS1ΔE10 is a mutation that, due to a splicing error, results in the deletion of the endoproteolytic cleavage site resulting in the accumulation of uncleaved protein and a pathogenic point mutation (C290S).[15] Neither PS1 FAD-linked point mutations nor the absence of endoproteolysis affected β-catenin binding or GSK3β recruitment in the complex.

We also addressed the question whether the absence of PS1 endoproteolysis and inhibition of γ-secretase activity due to D257A or D385A mutations might affect β-catenin/GSK3β/PS1 complex formation. Co-immunoprecipitation (co-IP) experiments were performed using CHO naïve cells or CHO cell lines stably transfected with APP751 alone (7W) or in association with PS1 WT (WT-1, WT-2), PS1M146L

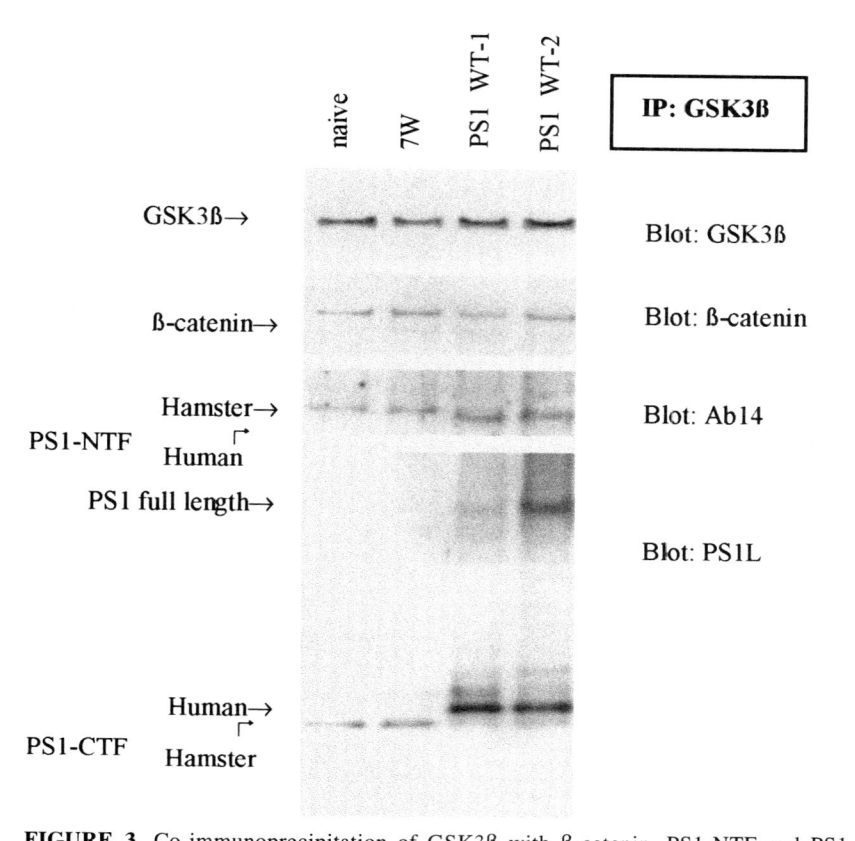

FIGURE 3. Co-immunoprecipitation of GSK3β with β-catenin, PS1-NTF and PS1-CTF in lysates from CHO naïve and cell lines overexpressing APP751 (7W) alone and in association with PS1 wild-type (PS1 WT-1 and PS1 WT-2). Western blot with anti-GSK3β antibody, anti-β-catenin antibody, Ab14 antibody, and αPS1 Loop antibody.

(ML-1, ML-2), or PS1D257A, PS1D385A[4,16] (FIG.2). The presence of the M146L FAD mutation or dominant negative aspartate mutations did not affect β-catenin binding or GSK3β recruitment. PS1 was co-immunoprecipitated with both β-catenin and GSK3β in naïve CHO cells (IP with αPS1 Loop antibody). In the reverse experiment (IP with anti-GSK3β antibody; Transduction Laboratories), GSK3β was co-immunoprecipitated with β-catenin, and with both PS1-NTF and PS1-CTF (FIG. 3). In CHO cells overexpressing PS1 WT, GSK3β also bound full-length PS1 (FIG. 3).

CONCLUSIONS

Our findings show that endogenously GSK3β is part of a tetrameric complex with PS1-CTF/NTF and β-catenin at endogenous level. The absence of PS1 endoproteolysis due to D257A/D385A or ΔE10 mutations does not interfere with β-catenin/

GSK3β/PS1 complex formation. PS1D257A/D385A and FAD-linked (ΔE10, M146L, A246E, L286V) mutations do not affect β-catenin/PS1 binding or GSK3β recruitment in both CHO and H4 cell lines. Further studies will be necessary to determine the physiological role of PS1 in the β-catenin pathway and how FAD-linked mutations might affect GSK3β and β-catenin functions.

ACKNOWLEDGMENTS

G.T. is a recipient of a The John Douglas French Foundation/Extendicare fellowship. This work was supported by grants from NIA and NINDS.
We thank Drs. S. Gandy and M. Seeger for the generous gift of Ab14 antibody, Drs. S. Sisodia and G. Thinakaran for the αPS1 Loop antibody, Drs. D.J. Selkoe and W. Xia for the CHO cell lines, Dr. D.M. Kovacs for H4 cell lines, and Dr. T.-W. Kim for helpful discussion.

REFERENCES

1. TANZI, R.E. 1999. A genetic dichotomy model for the inheritance of Alzheimer's disease and common age-related disorders. J. Clin. Invest. **104:** 1175–1179.
2. ANNAERT, W. & B. DE STROOPER. 1999. Presenilins: molecular switches between proteolysis and signal transduction. Trends Neurosci. **22:** 439–443.
3. DE STROOPER, B., P. SAFTIG, K. CRAESSAERTS, et al. 1998 Deficiency of presenilin-1 inhibits the normal cleavage of amyloid precursor protein. Nature **391:** 387–390.
4. WOLFE, M.S., W. XIA, B.L. OSTASZEWSKI, et al. 1999. Two transmembrane aspartates in presenilin-1 required for presenilin endoproteolysis and gamma-secretase activity. Nature **398:** 513–517.
5. ZHOU, J., U. LIYANAGE, M. MEDINA, et al. 1997. Presenilin 1 interaction in the brain with a novel member of the Armadillo family. Neuroreport **8:** 2085–2090.
6. TESCO, G., T.W. KIM, A. DIEHLMANN, K. BEYREUTHER & R.E. TANZI. 1998. Abrogation of the presenilin 1/β-catenin interaction and preservation of the heterodimeric presenilin 1 complex following caspase activation. J. Biol. Chem. **273:** 33909–33914.
7. YU, G., F. CHEN, G. LEVESQUE, et al. 1998. The presenilin 1 protein is a component of a high molecular weight intracellular complex that contains β-catenin. J. Biol. Chem. **273:** 16470–16475.
8. ZHANG, Z., H. HARTMANN, V.M. DO, et al. 1998. Destabilization of β-catenin by mutations in presenilin-1 potentiates neuronal apoptosis. Nature **395:** 698–702.
9. MURAYAMA, M., S. TANAKA, J. PALACINO, et al. 1998. Direct association of presenilin-1 with β-catenin. FEBS Lett. **433:** 73–77.
10. LEVESQUE, G., G. YU, M. NISHIMURA, et al. 1999. Presenilins interact with armadillo proteins including neural-specific plakophilin-related protein and β-catenin. J. Neurochem. **72:** 999–1008.
11. KANG, D.E., S. SORIANO, M.P. FROSCH, et al. 1999. Presenilin 1 facilitates the constitutive turnover of β-catenin: differential activity of Alzheimer's disease-linked PS1 mutants in the β-catenin-signaling pathway. J. Neurosci. **19:** 4229–4237.
12. BARTH, A.I., I.S. NÄTHKE & W.J. NELSON. 1997. Cadherins, catenins and APC protein: interplay between cytoskeletal complexes and signaling pathways. Curr. Opin. Cell Biol. **9:** 683–690.
13. TAKASHIMA, A., M. MURAYAMA, O. MURAYAMA, et al. 1998. Presenilin 1 associates with glycogen synthase kinase-3β and its substrate tau. Proc. Natl. Acad. Sci. USA **95:** 9637–9641.
14. KOVACS, D.M., R. MANCINI, J. HENDERSON, et al. 1999. Staurosporine-induced activation of caspase-3 is potentiated by presenilin 1 familial Alzheimer's disease mutations in hu man neuroglioma cells. J. Neurochem. **73:** 2278–2285.

15. STEINER, H., H. ROMIG, M.G. GRIM, *et al.* 1999. The biological and pathological function of the presenilin-1 Deltaexon 9 mutation is independent of its defect to undergo proteolytic processing. J. Biol. Chem. **274:** 7615–7618.
16. XIA, W., J. ZHANG, R. PEREZ, E.H. KOO & D.J. SELKOE. 1998. Interaction between amyloid precursor protein and presenilins in mammalian cells: implications for the pathogenesis of Alzheimer disease. Proc. Natl. Acad. Sci. USA **94:** 8208–8213.

An Empirical Model of γ-Secretase Activity

M.P. MURPHY,[a] R. WANG,[b] P.E. FRASER,[c] A. FAUQ,[a] AND T.E. GOLDE[a,d]

[a]*Mayo Clinic Jacksonville, Department of Pharmacology, Jacksonville, Florida, USA*

[b]*The Rockefeller University, Laboratory for Mass Spectrometry, New York, New York*

[c]*The University of Toronto, Toronto, Ontario, Canada M5S 3H2*

ABSTRACT: γ-Secretase catalyzes the cleavage at the carboxyl terminus of Aβ to release it from the APP. While γ-secretase is a major therapeutic drug target for the treatment of Alzheimer's disease (AD), it appears to be an unusual proteolytic activity, and, to date, no protease responsible for this activity has been identified. Based on studies of APP transmembrane domain (TMD) mutants, it is apparent that there are multiple pharmacologically distinct γ-secretase activities that are spatially restricted and that presenilins (PS) regulate cleavage by γ-secretases in a protease independent fashion. Based on these studies, we propose a multiprotease model for γ-secretase activity and predict that the γ-secretases are likely to be closely related proteases.

INTRODUCTION

Generation of the 4 kDa amyloid β protein (Aβ) from the amyloid β protein precursor (APP) requires two sequential proteolytic events:[1–3] an initial cleavage at the amino terminus of the Aβ sequence referred to as β-secretase[4] and a subsequent cleavage at the carboxyl terminus known as γ-secretase. Recently, a membrane-bound aspartic protease, BACE, has been implicated as a β-secretase.[5,6–8] However, the protease(s) responsible for γ-secretase cleavage have not been identified. In addition, a third proteolytic activity referred to as α-secretase cleaves within the Aβ sequence to release a large secreted derivative (sAPPα), thus precluding formation of full-length Aβ.

γ-Secretase catalyzed cleavages are of particular interest for a number of reasons. First, γ-secretase is predicted to cleave a substrate that lies within the transmembrane domain (TMD), and rather than primary amino acid sequence, position of the γ-cleavage site with respect to the membrane appears to be the prime determinant of cleavage with the length of the lumenal TMD determining that position.[9] Whether γ-secretase actually cleaves residues within the membrane is a subject of much controversy. To date, no definitive evidence exists to show that *any* protease can cleave bonds buried within a TMD. Second, altered γ-secretase cleavage is implicated in the development of AD (reviewed in Ref. 10). FAD-linked mutations in APP, PS1, and PS2 alter γ-secretase activity by increasing the amount of a minor Aβ species (the more amyloidogenic Aβ$_{42}$) without significantly altering total Aβ production. Al-

---

[d]Address for correspondence: T.E. Golde, Mayo Clinic Jacksonville, Department of Pharmacology, 4500 San Pablo Road, Jacksonville, Florida 32224. Tel.: (904) 953-2538; fax: (904) 953-7370.

e-mail: tgolde@mayo.edu

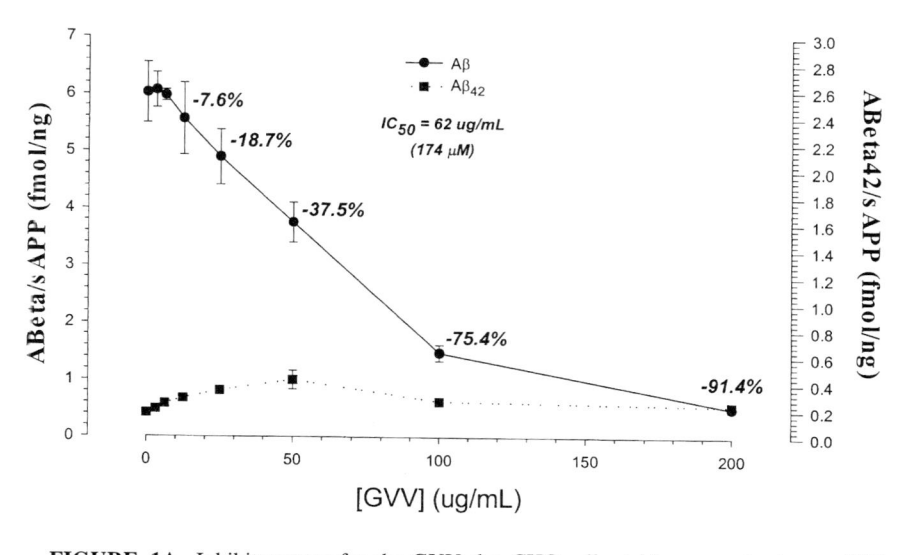

FIGURE 1A. Inhibitor curve for cbz-GVV-cho. CHO cells stably expressing human WT βAPP were treated overnight with the indicated concentrations of cbz-GVV-cho in 2% DMSO, serum-free conditioned media samples were collected and assayed by ELISA. Total Aβ production is inhibited in a dose-dependent manner, whereas Aβ$_{42}$ is slightly increased at lower concentrations and relatively unaffected at concentrations which nearly eliminate production of shorter Aβ species. Total sAPP is unaffected by treatment. Results shown are averaged from three experiments, and all ELISA measurements were performed in duplicate.

though the mechanism through which mutations in APP or presenilins (PS) shift γ-secretase cleavage remains unknown, it is clear that PS somehow regulate γ-secretase activity. Both PS1 knockout and PS aspartate mutants decrease γ-secretase cleavage.[11–13] Third, APP CTFs are not the only substrate for γ-secretase activity. The cell surface receptor Notch undergoes processing similar to APP. Cleavage of Notch in the extracellular domain is followed by cleavage of residues near the cyto-plasm/membrane junction mediated by a γ-secretase-like activity.[14–16] Finally, be-cause γ-secretase cleavage is the final step in the generation of Aβ, it remains a major therapeutic target for strategies designed to lower Aβ production. Thus, γ-secretase is not only an unusual proteolytic event, but its activity has important biological con-sequences in both the normal state and with respect to the pathogenesis and treat-ment of AD. Described below are several observations that provide further insight into the activities of γ-secretases that generate the Aβ.

SUBSTRATE-BASED PEPTIDE ALDEHYDE INHIBITORS: EVIDENCE THAT γ-40 AND γ-42 ACTIVITIES ARE SPATIALLY AND PHARMACOLOGICALLY DISTINGUISHABLE

We have recently synthesized a substrate-based peptide aldehyde cbz-GVV-CHO that selectively inhibits Aβ$_{40}$ cleavage (FIG. 1A). Like pepstatin, this inhibitor also

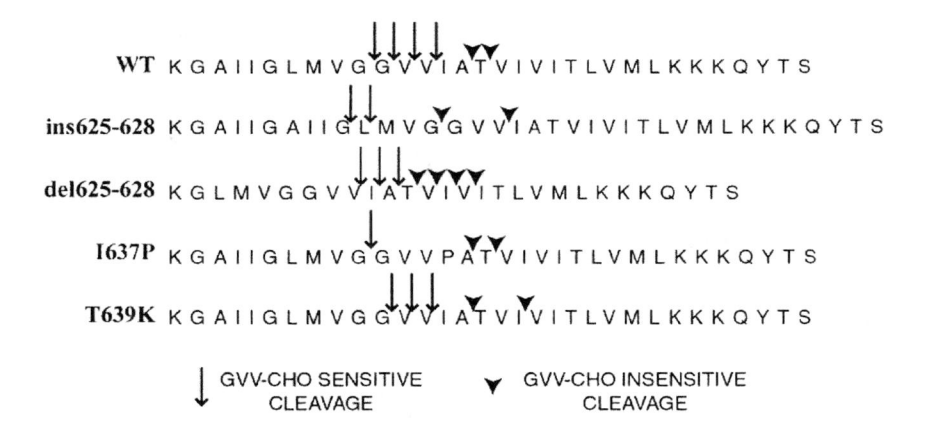

FIGURE 1B. Effects of 250 μM cbz-GVV-cho on γ-secretase cleavage in APP TMD mutants. The schematic represents the effects of 250 μM cbz-GVV-cho on the various γ-secretase in several APP TMD mutants. Mass spectral analysis and data interpretation were performed as previously described.[9] The *arrows* indicate those cleavages that are inhibited by treatment with this concentration. *Arrowheads* indicate cleavages that are either unaffected or increased by this treatment. Note that proximal cleavages are inhibited while distal cleavages are not.

differentially inhibits cleavages of APP TMD mutants (I637P, T639K ins625-628, and del625-628).[9] Shown in FIGURE 1B are the cbz-GVV-CHO sensitive and insensitive γ-secretase cleavages. Analysis of these cleavages reveals several interesting features. First, cbz-GVV-CHO sensitive cleavages and cbz-GVV-CHO insensitive cleavages are separable by distance with the more proximal cleavages being sensitive to cbz-GVV-CHO and the more distal cleavages insensitive. Second, this sensitivity is not dependent on primary sequence as the $A\beta_{42}$ cleavage that is insensitive to cbz-GVV-CHO in APP695NL is sensitive to cbz-GVV-CHO in the del625-628 construct. Instead, it appears that membrane positioning appears to be the primary determinant of whether a site is cleaved by the cbz-GVV-CHO and pepstatin sensitive γ-secretase or by a γ-secretase insensitive to these compounds. Like our previous work with pepstatin, these data support the notion that there are multiple γ-secretase activities, and extend those observations by demonstrating that these two activities appear to be spatially constrained.

PS REGULATE MULTIPLE γ-SECRETASE ACTIVITIES

Many disparate roles have been hypothesized to account for the observed effects of PS on γ-secretase cleavage. PS have been implicated in intracellular trafficking,[17] as co-factors for γ-secretase activity,[11] or as γ-secretase themselves.[12] This later notion that PS may be γ-secretase gained further support from a study that demonstrated that mutation of either of two aspartate residues potentially lying in opposing transmembrane domains decreases γ-secretase activity. Thus, it was proposed that

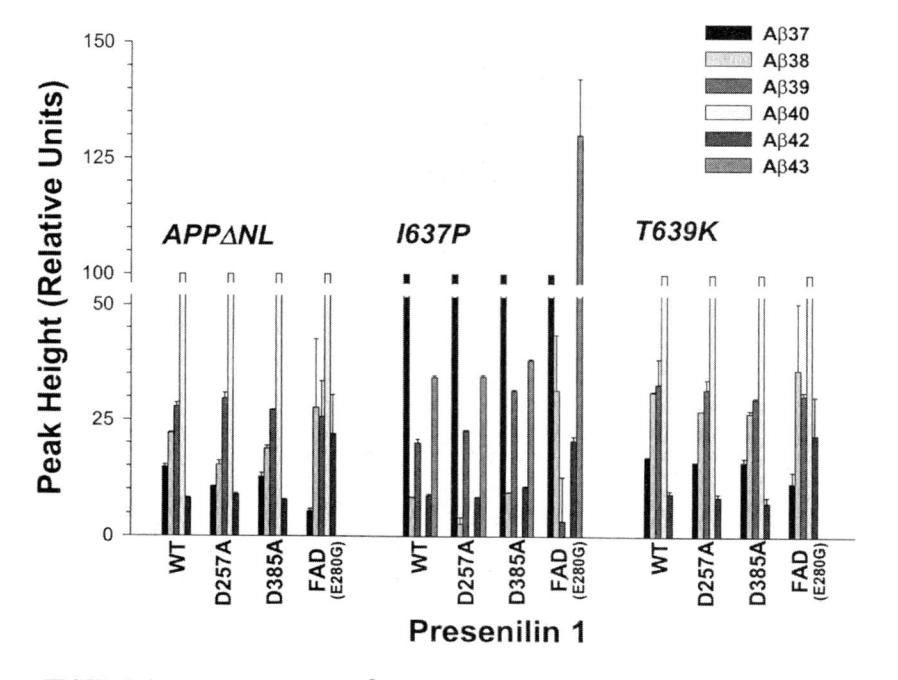

FIGURE 2. IP/MS analysis of Aβ produced from APP TMD mutants transiently trans-fected into pooled stable PS1 cell lines (WT, D257A, D385A, and the FAD-linked E280G). No differences were seen between the MS profiles of the PS1 aspartate mutant lines (com-pared to PS1wt) in any of the APP TMD constructs (ins625-8 and del625-8 not shown); in-creases in the relative amounts of 42 (or 43 for I637P) can be seen for the E280G mutant. Even though all γ-cleavage(s) are inhibited equally by mutation of the PS1 aspartate resi-dues, both I637P and T639K have sites that are insensitive to inhibition by the aspartic pro-tease inhibitor pepstatin and to the peptide aldehyde, cbz-GVV-cho.

PS may be novel intramembranous aspartyl proteases with the intramembranous as-partates functioning as the catalytic residues. Consistent with this hypothesis, treat-ment of cultured cells with either pepstatin,[9] a prototypic aspartyl protease inhibitor, or a difluoro ketone compound which inhibits aspartyl proteases,[18] reduces Aβ pro-duction to a similar extent as seen in PS knockout cell lines. In all of these cases Aβ production is not completely abolished, indicating that more than one protease likely contributes to γ-secretase activity, a notion which has been suggested by numerous studies showing differential inhibition of the γ-40 and γ-42 activities.[9,19–22] Recent-ly we have shown that PS regulate multiple pharmacologically distinct γ-secretases as well as inducible α-secretase activity (FIG. 2). This finding is difficult to reconcile with the hypothesis that PS are γ-secretases with active site residues, D257 and D385E. It is possible to speculate that PS are novel proteases with multiple pro-teolytic activities; however, such a speculation would imply that PS themselves have multiple active sites responsible for the various γ-secretase activities we and other

TABLE 1. Effects of P_1–P_4 mutations on γ-secretase activity

Construct	Total Aβ fmol/ml	Aβ$_{1-40}$ fmol/ml	Aβ$_{1-42}$ fmol/ml	sAPP ng/ml
V632A	>6000	522	70	3463
G633A	>6000	4731	0	4640
G634A	>6000	0	0	3567
V635A	>6000	1776	134	4499
V636A	>6000	3657	255	3820
V632C	>6000	981	0	2800
G634C	>6000	0	0	5926
V635C	>6000	1501	3	3026
V636C	>6000	11.2	210	3652
V632F	>6000	490	0	4944
G633F	>6000	0	0	2428
G634F	>6000	34	0	3069
V635F	>6000	762	65	3197
V636F	>6000	492	97	3567
NL	>6000	4302	187	2800

Mutant nomenclature based on APP695, NL refers to the KM to NL Swedish mutant. Aβ residues modified: $632 = Aβ_{36}$; $633 = Aβ_{37}$; $634 = Aβ_{38}$; $635 = Aβ_{39}$; $636 = Aβ_{40}$.

have described. Based on the fact that PS have no homology to any known protease, and γ-secretase activity is inhibited by several classical protease inhibitors (e.g., pepstatin, ALLN) that interact with typical proteases, we feel that in light of our data it is almost certain that PS themselves do not contain the active site(s) of γ-secretase. Instead, it is clear that PS somehow function as regulators of several proteolytic activities that act on membrane proteins.

FURTHER ANALYSIS OF γ-SECRETASE CLEAVAGE SPECIFICITY

Previous studies have not explored the effect of mutation in substrate positions P_1–P_4 (Aβ$_{40}$–Aβ$_{36}$, based on Aβ$_{40}$ cleavage) on generation of Aβ. Shown in TABLE 1 are the effects of systematic mutations to the P_1–P_4 residues on sAPP, total Aβ, Aβ$_{1-40}$, and Aβ$_{1-42}$ as assessed by ELISA. As alterations in these residues may alter reactivity of the Aβ peptides in the Aβ$_{1-40}$ and Aβ$_{1-42}$ ELISAs, IP/MS studies will be needed to determine the exact effects on γ-secretase cleavage; however, while total Aβ levels for most of the constructs are only slightly altered, many appear to shift the site of cleavage. These studies further confirm the loose sequence specificity of γ–secretase by showing that mutations of the P_1–P_4 residues of APP do not prevent γ-secretase cleavage.

EPOXIDE BASED γ-SECRETASE INHIBITORS

Because of the unusual nature of γ-secretase, it is likely to be very difficult to purify the protease or proteases responsible for the activity based on traditional activity-based biochemical approaches. Although genomics-based approaches might also be considered, these are only likely to work if there is some certainty as to the class of protease being studied. In the case of γ-secretase, there is some evidence that it may be an aspartyl protease because multiple protease inhibitors that inhibit γ-secretase are known to inhibit aspartyl proteases at the concentrations used (e.g., pepstatin, haloperidol, difluoro ketone compounds, and ALLN). However, despite the recent intensive studies of aspartic proteases that lead to the identification of BACE, so far no novel aspartic proteases have been identified as a candidate γ-secretase. A more certain approach might be to develop tagged irreversible inhibitors that can be used to purify the γ-secretase activity. To that end, we have synthesized a dipeptide epoxide (cbz-IL-epoxide) that is based on the moderately potent $A\beta_{40}$ selective disuccinamide-IL-CHO inhibitor recently reported by Higaki *et al.*[21] As shown in FIGURE 3, cbz-IL-epoxide is a potent inhibitor of Aβ. Ongoing studies will determine whether this inhibitor is irreversible and whether it can be used to tag γ-secretase for purification.

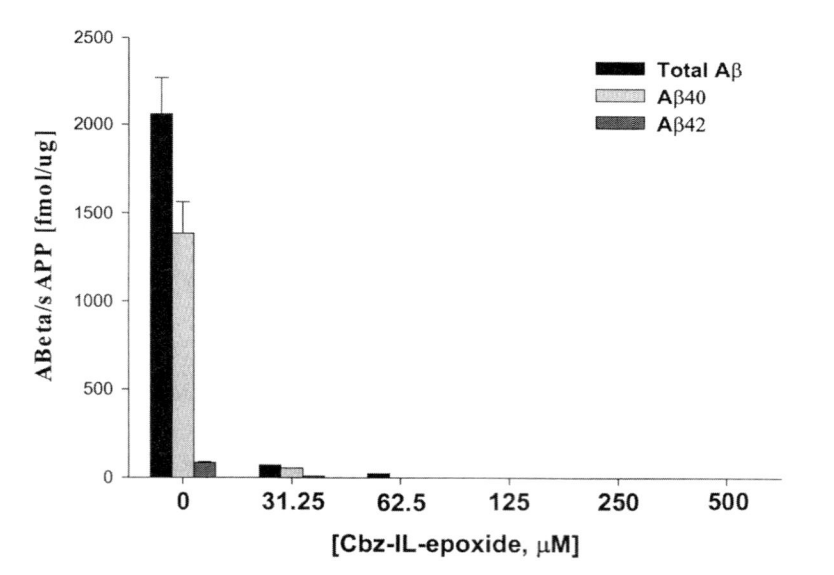

FIGURE 3. Inhibitor curve for cbz-IL-epoxide. CHO cells stably expressing human WT βAPP were treated overnight with the indicated concentrations of cbz-IL-cho (in 2% DMSO), serum- free conditioned media samples were collected (and assayed by ELISA). Total Aβ, $A\beta_{40}$ and $A\beta_{42}$ production are inhibited in a dose-dependent manner. The IC_{50} of this compound appears to be similar to the parent compound cbz-IL-cho (data not shown).

A MODEL FOR γ-SECRETASE CLEAVAGE

Clearly, speculation regarding the true nature of γ-secretase will hinge upon the ultimate cloning of the protease or proteases. However, based on the available data, it is possible to make some predictions as to the nature of the proteases responsible for γ-secretase activity. Inhibitor studies reveal that γ-40 cleavages can be selectively inhibited by low concentrations of moderately potent (μM IC_{50}s) protease inhibitors; yet, higher concentrations of the same compounds inhibit both γ-40 and γ-42 cleavages. Because several of these inhibitors are substrate based and have been shown to work in broken cell γ-secretase assays, it is likely that they are acting directly on γ-secretase. Other compounds with higher potency (nM IC_{50}s) appear to inhibit both activities equally. If these more potent inhibitors are directly acting on γ-secretase, then these data are all consistent with a model in which two or more closely related proteases contribute to the γ-activity. Since the active site of these molecules would be structurally similar, it is not surprising that the more potent small molecule inhibitors developed equally inhibit both activities whereas less potent molecules show some selectivity for the γ-40 secretase. Consistent with this multiprotease model is our finding that these activities appear to be not only pharmacologically separable, but also spatially separable (see FIG. 1). In this regard, both activities are consistent with many "secretase"-like enzymes, whose prime determinant of cleavage is not primary amino acid sequence, but distance from the membrane.[23]

ACKNOWLEDGMENTS

This work was supported by a Beeson Award from AFAR and an Ellison Medical Foundation New Scholars award (T.E.G.), NIH/NIA AG-16065 (R.W.), and the Alzheimer's Society of Ontario and MRC (P.E.F.). M.P.M. is a John Douglas French Alzheimer's Foundation Fellow.

REFERENCES

1. HAASS, C., M.G. SCHLOSSMACHER, A.Y. HUNG, *et al.* 1992. Amyloid β-peptide is produced by cultured cells during normal metabolism. Nature **359:** 322–325.
2. SHOJI, M., T.E. GOLDE, J. GHISO, *et al.* 1992. Production of the Alzheimer amyloid β protein by normal proteolytic processing. Science **258:** 126–129.
3. BUSCIGLIO, J., D.H. GABUZDA, P. MATSUDAIRA & B.A. YANKNER. 1993. Generation of β-amyloid in the secretory pathway in neuronal and nonneruonal cells. Proc. Natl. Acad. Sci. USA **90:** 2092–2096.
4. SEUBERT, P., T. OLTERSDORF, M.G. LEE, *et al.* 1993. Secretion of β-amyloid precursor protein cleaved at the amino terminus of the β-amyloid peptide. Nature **361:** 260–263.
5. VASSAR, R., B.D. BENNETT, S. BABU-KHAN, *et al.* 1999. Beta-secretase cleavage of Alzheimer's amyloid precursor protein by the transmembrane aspartic protease BACE. Science **286:** 735–740.
6. YAN, R., M.J. BIENKOWSKI, M.E. SHUCK, *et al.* 1999. Membrane-anchored aspartyl protease with Alzheimer's disease beta- secretase activity [In Process Citation]. Nature **402:** 533–537.
7. SINHA, S., J.P. ANDERSON, R. BARBOUR, *et al.* 1999. Purification and cloning of amyloid precursor protein beta-secretase from human brain [In Process Citation]. Nature **402:** 537–540.

3. HUSSAIN, I., D. POWELL, D.R. HOWLETT, *et al.* 1999. Identification of a novel aspartic protease (Asp 2) as beta-secretase. Mol. Cell. Neurosci. **14:** 419–427.

9. MURPHY, M.P., L.J. HICKMAN, C.B. ECKMAN, *et al.* 1999. γ-Secretase, evidence for multiple proteolytic activities and influence of membrane positioning of substrate on generation of amyloid beta peptides of varying length. J. Biol. Chem. **274:** 11914–11923.

10. HARDY, J. 1997. Amyloid, the presenilins and Alzheimer's disease. Trends Neurosci. **20:** 154–159.

11. DE STROOPER, B., P. SAFTIG, K. CRAESSAERTS, *et al.* 1998. Deficiency of presenilin-1 inhibits the normal cleavage of amyloid precursor protein [see comments]. Nature **391:** 387–390.

12. WOLFE, M.S., W. XIA, B.L. OSTASZEWSKI, *et al.* 1999. Two transmembrane aspartates in presenilin-1 required for presenilin endoproteolysis and gamma-secretase activity. Nature **398:** 513–517.

13. STEINER, H., K. DUFF, A. CAPELL, *et al.* 1999. A loss of function mutation of presenilin-2 interferes with amyloid-peptide production and Notch signaling. J. Biol. Chem. **274:** 28669–28673.

14. YE, Y.H., N. LUKINOVA & M.E. FORTINI. 1999. Neurogenic phenotypes and altered Notch processing in Drosophila presenilin mutants. Nature **398:** 525–529.

15. DE STROOPER, B. *et al.* 1999. A presenilin-1-dependent gamma-secretase-like protease mediates release of Notch intracellular domain. Nature **398:** 518–522.

16. STRUHL, G. & I. GREENWALD. 1999. Presenilin is required for activity and nuclear access of Notch in Drosophila. Nature **398:** 522–525.

17. NARUSE, S., G. TINAKARAN, J.J. LUO, *et al.* 1998. Effects of PS1 deficiency on membrane protein trafficking in neurons. Neuron **21:** 1213–1221.

18. WOLFE, M.S., M. CITRON, T.S. DIEHL, *et al.* 1998. A substrate-based difluoro ketone selectively inhibits Alzheimer's gamma-secretase activity. J. Med. Chem. **41:** 6–9.

19. CITRON, M., T.S. DIEHL, G. GORDON, *et al.* 1996. Evidence that the 42- and 40-amino acid forms of amyloid beta protein are generated from the beta-amyloid precursor protein by different protease activities. Proc. Natl. Acad. Sci. USA **93:** 13170–13175.

20. KLAFKI, H., D. ABRAMOWSKI, R. SWOBODA, *et al.* 1996. The carboxyl termini of beta-amyloid peptides 1–40 and 1–42 are generated by distinct gamma-secretase activities. J. Biol. Chem. **271:** 28655–28659.

21. HIGAKI, J., N.S. CHAKRAVARTY, C.M. BRYANT, *et al.* 1999. A combinatorial approach to the identification of dipeptide aldehyde inhibitors of beta-amyloid production. J. Med. Chem. **42:** 3889–3898.

22. WOLFE, M.S., W. XIA, C.L. MOORE, *et al.* 1999. Peptidomimetic probes and molecular modeling suggest that Alzheimer's gamma-secretase is an intramembrane-cleaving aspartyl protease. Biochemistry **38:** 4720–4727.

23. HOOPER, N.M., E.H. KARRAN & A.J. TURNER. 1997. Membrane protein secretases. Biochem. J. **321:** 265–279.

Overexpression of Presenilin-2 Enhances Apoptotic Death of Cultured Cortical Neurons

W. ARAKI,[a,c] K. YUASA,[b] S. TAKEDA,[b] K. SHIROTANI,[a] K. TAKAHASHI,[a] AND T. TABIRA[a]

[a]*Division of Demyelinating Disease and Aging, and [b]Division of Molecular Genetics, National Institute of Neuroscience, NCNP, Kodaira, Tokyo 187-8502, Japan*

ABSTRACT: Presenilin-2 (PS2) is a gene of unknown function linked with some forms of familial Alzheimer's disease. To investigate the biological role of PS2 in neurons, we overexpressed PS2 in primary cortical neurons using recombinant adenoviral vectors. Western blot and immunohistochemical analyses showed enhanced expression of PS2 proteins in infected neurons after infection of recombinant adenoviruses containing the human wild-type or mutant PS2 gene. Neuronal survival was decreased by approximately 30% in cultures infected with adenovirus expressing either wild-type or mutant PS2, as compared with those infected with adenovirus expressing the LacZ gene. Fragmented nuclei were frequently observed in dying neurons. These data suggest that apoptotic death of cultured cortical neurons is enhanced by PS2 overexpression.

INTRODUCTION

Presenilin-1 (PS1) and presenilin-2 (PS2) are homologous genes associated with familial Alzheimer's disease (FAD), and encode integral membrane proteins with multiple transmembrane domains and a large hydrophilic loop domain.[1,2] An interesting characteristic of the metabolism of presenilins (PSs) is that presenilin holoproteins are normally processed to generate stable N- and C-terminal fragments.[3] Recent studies have indicated that PSs are involved in such cellular processes as Notch signaling and β-amyloid production.[4] Several lines of evidence have also suggested that PSs play a role in cell death. For example, overexpression of PS2 increased apoptosis in PC12 cells and HeLa cells;[5,6] ALG-3, a truncated homologue of PS2, and antisense PS2 protect PC12 cells from glutamate-induced death;[7] PSs are cleaved by caspase 3 during apoptosis;[8] and neuron death is increased in the brain of aged transgenic mice expressing mutant PS1.[9] In the present study, we used primary cortical neurons to study the biological role of PS2. We overexpressed PS2 in cultured neurons using recombinant adenoviral vectors, and investigated the effects of PS2 overexpression on the neurons.

[c]Address for correspondence: W. Araki, Division of Demyelinating Disease and Aging, National Institute of Neuroscience, NCNP, Kodaira, Tokyo 187-8502, Japan. Tel.: 81-423-41-2711 ext. 5163; fax: 81-423-46-1747.

e-mail: araki@ncnp.go.jp

METHODS

Recombinant adenoviruses expressing human wild-type or FAD-associated N141I mutant PS2 were constructed by the COS/TPC method.[10] In brief, the PS2 cDNA was introduced into a cassette cosmid bearing the full-length adenovirus genome with deletions of E1 and E3 regions. This cassette cosmid was co-transfected into human kidney 293 cells together with the adenovirus DNA-terminal protein complex, and the recombinant adenovirus was generated through homologous recombination. The recombinant adenovirus was purified by discontinuous CsCl density gradient centrifugation and dialysis against phosphate-buffered saline (PBS) containing 10% glycerol.[11] The adenoviruses expressing wild-type and mutant PS2 were named AxCAPS2wt and AxCAPS2mu, respectively. The adenovirus containing the *E. coli* LacZ gene, AxCALacZ, was prepared as above, and used as a control.

Cerebral cortical neurons were obtained from 17-day rat embryos and cultured in serum-free medium by the previously described method.[12] Seven or eight days after plating, cells were infected with the recombinant adenoviruses. The efficiency of adenovirus infection was very high, because >90% were positive for β-galactosidase staining after infecting cells with AxCALacZ.

For immunoblot analysis of PS2 proteins, cells were lysed in RIPA (radioimmunoprecipitation assay) buffer containing protease inhibitors. Proteins were separated on 12% polyacrylamide gel, blotted on PVDF membranes, and probed with anti-PS2 antibodies. We used two polyclonal antibodies, Ab555C and Ab333, which were raised against glutathione-S-transferase fusion proteins containing residues 1–71 and 277–387 of PS2, respectively.[13]

For immunohistochemistry, cells on glass coverslips were fixed in 4% paraformaldehyde in PBS, and immunostained with anti-PS2 antibodies or anti-microtubule associated protein 2 (MAP2) antibody (Roche Diagnostics), using a peroxidase-based ABC kit (Vecstatin).

RESULTS AND DISCUSSION

To examine PS2 protein expression in rat primary cortical neuron cultures infected with the recombinant adenovirus, we performed Western blots of cell lysates two days after adenovirus infection at multiplicity of infection (moi) of 10. In cells infected with AxCAPS2wt or AxCAPS2mu, the 55 kDa full-length form of PS2, high molecular weight forms of PS2, the 23 kDa C-terminal fragment (CTF), and a weak band of 18 kDa CTF probably derived from caspase cleavage were detected with the PS2 loop antibody, while the full-length and high molecular weight forms of PS2 as well as the 35 kDa N-terminal fragment (NTF) were detected with the PS2 N-terminal antibody. In contrast, the endogenous 23 kDa CTF and 35 kDa NTF, but not the full-length PS2, were detected in noninfected cells, and the levels of these bands were very low, compared with those of the PS2-infected cells. Wild-type and mutant PS2-infected cells exhibited almost identical levels of full-length PS2, PS2 NTF and CTF, but the intensity of the alternative CTF appeared to be slightly increased in mutant PS2 cells relative to wild-type PS2 cells. During the time course after infection of AxCAPS2wt, the levels of full-length and high molecular weight forms of PS2 were maximum at day 1 and decreased thereafter, while the levels of normal NTF and CTF increased until the third day, and remained comparable by the fifth day. This indicates that the normal PS2 NTF and CTF are highly stable and tend to accumulate in the cells.

We also examined PS2 expression in the cultured neurons by immunohistochemical staining with the PS2 loop antibodies. Compared with the control noninfected neurons, which were only weakly stained, neurons infected with AxCAPS2wt or AxCAPS2mu showed increased immunoreactivity for PS2, although the staining intensity was variable among cells. The PS2 immunoreactivity was localized in cell bodies and proximal neurites. No difference in the staining pattern was observed between cells expressing wild-type PS2 and those expressing mutant PS2.

To determine whether PS2 overexpression affects cellular viability of the neurons, we evaluated neuronal survival by counting the number of MAP2-positive neurons. Four days after adenovirus infection at moi of 10, the number of surviving neurons appeared to be decreased in the cultures infected with AxCAPS2wt or AxCAPS2mu, compared with the noninfected cultures or the cultures infected with AxCALacZ. Quantitation of MAP2-positive neurons revealed that neuronal survival was decreased significantly by approximately 30% in the cultures infected with either AxCAPS2wt or AxCAPS2mu, compared with the control cultures. In addition, Hoechst33342-positive fragmented nuclei were frequently seen in dying neurons, indicating that they were undergoing apoptosis. Taken together, these results indicate that apoptotic death of cultured neurons is enhanced by overexpression of PS2. We are currently examining whether PS2-expressing neurons show altered sensitivity to apoptotic stimuli. Our preliminary data suggest that PS2 overexpression increases the susceptibility of cultured neurons to apoptotic stimulation with staurosporin. Our present data appear to be consistent with previous studies showing that apoptosis of PC12 cells and HeLa cells was induced by PS2 overexpression,[5,6] and suggest that PS2 may have an important function in the regulation of neuronal cell death. Our *in vitro* system will be useful for further investigating the molecular mechanism of neurodegeneration caused by PS mutations.

REFERENCES

1. SHERRINGTON, R., E.I. ROGAEV, Y. LIANG, E.A. ROGAEVA, G. LEVESQUE, M. IKEDA, H. CHI, C. LIN, G. LI, K. HOLMAN, T. TSUDA, L. MAR, J.-F. FONCIN, A.C. BRUNI, M.P. MONTESI, S. SORBI, I. RAINERO, L. PINESSI, L. NEE, I. CHUMAKOV, D. POLLEN, A. BROOKES, P. SANSEAU, R.J. POLINSKY, W. WASCO, H.A. DA SILVA, J.L. HAINES, M.A. PERICAK-VANCE, R.E. TANZI, A.D. ROSES, P.E. FRASER, J.M. ROMMENS & P.H. ST GEORGE-HYSLOP. 1995. Cloning of a gene bearing missense mutations in early-onset familial Alzheimer's disease. Nature **375**: 754–760.
2. EPHRAT, L.-L., W. WASCO, P. POORKAJ, D.M. ROMANO, J. OSHIMA, W.H. PETTINGELL, C.-E. YU, P.D. JONDRO, S.D. SCHMIDT, K. WANG, A.C. CROWLEY, Y.-H. FU, S.Y. GUENETTE, D. GALAS, E. NEMENS, E.M. WIJSMAN, T.D. BIRD, G.D. SCHELLENBERG & R.E. TANZI. 1995. Candidate gene for the chromosome 1 familial Alzheimer's disease locus. Science **269**: 973–977.
3. THINAKARAN, G., D.R. BORCHELT, M.K. LEE, H.H. SLUNT, L. SPITZER, G. KIM, T. RATOVITSKY, F. DAVENPORT, C. NORDSTEDT, M. SEEGER, J. HARDY, A.I. LEVEY, S.E. GANDY, N.A. JENKINS, N.G. COPELAND, D.L. PRICE & S.S. SISODIA. 1996. Endoproteolysis of presenilin 1 and accumulation of processed derivatives *in vivo*. Neuron **17**: 181–190.

4. ANNAERT, W. & B. DE STROOPER. 1999. Presenilins: molecular switches between proteolysis and signal transduction. Trends Neurosci. **22:** 439–443.
5. WOLOZIN, B., K. IWASAKI, P. VITO, J.K. GANJEI, E. LACANÀ, T. SUNDERLAND, B. ZHAO, J.W. KUSIAK, W. WASCO & L. D'ADAMIO. 1996. Participation of presenilin 2 in apoptosis: enhanced basal activity conferred by an Alzheimer mutation. Science **274:** 1710–1713.
6. JANICKI, S. & M.J. MONTEIRO. 1997. Increased apoptosis arising from increased expression of the Alzheimer's disease-associated presenilin-2 mutation (N141I). J. Cell Biol. **139:** 485–495.
7. VITO, P., B. WOLOZIN, J.K. GANJEI, K. IWASAKI, E. LACANÁ & L. D'ADAMIO. 1996. Requirement of the familial Alzheimer's disease gene PS2 for apoptosis: Opposing effect of ALG-3. J. Biol. Chem. **271:** 31025–31028.
8. KIM, T.-W., W.H. PETTINGELL, Y.-K. JUNG, D.M. KOVACS & R.E. TANZI. 1997. Alternative cleavage of Alzheimer-associated presenilins during apoptosis by a caspase-3 family protease. Science **277:** 373–376.
9. CHUI, D.-H., H. TANAHASHI, K. OZAWA, S. IKEDA, F. CHECLER, O. UEDA, H. SUZUKI, W. ARAKI, H. INOUE, K. SHIROTANI, K. TAKAHASHI, F. GALLYAS & T. TABIRA. 1999. Transgenic mice with Alzheimer presenilin 1 mutations show accelerated neurodegeneration without amyloid plaque formation. Nature Med. **5:** 560–564.
10. MIYAKE, S., M. MAKIMURA, Y. KANEGAE, S. HARADA, Y. SATO, K. TAKAMORI, C. TOKUDA & I. SAITO. 1996. Efficient generation of recombinant adenoviruses using adenovirus DNA-terminal protein complex and a cosmid bearing the full-length virus genome. Proc. Natl. Acad. Sci. USA **93:** 1320–1324.
11. KANEGAE, Y., M. MAKIMURA & I. SAITO. 1994. A simple and efficient method for purification of infectious recombinant adenovirus. Jpn. J. Med. Sci. Biol. **47:** 157–166.
12. BREWER, G.J., J.R. TORRICELLI, E.K. EVEGE & P.J. PRICE. 1993. Optimized survival of hippocampal neurons in B27-supplemented Neurobasal™, a new serum-free medium combination. J. Neurosci. Res. **35:** 567–576.
13. SHIROTANI, K., K. TAKAHASHI, K. OZAWA, T. KUNISHITA & T. TABIRA. 1997. Determination of a cleavage site of presenilin 2 protein in stably transfected SH-SY5Y human neuroblastoma cell lines. Biochem. Biophys. Res. Commun. **240:** 728–731.

α1-Antichymotrypsin Inhibits
Aβ Degradation *in Vitro* and *in Vivo*

CARMELA R. ABRAHAM,[a] WALKER T. McGRAW,
FRANCHOT SLOT, AND RINA YAMIN

*Department of Biochemistry, Boston University School of Medicine,
Boston, Massachusetts 02118, USA*

ABSTRACT: The neuropathology of Alzheimer's disease (AD) is characterized by extensive deposition of the toxic amyloid β peptide (Aβ) in selected regions of the brain and brain vasculature (Selkoe, 1999). Thus, lowering the levels of Aβ may be beneficial for AD patients. Aβ is a proteolytic fragment derived from the amyloid precursor protein (APP). The mechanisms of Aβ formation from its precursor have been studied extensively; however, considerably less effort has been invested into studying Aβ clearance. We find that the degradation of Aβ in our system is dependent upon the presence of a metallopeptidase E.C.3.4.24.15 (MP24.15) (Yamin *et al.*, 1999). We have previously purified MP24.15 to homogeneity from AD brain and identified it as an APP-processing protease *in vitro* (Papastoitis, 1994). To confirm its role in cell culture, we transfected SKNMC neuroblastoma cells with sense and antisense cDNAs of MP24.15 and with a mock construct. Compared to mock conditioned media (CM), CM of MP24.15-overexpressing cells had very high Aβ-degrading activity. Conversely, CM of antisense-expressing cells lacked Aβ-degrading activity. These results suggested that MP24.15 is involved in Aβ degradation. Characterization of the proteolytic activity directly responsible for Aβ degradation using a spectrum of protease inhibitors revealed that only serine protease inhibitors completely blocked Aβ degradation. Therefore, MP24.15 appears to activate a serine protease, which then cleaves Aβ. Interestingly, α1-antichymotrypsin (ACT) which we discovered to be highly elevated in AD brain (Abraham, *et al.*, 1988) also inhibited Aβ degradation. To our delight, ACT proved to be an inhibitor of Aβ degradation *in vivo* as well. When we crossed transgenic mice expressing human ACT with plaque-producing mice expressing human APP, the doubly transgenic mice had twice as many plaques at 20 months of age as the APP mice (Mucke *et al.*, 2000). Successful completion of this study could lead to the design of reagents that would reduce the amyloid load in AD patients.

INTRODUCTION

The major protein component of amyloid plaques is the amyloid β peptide (Aβ), a 40–42 amino acid peptide proteolytically derived from the amyloid precursor protein (APP). In solution $A\beta_{1-42}$ forms fibrils readily within hours, while $A\beta_{1-40}$ is less amyloidogenic and only becomes fibrillar within days.

[a]Address for correspondence: Dr. Carmela R. Abraham, Department of Biochemistry, Boston University School of Medicine, 715 Albany Street, K6, Boston, MA 02118. Tel.: (617) 638-4308; fax: (617) 638-5339.
e-mail: cabraham@bu.edu

Extracellular Aβ can be cleared by at least two mechanisms: 1) proteolytic degradation, and 2) receptor-mediated internalization. Three proteolytic systems have been described recently that degrade Aβ. These involve a proteolytic cascade, which we have demonstrated,[2] as well as mechanisms surrounding the insulin degrading enzyme (IDE)[6] and neprilysin (E.C.3.4.24.11).[7] Our cascade has been shown to be comprised of a metallopeptidase E.C.3.4.24.15 (MP24.15), which is also known as thimet oligopeptidase and Pz peptidase (for review, see Ref. 8), and an incompletely characterized serine protease.

The role that α1-antichymotrypsin (ACT) plays in Alzheimer's disease (AD) has remained an enigma since the discovery of its association with the disease over a decade ago. We found that ACT RNA and protein are highly elevated in AD brain and that ACT is closely associated with amyloid plaques.[4] The same association of ACT with Aβ is also seen in the brains of normal aged humans,[9] aged rhesus monkeys,[10] and APP/ACT doubly transgenic mice.[5,20]

ACT is a serine protease inhibitor of the serpin family and an acute phase protein.[11] ACT is mostly produced and secreted by the liver, and its expression is low in the normal brain.[9] In AD, however, reactive astrocytes in the gray matter are the major producers of ACT.[12,13] This overexpression of ACT suggested that an inflammatory process occurs in AD brain. It has been shown that Aβ can activate microglia, which in turn secrete a variety of cytokines, including IL-1 and IL-6. These two cytokines induce the expression of ACT in astrocytes.[14] Thus, it appears that ACT expression by reactive astrocytes is a secondary phenomenon to Aβ deposition, but ACT association with Aβ can render it insoluble. Indeed, several studies have demonstrated that ACT enhanced amyloid fibril formation[15,16] when the interaction of ACT and Aβ was tested *in vitro*. This issue remains controversial, since in two other studies ACT caused Aβ fibril dissagregation.[17,18] The discrepancy between these studies may be explained by the different stoichiometry of Aβ to ACT.

RESULTS AND DISCUSSION

The discovery of the protease inhibitor ACT in the AD plaques prompted us to search for proteases responsible for the formation of Aβ, or for proteases that degrade Aβ and are inhibited by ACT. Over the past ten years we have searched for such proteinases in the hope that an inhibitor of an Aβ-producing protease or an activator of an Aβ-degrading protease would yield pharmaceutical compounds for the treatment of AD.[2] We have recently described a proteolytic cascade in a variety of cell types in which a serine protease degrades extracellular Aβ. To our great satisfaction, ACT inhibited the degradation of Aβ. Since ACT is known to produce SDS-insoluble complexes with the enzymes it inhibits,[2] we searched for such complexes in the CM of the neuroblastoma cells used in our experiments. Interestingly, when CM of MP24.15-overexpressing cells was incubated with purified ACT, an SDS-resistant, ACT-containing complex was detected, which suggested that an interaction occurs between ACT and an active serine protease present in the medium. Furthermore, we demonstrated by ^{14}C-DFP labeling that a 28-kDa and several >200-kDa active serine proteases are present in the CM of MP24.15-overexpressing cells at a higher concentration than in the CM of mock-transfected cells. This result indicates a direct correlation between the amount of MP24.15 present in the cells and the amount of active serine proteases in these cells.[2] Work is in progress to isolate and characterize the serine protease that degrades Aβ and to identify the mechanism of its activation.

Since ACT inhibits Aβ degradation *in vitro*, we analyzed its role in APP/ACT doubly transgenic mice to determine whether the presence of ACT leads to a heavier load of Aβ in these mice compared to the APP in singly transgenic mice.[19] Indeed, as expected, APP/ACT doubly transgenic mice exhibited a significantly greater load of plaques at 14 and 20 months than APP mice alone.[5,20] At this time it is unclear whether ACT causes accumulation of Aβ by directly inhibiting an Aβ-degrading enzyme or by binding to Aβ and rendering it protease resistant.[2]

Finally, ACT, an acute phase protein, participates in the inflammatory process that occurs in the AD brain. Therefore, an additional rationale for the use of antiinflammatory drugs in AD patients would be to reduce the ACT levels produced by reactive astrocytes. This reduction in ACT levels would be beneficial, since it will result in enhanced Aβ degradation. Elucidation of the mechanism by which ACT inhibits Aβ degradation is of primary importance to understanding the mechanisms of Aβ degradation.

ACKNOWLEDGMENTS

This work was supported by the Alzheimer's Association and by NIH grant AG09905 to C.R.A. The authors wish to thank Drs. Lennart Mucke and Eliezer Masliah for the production and characterization of the transgenic mice.

REFERENCES

1. SELKOE, D.J. 1999. Translating cell biology into therapeutic advances in Alzheimer's disease. Nature **399:** A23–A31.
2. YAMIN, R., E. MALGERI, W.T. MCGRAW *et al.* 1999. Metalloendopeptidase E.C.3.4.24.15 is necessary for Alzheimer's amyloid β peptide degradation. J. Biol. Chem. **274:** 17777–17784.
3. PAPASTOITSIS, G., R. SIMAN, R. SCOTT & C.R. ABRAHAM. 1994. Indentification of a metalloprotease from Alzheimer's disease brain able to degrade the β-amyloid precursor protein and generate amyloidogenic fragments. Biochemistry **33:** 192–199.
4. ABRAHAM, C.R., D.J. SELKOE & H. POTTER. 1988. Immunochemical identification of the serine protease inhibitor α_1-antichymotrypsin in the brain amyloid deposits of Alzheimer's disease. Cell **52:** 487–501.
5. MUCKE, L., G.-Q. YU, C.R. ABRAHAM *et al.* 1999. Potential roles of α1-antichymotrypsin and α-synuclein in Alzheimer's pathogenesis assessed in bigenic mice expressing human amyloid precursor protein. Soc. Neurosci. Abstr. **25:** 122.10.
6. QIU, W.Q., D.M. WALSH, Z. YE *et al.* 1998. Insulin-degrading enzyme regulates extracellular levels of amyloid beta-protein by degradation. J. Biol. Chem. **273:** 32730–32738.
7. HOWELL, S., J. NALBANTOGLU & P. CRINE. 1995. Neutral endopeptidase can hydrolyze beta-amyloid(1–40) but shows no effect on beta-amyloid precursor protein metabolism. Peptides **16:** 647–652.
8. TISLJAR, U. 1993. Thimet oligopeptidase: a review of a thiol dependent metallo-endopeptidase also known as Pz-peptidase, endopeptidase 24.15 and endo-oligopeptidase. Biol. Chem. Hoppe-Seyler **374:** 91–100.
9. ABRAHAM, C.R., T. SHIRAHAMA & H. POTTER. 1990. The protease inhibitor α_1-antichymotrypsin is associated solely with amyloid deposits containing the β-protein and is

localized in specific cells of both normal and diseased brain. Neurobiol. Aging **11:** 123–129.

10. ABRAHAM, C.R., D.J. SELKOE, H. POTTER *et al.* 1989. α_1-Antichymotrypsin is present together with the β-protein in monkey brain amyloid deposits. Neuroscience **32:** 715–720.

11. TRAVIS, J. & G. SALVESEN. 1983. Human plasma protease inhibitors. Annu. Rev. Biochem. **52:** 655–709.

12. PASTERNACK, J.M., C.R. ABRAHAM, B. VAN DYKE *et al.* 1989. Astrocytes in Alzheimer's disease gray matter express α_1-antichymotrypsin mRNA. Am. J. Pathol. **135:** 827–834.

13. KOO, E.H., C.R. ABRAHAM, H. POTTER *et al.* 1991. Developmental expression of α1-antichymotrypsin in brain may be related to astrogliosis. Neurobiol. Aging **12:** 495–501.

14. DAS, S. & H. POTTER. 1995. Expression of Alzheimer amyloid-promoting factor antichymotrypsin is induced in human astrocytes by IL-1. Neuron **14:** 447–456.

15. MA, J., A. YEE, B. BREWER, JR. *et al.* 1994. Amyloid-associated proteins alpha 1-antichymotrypsin and apolipoprotein E promote assembly of Alzheimer beta-protein into filaments. Nature **372:** 92–94.

16. JANCIAUSKIENE, S., S. ERIKSSON & H.T. WRIGHT. 1996. A specific structural interaction of Alzheimer's peptide A beta 1–42 with alpha 1-antichymotrypsin. Nat. Struct. Biol. **3:** 668–671.

17. FRASER, P.E., J.T. NGUYEN, D.R. MCLACHLAN *et al.* 1993. α_1-Antichymotrypsin binding to synthetic Alzheimer βA4 amyloid peptides is sequence-specific and induces fibril disaggregation *in vitro*. J. Neurochem. **61:** 298–305.

18. ERIKSSON, S., S. JANCIAUSKIENE & L. LANNFELT. 1995. Alpha 1-antichymotrypsin regulates Alzheimer beta-amyloid peptide fibril formation. Proc. Natl. Acad. Sci. USA **92:** 2313–2317.

19. GAMES, D., D. ADAMS, R. ALESSANDRINI *et al.* 1995. Alzheimer-type neuropathology in transgenic mice overexpressing V717F beta-amyloid precursor protein. Nature **373:** 523–527.

20. MUCKE, L., G.-Q. YU, L. MCCONLOGUE *et al.* 2000. Astroglial expression of human α1-antichymotrypsin enhances Alzheimer's pathology in amyloid protein precursor transgenic mice. Am. J. Pathol. **157.**

Activated Mitogenic Signaling Induces a Process of Dedifferentiation in Alzheimer's Disease That Eventually Results in Cell Death

THOMAS ARENDT,[a] MAX HOLZER, ANDREA STÖBE, ULRICH GÄRTNER, HANS-JOACHIM LÜTH, MARTINA K. BRÜCKNER, AND UWE UEBERHAM

Paul Flechsig Institute for Brain Research, Department of Neuroanatomy, University of Leipzig, Leipzig, Germany

ABSTRACT: Neurodegeneration in Alzheimer's disease (AD) is associated with the appearance of dystrophic neuronal growth profiles that most likely reflect an impairment of neuronal reorganization. This process of morphodysregulation, which eventually goes awry and becomes a disease itself, might be triggered either by a variety of life events that place an additional burden on the plastic capability of the brain or by genetic pertubations that shift the threshold for decompensation. This paper summarizes recent evidence that impairment of the p21ras intracellular signal transduction, which is is mediated by a hierarchy of phosphorylation signals and eventually results in loss of differentiation control and an attempt of neurons to re-enter the cell-cycle, is critically involved in this process. Neurodegeneration might thus be viewed as an alternative effector pathway of those events that in the dividing cell would lead to cellular transformation. This hypothesis might be of heuristic value for the development of a therapeutic strategy.

MITOGENIC SIGNALING IN AD

Neurodegeneration in Alzheimer's disease (AD) is associated with the appearance of aberrant neuritic growth profiles that precede formation of paired helical filaments,[1,2] making a primary pathogenetic role of aberrancies of growth and proliferation regulating mechanisms in neurons very likely.

Numerous neurotrophic and potentially mitogenic compounds are elevated early in the course of the disease. These factors might activate an intracellular cascade of mitogenic signaling involving the mitogen-activated protein kinase (MAPK) pathway that potentially modulates the expression and posttranslational processing of APP and tau protein.[3-5] The activation of cell surface receptors of these trophic factors is linked to the downstream MAPK-cascade by p21ras, a small G protein also activated by nitric oxide (NO) and intermediates generated through oxidative stress.[6]

During brain development, p21ras is involved in the regulation of the G_0/G_1 transition of the cell cycle and thus might be a critical regulator for cellular proliferation

[a]Address for correspondence: Thomas Arendt, Paul Flechsig Institute for Brain Research, Department of Neuroanatomy, University of Leipzig, 04109 Leipzig, Germany. Tel.: +49/341/9725721; fax: +49/341/2114397.
e-mail: aret@medizin.uni-leipzig.de

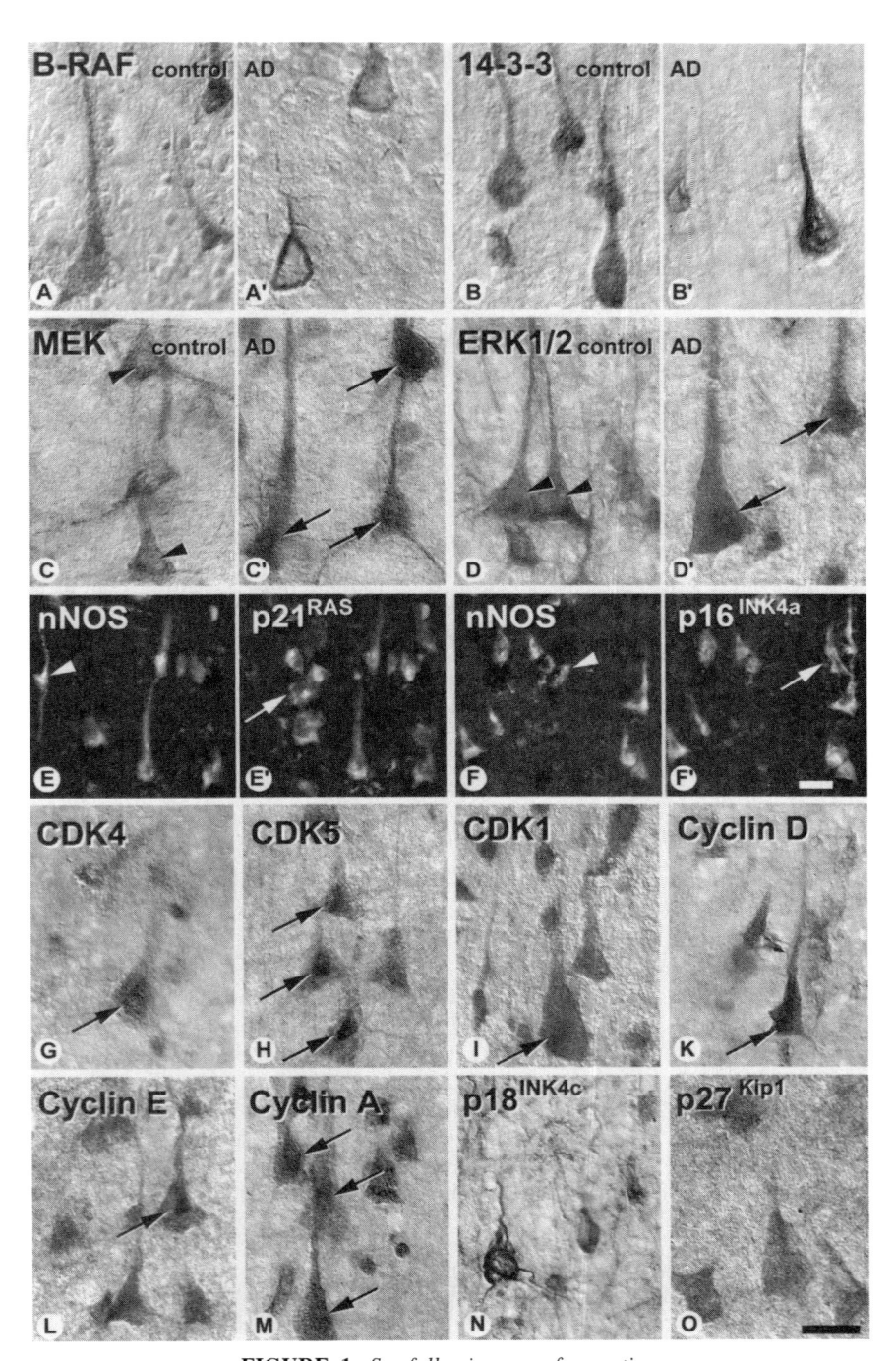

FIGURE 1. *See following page for caption.*

and differentiation.[7,8] In AD, the p21ras-protein as well as major identified downstream elements of the MAPK-cascade, such as Raf-kinase, p14-3-3, mitogen-activated protein kinase kinase (MAPKK, MEK) and the MAP-kinases ERK1 and EKR2 are elevated at very early stages of the disease.[9,10] The strong expression of these kinases associated with neurofibrillary degeneration, as well as the subcellular translocation of MEK, ERK1, and ERK2 (FIG. 1, A to D'), indicating their activation, suggests that a developmentally immature condition of neurons might be of critical importance in the pathomechanism.

DEDIFFERENTIATION IN AD

The re-expression of developmentally regulated genes, as well as the induction of posttranslational modifications and accumulation of gene products to an extent which goes beyond those observed during regeneration, has been demonstrated in AD by a number of groups, and is indicative of a process of de-differentiation. Recent evidence for a dysfunction of cell-cycle regulation in AD in various cell types including neurons[11–18] supports the original suggestion of a link between neurodegeneration in AD and cell-cycle related events.[19,20]

Expression of the cyclin-dependent kinases cdk4 and cdk6, as well as their inhibitors of the INK4-family that are critical regulators of the orderly progression through the cell cycle, is elevated in AD (FIG. 1, G to O). Furthermore, observations of an increased expression of the protooncogene p21ras in AD are paralleled by experimental *in vitro* studies showing that expression of p21ras in primary human or rodent cells results in a permanent G1 arrest. This arrest induced by p21ras is accompanied by accumulation of p16[INK4a], and is phenotypically identical to premature cellular senescence.[21] Induction of dominant-inhibitory p21ras, furthermore, can rescue neuronally differentiated PC12 cells from death caused by NGF withdrawal, implying a relationship between proliferative capacity and cell death. Recent studies have indeed shown that a high degree of structural neuronal plasticity might predispose neurons to neurofibrillary degeneration and cell death in AD.[22,23]

FIGURE 1. Immunohistochemical detection of molecular components associated with mitogenic signaling and cell-cycle regulation in the temporal cortex (Brodmann area 22) in Alzheimer's disease. **A/A′ to D/D′:** Elements of the MAP-kinase cascade. (A/A′ and B/B′) The high expression of B-Raf and p 14-3-3 is associated with tangle formation. C/C' and D/D') In controls, MEK and ERK1/2 are localized to the cytoplasm and are not found in nuclei (*arrowheads*). Their nuclear translocation in AD (*arrows*) indicates an activation of these kinases. **E/E′ to F/F′:** Double immunofluorescence demonstrating the co-localization between nNOS and p21ras and p16[INK4a], respectively. While nNOS reactive interneurons (*arrowheads*) are generally free of p21ras and p16[INK4a] expression, most pyramidal neurons prone to neurofibrillary degeneration clearly show double immunoflourescence. Only a minor subset of pyramidal cells do not express nNOS (arrows). **G to O:** Regulators of the activation and orderly progression through the cell cycle are highly expressed in pyramidal neurons in AD. They are preferentially found in nuclei (*arrows*). Scale bars: F′ refers to E–F′; O, refers to all others: 20 μm.

SELF-PERPETUATION OF NEURODEGENERATION

Nitric oxide (NO) might be a key mediator linking cellular activity to gene expression and long-lasting neuronal responses through activating p21ras by redox-sensitive modulation.[24] In AD, nNOS can be detected in pyramidal neurons containing neurofibrillary tangles or even unaffected by neurofibrillary degeneration. Expression of nNOS in these neurons is highly co-localized with p21ras and p16[INK4a] (FIG. 1, E to F').[25]

Thus, an autocrine loop may exist within cells, whereby NO activates p21ras which in turn leads to cellular activation and stimulation of NOS expression.[26] The co-expression of NOS and p21ras in neurons vulnerable to neurofibrillary degeneration early in the course of AD clearly provides the basis for a feedback mechanism that might exacerbate the progression of neurodegeneration in a self-propagating manner. This self-perpetuation of a process likely associated with limited prospects of physiological control and termination might be the critical switch converting two potentially neuroprotective mechanisms such as NO and p21ras dependent signaling into a disease process leading to slowly, but continuously progressing neuronal death (FIG. 2).

SUMMARY AND CONCLUSION

Research on the etiology of Alzheimer's disease (AD) increasingly provides evidence that AD is a heterogenous disorder characterized by a defective process of neuronal plasticity and repair that involves complex interactions between genetic and environmental factors. Compensatory mechanisms of both functional and structural adaptation, which are activated in the normal adult nervous system in response to injury, serving to regain much of the functional integrity of a neuronal population in the presence of cell loss, are defective in AD. These aberrancies in the neuronal response to degenerative stimuli might affect neuronal viability and might directly contribute to a self-perpetuating cascade of neurodegenerative events leading to the formation of PHFs, β/A4-amyloid and progressive cell loss. Minor neuronal damage due to a variety of life events associated with oxidative stress, mechanical injury, chronic intoxication, metabolic imbalances, latent infections or other damaging influences or genetic pertubations that are usually compensated in the normal adult brain by adaptation and repair might thus be amplified and accumulated, eventually resulting in progressive neurodegeneration.

Aberrancies in mitogenic signaling might be a key element in this pathogenetic chain. Challenging the mitogenic signal transduction pathways through liberation of growth factors, cytokines, and other molecules such as nitric oxide, oxygen free radicals or lipid peroxidation products leads to a mitogenic overstimulation of neurons. As a result, a condition of dedifferentiation is induced, which involves the activation of those molecular events that in dividing cell populations would lead to cellular transformation. Within terminally differentiated cells that are blocked from a complete progression through the cell cycle, however, these molecular events alternatively lead to cell death.

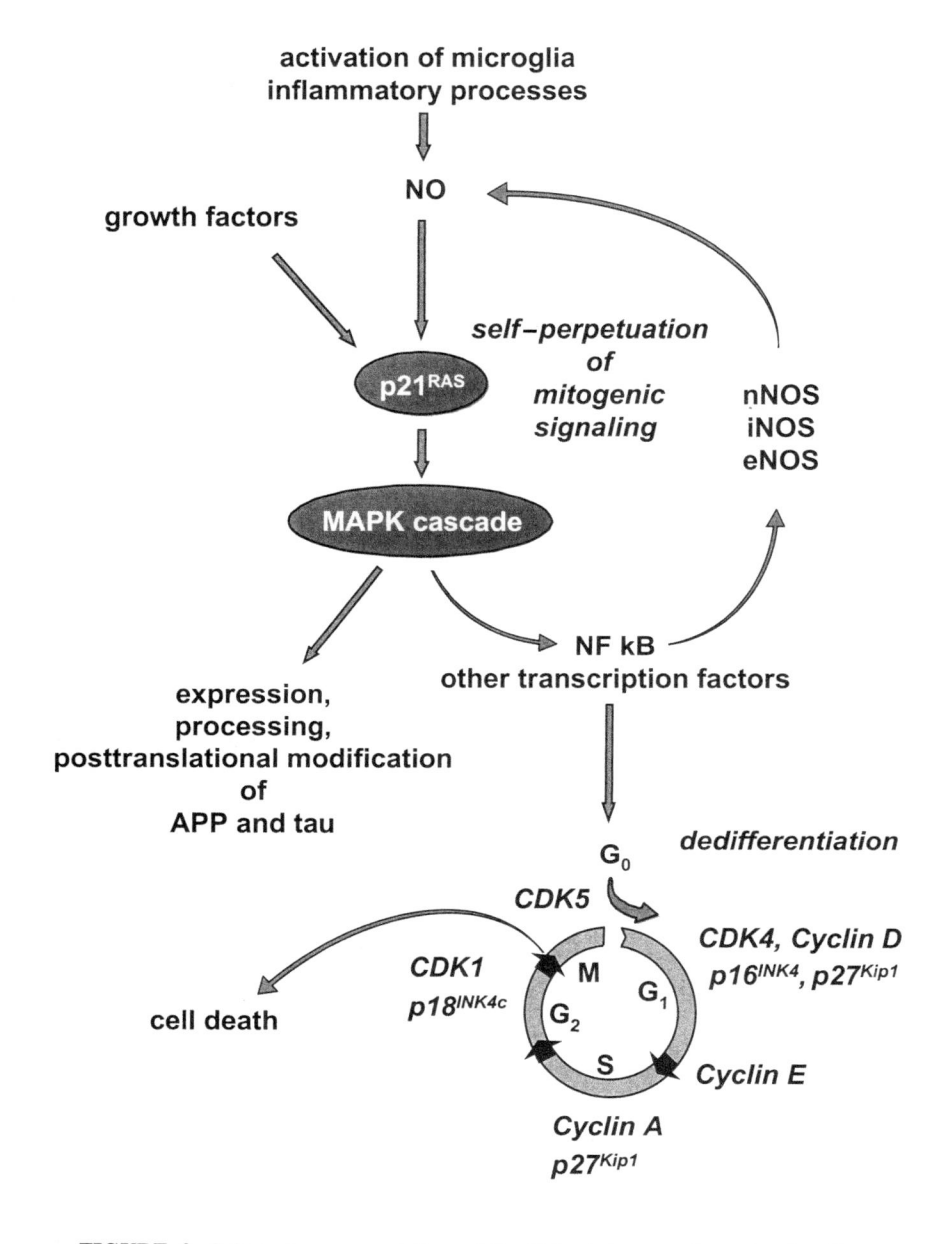

FIGURE 2. Schematic representation of the links between mitogenic signaling, expression and processing of APP and tau, dedifferentiation and cell death in AD. The immunohistochemical localization of major molecular components involved in these processes are shown in FIGURE 1.

ACKNOWLEDGMENT

This study was supported by the Bundesministerium für Bildung, Forschung und Technologie (BMBF), Interdisziplinäres Zentrum für Klinische Forschung (IZKF) at the University of Leipzig (01KS9504, Project C1).

REFERENCES

1. ARENDT, TH., C. SCHINDLER, M.K. BRÜCKNER, et al. 1997. Plastic neuronal remodeling is impaired in patients with Alzheimer's disease carrying apolipoprotein epsilon 4 allele. J. Neurosci. **17:** 516–529.
2. ARENDT, TH., H.G. ZVEGINTSEVA & T.A. LEONTOVICH. 1986. Dendritic changes in the basal nucleus of Meynert and in the diagonal band nucleus in Alzheimer's disease— a quantitative Golgi investigation. Neuroscience **19:** 1265–1278.
3. GREENBERG, S.M., E.H. KOO, D.J. SELKOE, W.Q. QIU & K.S. KOSIK. 1994. Secreted beta amyloid precursor protein stimulates mitogen activated protein kinase and enhances tau phosphorylation. Proc. Natl. Acad. Sci. USA **91:** 7104–7108.
4. MILLS, J., D.L. CHAREST, F. LAM, et al. 1997. Regulation of amyloid precursor protein catabolism involves the mitogen-activated protein kinase signal transduction pathway. J. Neurosci. **17:** 9415–9422.
5. SADOT, E., H. JAARO, R. SEGER & I. GINZBURG. 1998. Ras-signaling pathways: positive and negative regulation of tau expression in PC12 cells. J. Neurochem. **70:** 428–431.
6. YUN, H.Y., M. GONZALEZ-ZULUETA, V.L. DAWSON & T.M. DAWSON. 1998. Nitric oxide mediates N-methyl-D-aspartate receptor induced activation of p21ras. Proc. Natl. Acad. Sci. USA **95:** 5773–5778.
7. BORASIO, G.D., A. MARKUS, R. HEUMANN, et al. 1996. Ras p21 protein promotes survival and differentiation of human embryonic neural crest-derived cells. Neuroscience **73:** 1121–1127.
8. FERRARI, G. & L.A. GREENE. 1994. Proliferative inhibition by dominant-negative Ras rescues naive and neuronally differentiated PC12 cells from apoptotic death. EMBO J. **13:** 5922–5928.
9. ARENDT, TH., M. HOLZER, A. GROSSMANN, D. ZEDLICK & M.K. BRÜCKNER. 1995. Increased expression and subcellular translocation of the mitogen-activated protein kinase kinase and mitogen-activated protein kinase in Alzheimer's disease. Neuroscience **68:** 5–18.
10. GÄRTNER, U., M. HOLZER & TH. ARENDT. 1999. Elevated expression of p21^{ras} is an early event in Alzheimer's disease and precedes neurofibrillary degeneration. Neuroscience **91:** 1–5.
11. ARENDT, TH., M. HOLZER, U. GÄRTNER & M.K. BRÜCKNER. 1998. Aberrancies in signal transduction and cell cycle related events in Alzheimer's disease. J. Neural Transm. Suppl. **54:** 147–158.
12. ARENDT, TH., L. RÖDEL, U. GÄRTNER & M. HOLZER. 1996. Expression of the cyclin-dependent kinase inhibitor p16 in Alzheimer's disease. Neuroreport **7:** 3047–3049.
13. NAGY, Z., M.M. ESIRI, A.M. CATO & A.D. SMITH. 1997. Cell cycle markers in the hippocampus in Alzheimer's disease. Acta Neuropathol. **94:** 6–15.
14. NAGY, Z., M.M. ESIRI & A.D. SMITH. 1997. Expression of cell division markers in the hippocampus in Alzheimer's disease and other neurodegenerative conditions. Acta Neuropathol. **93:** 294–300.
15. SMITH, T.W. & C.F. LIPPA. 1995. Ki-67 immunoreactivity in Alzheimer's disease and other neurodegenerative disorders. J. Neuropathol. Exp. Neurol. **54:** 297–303.
16. VINCENT, I., M. ROSADO & P. DAVIES. 1996. Mitogenic mechanisms in Alzheimer's disease? J. Cell. Biol. **132:** 413.
17. BUSSER, J., D.S. GELDMACHER & K. HERRUP. 1998. Ectopic cell cycle proteins predict the sites of neuronal cell death in Alzheimer's disease brain. J. Neurosci. **18:** 2801–2807.

18. ZHU, X.W., A.K. RAINA & M.A. SMITH. 1999. Cell cycle events in neurons—proliferation or death? Am. J. Pathol. **155:** 327–329.
19. HEINTZ, N. 1993. Cell-death and the cell-cycle—a relationship between transformation and neurodegeneration. Trends Biochem. Sci. **18:** 157–159.
20. ARENDT, TH. 1993. Neuronal dedifferentiation and degeneration in Alzheimer's disease. Biol. Chem. Hoppe-Seyler **374:** 911–912.
21. SERRANO, M., A.W. LIN, M.E. MCCURRACH, D. BEACH & S.W. LOWE. 1997. Oncogenic ras provokes premature cell senescence associated with accumulation of p53 and p16INK4a. Cell **88:** 593–602.
22. ARENDT, TH., M.K. BRÜCKNER, V. BIGL & L. MARCOVA. 1995. Dendritic reorganisation in the basal forebrain under degenerative conditions and its defects in Alzheimer's disease II. Aging, Korsakoff's disease, Parkinson's disease and Alzheimer's disease. J. Comp. Neurol. **151:** 189–222.
23. ARENDT, TH., M.K. BRÜCKNER, H.-J. GERTZ & L. MARCOVA. 1998. Cortical distribution of neurofibrillary tangles in Alzheimer's disease matches the pattern of neurones that retain their capacity of plastic remodelling in the adult brain. Neuroscience **83:** 991–1002.
24. DAWSON, T.M., M. SASAKI, M. GONZALES-ZULUETA & V.L. DAWSON. 1998. Regulation of neuronal nitric oxide synthase and identification of novel nitric oxide signaling pathways, Prog. Brain Res. **118:** 3–11.
25. LÜTH, H.J., M. HOLZER, H.-J. GERTZ & TH. ARENDT. 2000. Aberrant expression of nNOS in pyramidal neurons in Alzheimer's disease is highly co-localized with $p21^{ras}$ and $p16^{INK4a}$. Brain Res. **852:** 45–55.
26. LANDER, H.M., J.S. OGISTE, S.F.A. PEARCE, R. LEVI & A. NOVOGRODSKY. 1995. Nitric oxide-stimulated guanine nucleotide exchange on p21 ras. J. Biol. Chem. **270:** 7017–7020.

Inhibition of the Neuronal Insulin Receptor

An *in Vivo* Model for Sporadic Alzheimer Disease?

SIEGFRIED HOYER,[a,c] SAE KYUNG LEE,[a] THOMAS LÖFFLER,[b] AND REINHARD SCHLIEBS[b]

[a]*Department of Pathochemistry & General Neurochemistry, University of Heidelberg, Heidelberg, Germany*

[b]*Paul-Flechsig-Institute for Brain Research, University of Leipzig, Leipzig, Germany*

ABSTRACT: It has been hypothesized that a central event in the early pathogenesis of sporadic Alzheimer disease (SAD) is the dysfunction of the neuronal insulin receptor signal transduction. To prove this, this receptor was inhibited by a triplicate icv application of STZ. Insulin binding sites were upregulated as in SAD. With respect to glucose transport proteins, detailed investigations are necessary.

INTRODUCTION

Sporadic Alzheimer disease (SAD) is as yet of unknown etiology. Its pathogenesis, however, is multifactorial. An early and central abnormality was found in cerebral glucose/energy metabolism[1,2] which was assumed to be caused by a functional damage of the neuronal insulin receptor signal transduction comparable to diabetes mellitus II.[3,4] To mimic these abnormalities, an animal model was established in which the function of the neuronal insulin receptor was inhibited by the intracerebroventricularly (icv) injected diabetogenic substance streptozotocin (STZ). Both short- and long-term studies yielded abnormalities in oxidative/energy metabolism, phospholipid composition of membranes, cholinergic and catecholaminergic functions, and in learning, memory, and cognition (for review see Refs. 5 and 6). All abnormalities found as yet resembled ones also seen in SAD. In the present study, we were interested to study the binding sites of both insulin receptor and sulfonylurea receptor, (total) glucose transporter protein, and the expression of glucose transport protein 3 (GLUT3) mRNA. The area of interest was the hippocampus (CA1 to CA4). The animals were divided as good performers (GP) and poor performers (PP).

RESULTS AND CONCLUSIONS

The effects of a triplicate icv STZ-application on various glucose metabolism-related markers are listed in TABLES 1–4. After STZ induced damage of the neuronal

---

[c]Address for correspondence: Siegfried Hoyer, Department of Pathochemistry & General Neurochemistry, University of Heidelberg, Im Neuenheimer Feld 220/221, D-69120 Heidelberg, Germany. Tel.: +49-6221-562618; fax: +49-6221-564228.
e-mail: siegfried_hoyer@med.uni-heidelberg.de

TABLE 1. [^{125}I] Insulin binding in brain sections to the insulin receptor using semiquantitative receptor autoradiography

Region	GP	PP	Ratio
CA1	120.4 ± 3.5*	110.8 ± 2.7*	1.087[+]
CA2	122.0 ± 4.2*	110.0 ± 3.2*	1.109[+]
CA3	122.1 ± 3.7*	108.2 ± 3.2	1.128[+]
CA4	117.0 ± 2.9*	101.0 ± 4.2	1.158[+]

NOTE: Data are given as percentage of control value (control = 100%) and represent mean values ± SEM obtained from five independent experiments. *$p < 0.05$ vs. control, Student's t test; [+]$p < 0.05$ between GP and PP.

TABLE 2. [^{3}H] Glyburide binding in rat brain sections to sulfonylurea binding sites using semiquantitative receptor autoradiography

Region	GP	PP	Ratio
CA1	109.7 ± 6.0	103.7 ± 10.7	1.058
CA2	113.3 ± 5.6	103.3 ± 10.4	1.097
CA3	114.7 ± 7.5	103.7 ± 11.2	1.106
CA4	108.2 ± 5.5	104.5 ± 9.9	1.035

NOTE: Data are given as percentage of control value (control = 100%) and represent mean values ± SEM obtained from five independent experiments. No statistically significant differences were found.

TABLE 3. [^{3}H]Cytochalasin-B binding to rat brain sections to the total population of glucose transporter using semiquantitative receptor autoradiography

Region	GP	PP	Ratio
CA1	126.8 ± 11.1*	108.5 ± 5.2	1.169[+]
CA2	128.2 ± 9.9*	121.5 ± 2.5	1.055
CA3	133.8 ± 12.2*	119.9 ± 4.2	1.116
CA4	130.7 ± 16.2	101.2 ± 5.4	1.292[+]

NOTE: Data are given as percentage of control value (control = 100%) and represent mean values ± SEM obtained from five independent experiments.
*$p < 0.05$ vs. control, Student's t test.
[+]$p < 0.05$ between GP and PP.

TABLE 4. *In situ* hybridization in rat brain sections using [^{35}S]labeled subtype-specific riboprobe and autoradiography

Region	GP	PP	Ratio
CA1	86.4 ± 12.8	97.8 ± 13.4	0.88
CA2	95.2 ± 9.8	101.6 ± 10.9	0.94
CA3	91.5 ± 11.3	109.6 ± 10	0.83
CA4	81.0 ± 10.8	86.9 ± 9.2	0.93

NOTE: Data are given as percentage of control value (control = 100%) and represent mean values ± SEM obtained from five independent experiments. No statistically significant differences were found.

insulin receptor, its binding sites were found to be upregulated in both GP and PP. This corresponds to insulin receptor upregulation in SAD.[3] Interestingly, upregulation differs significantly between GP andPP.

Total glucose transporter protein is elevated in hippocampal CA1 and CA3 subfields in GP, also showing differences compared to PP. In contrast, the concentrations of glucose transporter proteins GLUT1 and GLUT3 were found to be diminished in SAD.[7,8] Because there was no change in GLUT3 mRNA, it will have to be investigated whether or not the increase in total glucose transporter protein is due to an increased activation of glial cells[9] and, thus, GLUT5, too.

REFERENCES

1. HOYER, S., R.M. NITSCH & K. OESTERREICH. 1991. Predominant abnormality in cerebral glucose utilization in late-onset dementia of the Alzheimer type: a cross-sectional comparison against advanced late-onset and incipient early-onset cases. J. Neural Transm. (PD-Sect.) **3:** 1–14.
2. HOYER, S. 1992. Oxidative energy metabolism in Alzheimer brain. Studies in early-onset and late-onset cases. Mol. Chem. Neuropathol. **16:** 207–224.
3. FRÖLICH, L., D. BLUM-DEGEN, H.G. BERNSTEIN, et al. 1998. Insulin and insulin receptor in the brain in aging and in sporadic Alzheimer's disease. J. Neural Transm. **105:** 423–438.
4. HOYER, S. 1998. Is sporadic Alzheimer disease the brain type of non-insulin dependent diabetes mellitus? A challenging hypothesis. J. Neural Transm. **105:** 415–422.
5. HOYER, S., D. MÜLLER & K. PLASCHKE. 1994. Desensitization of brain insulin receptor. Effect on glucose/energy and related metabolism. J. Neural Transm. (Suppl.) **44:** 259–268.
6. LANNERT, H. & S. HOYER. 1998. Intracerebroventricular administration of streptozotocin causes long-term diminutions in learning and memory abilities and in cerebral energy metabolism in adult rats. Behav. Neurosci. **112:** 1199–1208.
7. SIMPSON, J.A., K.R. CHUNDU, T. DAVIES-HILL, W.G. HONER & P. DAVIES. 1994. Decreased concentrations of GLUT1 and GLUT3 glucose transporters in the brains of patients with Alzheimer's disease. Ann. Neurol. **35:** 546–551.
8. HARR, S.D, N.A. SIMONIAN & B.T. HYMAN. 1995. Functional alterations in Alzheimer's disease: decreased glucose transporter 3 immunoreactivity in the perforant pathway terminal zone. J. Neuropathol. Exp. Neurol. **54:** 38–41.
9. PRICKAERTS, J., J. DE VENTE, W. HONIG, et al. 2000. Nitric oxide synthase does not mediate neurotoxicity after an i.c.v. injection of streptozotocin in the rat. J. Neural Transm. **107:** 745–766.

Cytoplasmic Presenilin Aggregates in Proteasome Inhibitor-treated Cells

L.A. MacKENZIE INGANO, K.M. LENTINI, I. KOVACS,
R.E. TANZI, AND D.M. KOVACS[a]

*Genetics and Aging Unit and Department of Neurology, Massachusetts General Hospital,
Harvard Medical School, Charlestown, Massachusetts 02129, USA*

Disease-specific protein aggregates are a distinguishing feature of neurodegenerative disorders. Protein deposits can result from failure of cellular proteolytic systems (proteasomes, calpains, and lysosomes) or from a structural change in protein substrates which renders them inaccessible to degradation or more prone to aggregation. These processes have all been shown to be promoted by aging. Aging, indeed, results in the impairment of most proteolytic systems,[1] and also in increased oxidative damage. Elevated ROS production in turn can promote unfolding of target proteins.[2] Interestingly, a large number of cellular inclusions in neurodegenerative diseases are ubiquitinated.[3] However, studies on decreased proteasomal function during the aging process are scarce.[4,5]

Neurofibrillary tangles (NFTs) represent the major ubiquitinated protein inclusions found in Alzheimer's disease (AD) brains,[3] but the ubiquitinated components of the NFTs have yet to be identified. Presenilin 1 (PS1) immunostaining in 35% of tangles in AD brains[6] points to this protein as a possible ubiquitin-conjugated substrate in NFTs.[7] Normally, PS1 mainly resides in the ER.[8] Two other membrane proteins in neurodegenerative diseases, the prion protein and the cystic fibrosis mutant CFTR protein, accumulate in the ER upon misfolding and have already been shown to exit the ER and form possibly toxic aggregates in the cytoplasm.[9,10]

Mammalian cells transfected with excessive amounts of either PS1 or mutant CFTR form cytoplasmic aggregates termed aggresomes.[11] Aggresomes are pericentriolar structures containing ubiquitinated aggregates of insoluble proteins, enmeshed by a vimentin cage. Aggresomes, containing the overexpressed membrane protein, form in response to proteasome inhibition or to exceedingly high levels of the transgenes. Recent studies have shown that these structures can also form in cells transfected with a cytosolic protein.[12] Aggresomes, therefore, can serve as a model for the formation of generic cytoplasmic protein aggregates.

For PS1, aggresome formation involves sequential steps. First, PS1 retrotranslocates from the ER membrane into the cytoplasm. It is likely that PS1 is ubiquitinated during this process and thereby is targeted for degradation by the ATP-dependent, ubiquitin/proteasome system. Given that proteasome activity is inhibited in this system, the eight hydrophobic regions of PS1 tend to form a hydrophobic core in the cytoplasm. Presenilin aggregates are then retrotransported along microtubules to

[a]Address for correspondence: Dora M. Kovacs, Ph.D., Genetics and Aging Unit, Massachusetts General Hospital East, Building 149, 13th St., Charlestown, MA 02129. Tel.: (617) 726-3668; fax: (617) 726-5677.
e-mail: kovacs@helix.mgh.harvard.edu

the centrosome, where proteasomes also accumulate at the same time.[13,14] During this process, vimentin collapses around the PS1 aggregates.

In our study, we used fluorescent confocal microscopy to detect aggresome formation in stably transfected wild-type and FAD mutant PS1 cell lines treated with the proteasome inhibitors MG132 and ALLN. Transfected Chinese hamster ovary (CHO) and human neuroblastoma SY5Y cells exhibited "classic" aggresomes. Generic cell stress did not result in aggresome formation, indicating that these structures specifically accumulate when the ATP-dependent ubiquitin/proteasome system is impaired. Surprisingly, aggresome formation in CHO cells did not induce apoptosis. Although extended treatment with proteasome inhibitors did eventually result in cell death, this was not potentiated by FAD PS1 mutations. We had previously found that staurosporine-induced apoptosis was elevated in neuroglioma cells stably transfected with FAD mutant PS1.[15] Given that PS1 is found in neurofibrillary tangles, additional studies are aimed at further exploring the propensity of wild-type and FAD mutant presenilins to get retrotransported into the cytoplasm and serve as a core for cytoplasmic inclusion formation before reaching the centrosome.

REFERENCES

1. CUERVO, A.M. & J.F. DICE. 1998. How do intracellular proteolytic systems change with age? Frontiers Biosci. **3:** d25–d43.
2. GRUNE, T., T. REINHECKEL & K.J. DAVIES. 1997. Degradation of oxidized proteins in mammalian cells. FASEB J. **11:** 526–534.
3. ALVES-RODRIGUES, A., L. GREGORI & M. E. FIGUEIREDO-PEREIRA. 1998. Ubiquitin, cellular inclusions and their role in neurodegeneration. Trends Neurosci **21:** 516–520.
4. HAYASHI, T. & S. GOTO. 1998. Age-related changes in the 20S and 26S proteasome activities in the liver of male F344 rats. Mech. Ageing Dev. **102:** 55–66.
5. BARDAG-GORCE, F., L. FAROUT, C. VEYRAT-DUREBEX et al. 1999. Changes in 20S proteasome activity during ageing of the LOU rat. Mol. Biol. Rep. **26:** 89–93.
6. CHUI, D.H., K. SHIROTANI, H. TANAHASHI et al. 1998. Both N-terminal and C-terminal fragments of presenilin 1 colocalize with neurofibrillary tangles in neurons and dystrophic neurites of senile plaques in Alzheimer's disease. J. Neurosci. Res. **53:** 99–106.
7. KIM, T.W., W.H. PETTINGELL, O.G. HALLMARK et al. 1997. Endoproteolytic cleavage and proteasomal degradation of presenilin 2 in transfected cells. J. Biol. Chem. **272:** 11006–11010.
8. KOVACS, D.M., H.J. FAUSETT, K.J. PAGE et al. 1996. Alzheimer-associated presenilins 1 and 2: neuronal expression in brain and localization to intracellular membranes in mammalian cells. Nat. Med. **2:** 224–229.
9. MA, J. & S. LINDQUIST. 1999. De novo generation of a PrPSc-like conformation in living cells. Nat. Cell Biol. **1:** 358–361.
10. XIONG, X., E. CHONG & W.R. SKACH. 1999. Evidence that endoplasmic reticulum (ER)-associated degradation of cystic fibrosis transmembrane conductance regulator is linked to retrograde translocation from the ER membrane. J. Biol. Chem. **274:** 2616–2624.
11. JOHNSTON, J.A., C.L. WARD & R.R. KOPITO. 1998. Aggresomes: a cellular response to misfolded proteins. J. Cell Biol. **143:** 1883–1898.
12. GARCIA-MATA, R., Z. BEBOK, E.J. SORSCHER & E.S. SZTUL. 1999. Characterization and dynamics of aggresome formation by a cytosolic GFP-chimera. J. Cell Biol. **146:** 1239–1254.
13. WIGLEY, W.C., R.P. FABUNMI, M.G. LEE et al. 1999. Dynamic association of proteasomal machinery with the centrosome. J. Cell Biol. **145:** 481–490.
14. FABUNMI, R.P., W.C. WIGLEY, P.J. THOMAS & G.N. DEMARTINO. 2000. Activity and regulation of the centrosome-associated proteasome. J. Biol. Chem. **275:** 409–413.
15. KOVACS, D.M., R. MANCINI, J. HENDERSON et al. 1999. Staurosporine-induced activation of caspase-3 is potentiated by presenilin 1 familial Alzheimer's disease mutations in human neuroglioma cells. J. Neurochem. **73:** 2278–2285.

Regulation of APP Synthesis and Secretion by Neuroimmunophilin Ligands and Cyclooxygenase Inhibitors

ROBERT K.K. LEE[a,c] AND RICHARD J. WURTMAN[b]

[a]Division of Health Sciences and Technology, Harvard University–Massachusetts Institute of Technology, E25-604 MIT, Cambridge, Massachusetts 02139, USA

[b]Department of Brain and Cognitive Sciences, E25-604 MIT, Cambridge, Massachusetts 02139, USA

ABSTRACT: We and others previously showed that both the synthesis of the amyloid precursor protein (APP) and its processing (i.e., to amyloidogenic Aβ peptides; soluble nonamyloidogenic APPs; and other APP fragments) are regulated by neurotransmitters. Transmitters that elevate cellular cAMP levels (like norepinephrine and prostaglandins, which act on β-adrenergic receptors and prostaglandin E$_2$ receptors respectively) enhance APP synthesis and the formation of amyloidogenic APP holoprotein. Transmitters that stimulate phosphatidylinositol hydrolysis (by activating muscarinic m1 or m3 receptors, serotoninergic 5HT2a or 5HT2c receptors, or metabotropic glutamate receptors of subtypes 1 or 5) increase the conversion of APP to soluble APPs, and decrease the formation of Aβ. These findings suggest that drugs that regulate the activity of neurotransmitter receptors might be useful in preventing the excessive formation of Aβ or other amyloid precursors in Alzheimer's disease.

We now show that neuroimmunophilin ligands (like cyclosporin A or FK-506) and nonsteroidal antiinflammatory agents (NSAIDs), including cyclooxygenase (COX)-2 inhibitors, can also prevent APP overexpression and the overproduction of amyloidogenic peptides. We observe that the enhancement of APP overexpression by prostaglandin E$_2$ is inhibited by neuroimmunophilin ligands like cyclosporin A or FK-506 (tacrolimus). We also find that the NSAIDs, which reduce prostaglandin synthesis by inhibiting COX-1 and -2 enzymes, might also be expected to lower APP levels. Our present data confirm that these drugs, as well as drugs that selectively inhibit COX-2, reduce the levels of amyloidogenic APP holoprotein in cultured neurons or in cultured astrocytes. We previously showed that elevations in cAMP, perhaps generated in response to prostaglandins, can suppress APPs secretion. The NSAIDs and COX inhibitors also increased levels of soluble APPs in the media of cultured astrocytes and neurons, perhaps acting by inhibition of prostaglandin production. Since APP holoprotein can be amyloidogenic, while APPs may be neurotrophic, our findings suggest that some neuroimmunophilin ligands, NSAIDs and COX-2 inhibitors might suppress amyloid formation and enhance neuronal regeneration in Alzheimer's disease.

[c]Address for correspondence: Robert K.K. Lee, E25-604, MIT, Cambridge, MA 02139. Tel.: (617) 253-8371/6733; fax: (617) 253-6882.
e-mail: rkklee@mit.edu

INTRODUCTION

Amyloid plaques found in the brains of patients with Alzheimer's disease (AD) consist primarily of aggregates of amyloid peptides (Aβ) that are derived from the much larger amyloid precursor protein (APP). There is abundant evidence that astrocytes express components of the classical complementary cascade, as well as of inflammatory cytokines and acute phase proteins, which might contribute to local inflammatory responses and to neurodegeneration in brain regions adjacent to amyloid plaques and, through glial processes, at distant locations.[1,2]

Astrocytes or microglia may contribute to the overexpression of APP and possibly the formation of amyloid in AD. Neurons express primarily the 695-amino acid isoform of APP. Astrocytes and microglia, in contrast, express APP751 (i.e., APP695 plus an additional 56-amino acid Kunitz-type Protease Inhibitor insert at the N-terminus) or APP770 (APP691 plus a KPI domain, plus a 19-amino acid OX-2 insert).[3] mRNA levels for APP751 and APP770 appear to be elevated in brains and fibroblasts of individuals with AD, and the APP751:APP695 ratio increases with age.[4–6] Increased amounts of KPI-containing APP have been also detected, post-mortem, in brains of AD patients,[7] and it is especially prominent in brain regions exhibiting neurodegeneration. In cell cultures, KPI-containing APP appears to be more amyloidogenic than APP695.[8] Furthermore, a positive relationship exists between KPI-containing APP immunoreactivity and plaque density in the brain.[9]

APP normally undergoes constitutive processing which disrupts Aβ formation, and causes secretion of a soluble APPs fragment that appears to have neurotrophic or neuroprotective functions.[10,11] In cultured cells, APP overexpression results in aberrant and amyloidogenic APP processing associated with increased production of Aβ peptides or neurotoxic APP fragments.[12] APP overexpression in transgenic mice similarly enhances Aβ formation, and is associated with neuronal dysfunction; synapse loss; astrogliosis; and cognitive decline.[13] Increased levels of Aβ have been detected in the plasmas of AD patients.[14] It might be expected that drugs that enhance APPs secretion, inhibit Aβ formation, or prevent APP overexpression might suppress the pathophysiologic processes underlying Alzheimer's disease.

NEUROTRANSMITTER AGONISTS REGULATE APP PROCESSING AND APP SYNTHESIS

Neurotransmitter agonists that increase phosphatidylinositol (PI) hydrolysis and/or the activation of protein kinase C (PKC) stimulate constitutive APP processing in a variety of stable cell lines expressing cloned neurotransmitter receptors,[15,16] in primary cultures of brain neurons or astrocytes,[17,18] and in rat brain slices.[19] Consequently, the secretion of potentially neuroprotective, nonamyloidogenic APPs is increased, and Aβ production is decreased (FIG. 1).

Brain injury is associated with elevated cAMP levels, and is also accompanied by increased prostaglandin levels and circulating levels of norepinephrine. Such elevations in cAMP can suppress APPs secretion in brain cells, and result in excessive Aβ production.[20–22] Activation of β-adrenergic receptors or of PGE_2 receptors in cultured astrocytes can, by stimulating cAMP formation, initiate a signaling cascade that includes activation of protein kinase A; phosphorylation of the cAMP response

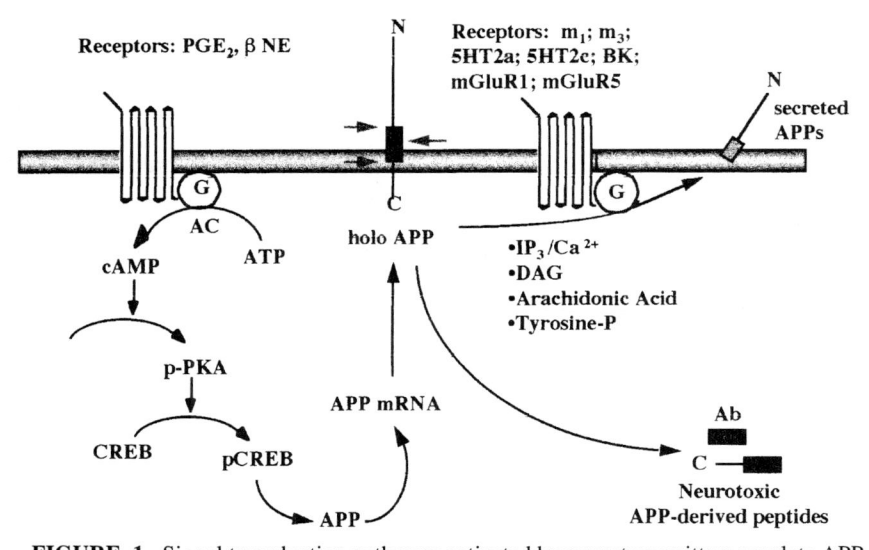

FIGURE 1. Signal transduction pathways activated by neurotransmitters regulate APP synthesis and metabolism of the amyloid precursor protein. Activation of neurotransmitters coupled to cAMP formation (e.g., β-adrenergic, β-NE, or prostaglandins, PGE_2) activates adenylate cyclase (AC) to produce cAMP, which phosphorylates protein kinase A (p-PKA). A putative cAMP response element binding protein (CREB) in the APP promoter may be phosphorylated to activate transcription. Increased APP mRNA or holoprotein can accelerate the formation of neurotoxic or amyloidogenic Aβ peptides. Neurotransmitter receptors coupled to inositol trisphosphate (IP_3), calcium mobilization (Ca^{2+}), diacylglycerol (DAG), arachidonic acid, or tyrosine phosphorylation (tyrosine-P), for example, muscarinic m1 or m3, serotoninergic $5HT_{2a}$ or $5HT_{2c}$, metabotropic glutamate receptor subtype 1 or 5 promote nonamyloidogenic processing of APP holoprotein such that soluble APPs is secreted and Aβ formation is reduced.

element binding transcription factor; and activation the APP gene leading to increased production of APP mRNA and elevated levels of APP holoprotein (FIG. 1).[21,23] Exposure of astrocytes to PGE_2 or norepinephrine also increases the immunoreactivity of astrocytic glial fibrillary acidic protein, and transforms quiescent astrocytes into process-bearing cells that are reminiscent of reactive astrocytes *in vivo*.[24] Thus, activation of neurotransmitter agonists coupled to cAMP formation can cause astrogliosis, and might also increase APP synthesis and exacerbate the formation of amyloid or the neuropathology of AD.

PROSTAGLANDIN E_2 STIMULATES APP OVEREXPRESSION: INHIBITION BY NEUROIMMUNOPHILIN LIGANDS

The early loss of synapses or neurons in AD is associated with astrogliosis and brain inflammation. Astrocytes are considered to be a major source of arachidonic acid in the brain, and may thereby, through arachidonate products, promote brain inflammation and accelerate amyloid formation in AD.[2] Analysis of postmortem brains from individuals with AD revealed that the activity of cytosolic phospholipase A_2, which releases arachidonic acid from membrane phospholipids, is elevated in brain astrocytes.[25] The release of arachidonic acid and its conversion, initiated by cyclooxygenase (COX), to prostaglandins can cause neurodegeneration and promote amyloid formation.[26]

We recently showed that prostaglandin E_2 stimulates overexpression of KPI-containing and amyloidogenic APP in cultured astrocytes, and that this stimulatory effect is inhibited by the immunosuppressants cyclosporin A or FK-506 (tacrolimus).[23] Both cyclosporin A and FK-506 activate neuroimmunophilin receptors to inhibit cAMP-mediated gene transcription. While cyclosporin A can cause severe liver toxicity and may not readily cross the blood-brain barrier, nonimmunosuppressive analogues of such neuroimmunophilin ligands have been synthesized.[27] These analogues appear also to have neurotrophic properties. Such neuroimmunophilin ligands, some of which also stimulate increased APPs secretion (H. Wood, R.J. Wurtman & R. K. Lee, in preparation) might thus have therapeutic potential in Alzheimer's disease.

NSAIDs AND COX-2 INHIBITORS STIMULATE APPs SECRETION

Epidemiologic and clinical data suggest that the use of NSAIDs delays the onset of AD and reduces the progression of pathologic symptoms in Alzheimer's disease.[2] NSAIDs, by inhibiting COX enzymes, might be expected to suppress both prostaglandin and cAMP production and, thereby, prevent APP overproduction or the excessive production of amyloidogenic and neurotoxic APP derivatives.

Aspirin, like most NSAIDs, prevents inflammation and pain by inhibiting both COX-1 and COX-2 enzymes. Resveratrol, a phenolic antioxidant and COX inhibitor found in grapes, inhibits prostaglandin production, and has anticancer and anti-inflammatory properties.[28] We treated cultured astrocytes or neurons with aspirin or resveratrol for 1 h (at nano- or micromolar range), and observed increases in the secretion of soluble APPs (as measured by Western blot analysis). The increase in APPs secretion caused by aspirin or resveratrol was accompanied by a decrease in the levels of cellular and amyloidogenic APP holoprotein (FIG. 2). Thus, NSAIDs appear to stimulate nonamyloidogenic APP processing *in vitro*.

Most traditional NSAIDs are more potent against COX-1 than COX-2. COX-1, which is essential for platelet thromboxane production, is constitutively expressed in most tissues, and regulates the production of essential prostaglandins in kidney and gastric mucosa. COX-2, by contrast, is rapidly inducible in response to cytokines, inflammation, and injury. The long-term use of nonspecific COX inhibitors such as aspirin and related NSAIDs can produce unacceptable renal or gastric side effects.[29,30] COX-2 mRNA is elevated in the postmortem brains of patients with AD.[31] Since COX-2 inhibitors may offer comparable efficacy to NSAIDs without their undesirable side effects, we examined the effect of several such compounds on APPs secretion and APP holoprotein levels.

DFU (5,5-dimethyl-3-(3-fluorophenyl)-4-(4-methylsulphonyl)phenyl-2(5H)-furanone) and DFP (3-(2-propyloxy)-(4-methylsulphonyl)-5,5-dimethylfuranone), which are highly selective, orally-active COX-2 inhibitors that prevent the conver-

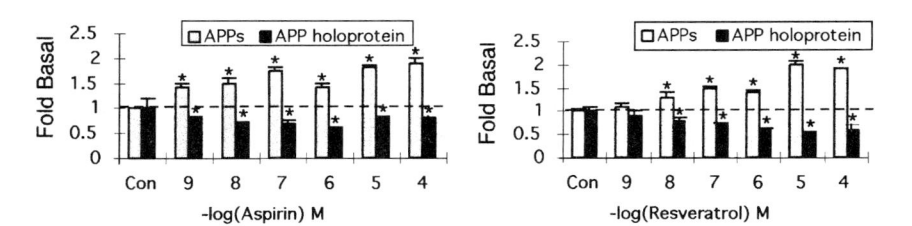

FIGURE 2. Effect of aspirin or resveratrol on APP expression and secretion in primary cultured astrocytes. Aspirin (**A**) or resveratrol (**B**) treatment promotes APPs secretion and decreases the levels of amyloidogenic APP holoprotein in cultured astrocytes. Similar results were obtained with aspirin or resveratrol treatment of primary cultured neurons (data not shown). Graph represents means, and standard errors were obtained from 4 independent experiments, (*, significantly different from control; $p < 0.05$).

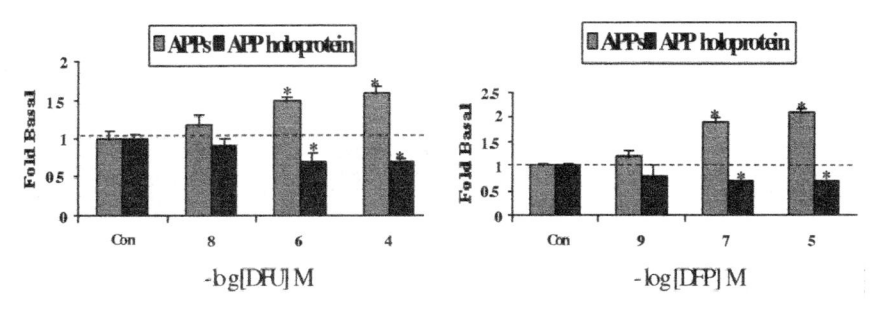

FIGURE 3. Effect of DFU or DFP on APP expression and secretion in primary cultured brain cells. Treatment of cultured astryctes with DFU (**A**) or of cultured neurons with DFP (**B**) promotes APPs secretion and decreases the levels of amyloidogenic APP holoprotein in cultured astrocytes (*, significantly different from control; $p < 0.05$).

sion of arachidonic acid to prostaglandins,[32] were kindly provided by Merck and Co., Inc. Treatment of cultured astrocytes with DFU or DFP (10^{-9}–10^{-3}M) for 1 h increased the secretion of soluble APPs and concurrently decreased the levels of cellular APP holoprotein (FIG. 3). Hence, specific COX-2 inhibitors can prevent the excessive accumulation of amyloidogenic APP, and also prevent the formation of amyloid, by enhancing the conversion of APP to form soluble APPs.

Although NSAIDs and selective COX-2 inhibitors stimulated APPs secretion and decreased the levels of amyloidogenic APP in cultured astrocytes and neurons, the biochemical basis underlying this stimulatory process is not known. NSAIDs and selective COX-2 inhibitors might, by reducing prostaglandin production, be expected also to suppress cAMP formation. We previously showed that elevations in cAMP can suppress APPs secretion and promote APP synthesis.[21] Therefore, the decreased levels of prostaglandins, and consequently of cAMP, caused by NSAIDs or selective COX-2 inhibitors, could be responsible for the increased APPs secretion and decreased levels of APP holoprotein observed in the astrocyte or neuronal cultures. Studies in progress are examining this possibility.

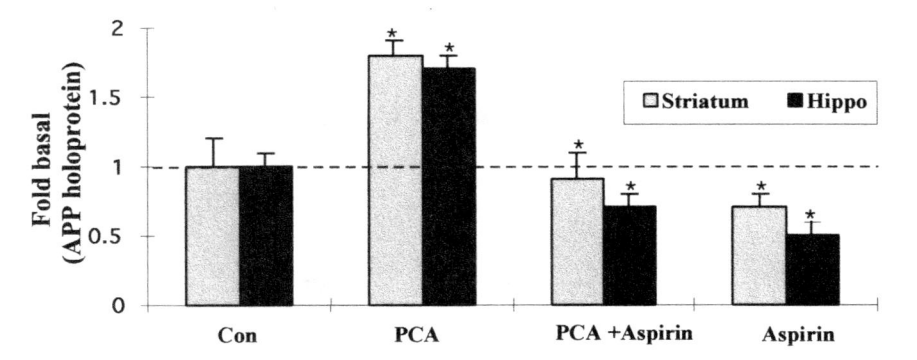

FIGURE 4. Effect of synapse loss induced by p-chloroamphetamine (PCA) on APP holoprotein levels in rats treated with or without aspirin. PCA induced significant increases in brain APP holoprotein levels, and this increase is attenuated by aspirin. Aspirin treatment alone also caused a small, but significant decrease in brain APP holoprotein levels (*, significantly different from control; $p < 0.05$).

ASPIRIN INHIBITS APP OVEREXPRESSION
CAUSED BY NEURONAL INJURY

Neuronal injury can stimulate prostaglandin production, and thereby stimulate APP overexpression. We injected rats chronically with para-chloroamphetamine (PCA), a neurotoxin which selectively damages serotonin-releasing brain neurons, and confirmed by subsequent microdialysis that serotonin release in the striatum had indeed been reduced.

Examination of brain tissue from the striatum or hippocampus revealed that the levels of APP holoprotein, as well as of KPI-containing APP isoforms, were increased by the PCA treatment (FIG. 4). In rats injected with both aspirin and PCA, levels of APP holoprotein did not differ from those of uninjected, control rats. Interestingly, injections of aspirin alone caused a significant decrease in levels of amyloidogenic APP holoprotein relative to control levels, an effect that is consistent with our *in vitro* studies with cultures of astrocytes or neurons. These data suggest that some NSAIDs may be useful in preventing APP overexpression in an *in vivo* model of AD. Inasmuch as the levels of glial fibrillary acidic protein (a marker for reactive astrocytes) were also elevated in the striatum and hippocampus following PCA injections, the increased APP levels in those brain regions may reflect APP synthesis by astrocytes responding to the PCA-induced loss of serotonin neurons.

SUMMARY

We previously showed that activation of neurotransmitter receptors coupled to the PI/PKC signaling cascade stimulate the nonamyloidogenic processing of APP and enhance the secretion of neurotrophic APPs. Drugs that activate such receptors may also enhance synaptic transmission and improve cognition in AD. We now show that neuroimmunophilin ligands or NSAIDs may be used to control the formation of amyloidogenic or neurotoxic APP fragments associated with APP overexpression; such compounds may also be beneficial for treating the immune or inflammatory processes associated with AD. An improved understanding of the roles of neurotransmitter signaling, immune, and inflammatory processes in AD will strengthen our rationale for prospective clinical trials. The feasibility of such drugs in protecting against the onset of AD, or in arresting the progression of neuropathology would represent a therapeutic breakthrough in AD.

ACKNOWLEDGMENTS

This work was supported by the National Institutes of Health (Grant No. MH-28783) and The Center for Brain Sciences and Metabolism Charitable Trust. We would like to thank Jeff Breu, Joanna Zarach, and Joy Portlock for technical assistance and data analysis. Merck & Co., Inc. kindly provided the selective cyclo-oxygenase-2 inhibitors (DFU and DFP) used in this study.

REFERENCES

1. EIKELENBOOM, P., S.-S. ZHAN, W.A. VAN GOOL & D. ALLSOP. 1994. Inflammatory mechanisms in Alzheimer's disease. Trends Pharmacol. **15:** 447–450.
2. MCGEER, P.L. & E.G. MCGEER. 1995. The inflammatory response system of brain: implications for therapy of Alzheimer and other neurodegenerative diseases. Brain Res. Rev. **21:** 195–218.
3. KITAGUCHI, N., Y. TAKAHASHI, Y. TOKUSHIMA et al. 1988. Novel precursor of Alzheimer's disease amyloid protein shows protease inhibitory activity. Nature **331:** 530–532.
4. TANZI, R.E., A.I. MCCLATCHEY, E.D. LAMPERTI et al. 1988. Protease inhibitor domain encoded by an amyloid protein precursor mRNA associated with Alzheimer's disease. Nature **331:** 528–530.
5. TANAKA, S., L. LIU, J. KIMURA et al. 1992. Age-related changes in the proportion of amyloid precursor protein mRNAs in Alzheimer's disease and other neurological disorders. Mol. Brain. Res. **15:** 303–310.
6. ROCKENSTEIN, E.M., L. MCCONLOGUE, H. TAN et al. 1995. Levels and alternative splicing of amyloid beta protein precursor (APP) transcripts in brains of APP transgenic mice and humans with Alzheimer's disease. J. Biol. Chem. **270:** 28257–28267.
7. MOIR, R.D., T. LYNCH, A.I. BUSH et al. 1998. Relative increase in Alzheimer's disease of soluble forms of cerebral Abeta amyloid protein precursor containing the Kunitz protease inhibitory domain. J. Biol. Chem. **273:** 5013–5019.
8. HO, L., K. FUKUCHI & S.G. YOUNKIN. 1996. The alternatively spliced Kunitz protease inhibitor domain alters amyloid protein precursor processing and amyloid protein production in cultured cells. J. Biol. Chem. **271:** 30929–30934.
9. ZHAN, S.S., R. SANDBRINK, K. BEYREUTHER & H.P. SCHMITT. 1995. APP with Kunitz type protease inhibitor domain (KPI) correlates with neuritic plaque density but not with cortical synaptophysin immunoreactivity in Alzheimer's disease and non-demented aged subjects: a multifactorial analysis. Clin. Neuropathol. **14:** 142–149.
10. ESCH, F.S., P.S. KEIM, E.C. BEATTIE et al. 1990. Cleavage of amyloid beta peptide during constitutive processing of its precursor. Science **248:** 1122–1124.
11. SMITH-SWINTOSKY, V.L., L.C. PETTIGREW, S.D. CRADDOCK et al. 1994. Secreted forms of beta-amyloid precursor protein protect against ischemic brain injury. J. Neurochem. **63:** 781–784.
12. YOSHIKAWA, K., T. AIZAWA & Y. HAYASHI. 1992. Degeneration in vitro of post-mitotic neurons overexpressing the Alzheimer amyloid protein precursor. Nature **359:** 64–67.

13. HSIAO, K.K., D.R. BORCHELT, K. OLSON et al. 1995. Age-related CNS disorder and early death in transgenic FVB/N mice overexpressing Alzheimer amyloid precursor proteins. Neuron 15: 1203–1218.
14. MAYEUX, R., M.X. TANG, D.M. JACOBS et al. 1999. Plasma amyloid beta-peptide 1–42 and incipient Alzheimer's disease. Ann. Neurol. 46: 412–416.
15. NITSCH, R.M., M. DENG, J.H. GROWDON & R.J. WURTMAN. 1996. Serotonin 5-HT2a and 5-HT2c receptors stimulate amyloid precursor protein ectodomain secretion. J. Biol. Chem. 271: 4188–4194.
16. NITSCH, R.M., R.J. WURTMAN & J.H. GROWDON. 1995. Regulation of proteolytic processing of the amyloid β-protein precursor by first messengers: a novel potential approach for the treatment of Alzheimer's disease. Drug Res. 45: 435–438.
17. LEE, R.K., R.J. WURTMAN, A.J. COX & R.M. NITSCH. 1995. Amyloid precursor protein processing is stimulated by metabotropic glutamate receptors. Proc. Natl. Acad. Sci. USA 92: 8083–8087.
18. LEE, R.K.K. & R.J. WURTMAN. 1997. Metabotropic glutamate receptors increase amyloid precursor protein processing in astrocytes: inhibition by cAMP. J. Neurochem. 68: 1830–1835.
19. ULUS, I.H., & R.J. WURTMAN. 1997. Metabotropic glutamate receptor agonists increase release of soluble amyloid precursor protein derivatives from rat brain cortical and hippocampal slices. J. Pharmacol. Exp. Ther. 281: 149–154.
20. EFTHIMIOPOULOS, S., S. PUNJ, M. PANGALOS et al. 1996. Intracellular cyclic AMP inhibits constitutive and phorbol ester-stimulated secretory cleavage of amyloid precursor protein. J. Neurochem. 67: 872–875.
21. LEE, R.K.K., W. ARAKI & R.J. WURTMAN. 1997. Stimulation of amyloid precursor protein synthesis by adrenergic receptors coupled to cAMP formation. Proc. Natl. Acad. Sci. USA 94: 5422–5426.
22. MARAMBAUD, P., N. CHEVALLIER, K. ANCOLIO & F. CHECLER. 1998. Post-transcriptional contribution of a cAMP-dependent pathway to the formation of a- and b/g-secretases-derived products of beta APP maturation in human cells expressing wild-type and Swedish mutated beta APP. Mol. Med. 4: 715–723.
23. LEE, R.K., S. KNAPP & R.J. WURTMAN. 1999. Prostaglandin E$_2$ stimulates amyloid precursor protein gene expression: inhibition by immunosuppressants. J. Neurosci. 19: 940–947.
24. YOUNG, M.J., R.K. LEE, S. JHAVERI & R.J. WURTMAN. 1999. Intracellular and cell-surface distribution of amyloid precursor protein in cortical astrocytes. Brain Res. Bull. 50: 27–32.
25. STEPHENSON, D.T., C.A. LEMERE, D.J. SELKOE & J.A. CLEMENS. 1996. Cytosolic phospholipase A$_2$ (cPLA$_2$) immunoreactivity is elevated in Alzheimer's disease brain. Neurobiol. Dis. 3: 51–63.
26. PRASAD, K.N., A.R. HOVLAND, F.G. LA ROSA & P.G. HOVLAND. 1998. Prostaglandins as putative neurotoxins in Alzheimer's disease. Proc. Soc. Exp. Biol. Med. 219: 120–125.
27. STEINER, J.P., M.A. CONNOLLY, H.L. VALENTINE et al. 1997. Neurotrophic actions of nonimmunosuppressive analogues of immunosuppressive drugs FK506, rapamycin and cyclosporin A. Nat. Med. 3: 421–428.
28. JANG, M., L. CAI, G.O. UDEANI et al. 1997. Cancer chemopreventive activity of resveratrol, a natural product derived from grapes. Science 275: 218–220.
29. ALLISON, M.C., A.G. HOWATSON, C.J. TORRANCE et al. 1992. Gastrointestinal damage associated with the use of nonsteroidal antiinflammatory drugs. N. Engl. J. Med. 327: 749–754.
30. WALLACE, J.L. 1994. Mechanisms of nonsteroidal anti-inflammatory drug (NSAID) induced gastrointestinal damage: potential for development of gastrointestinal tract safe NSAIDs. Can. J. Physiol. Pharmacol. 72: 1493–1498.
31. PASINETTI, G.M. & P.S. AISEN. 1998. Cyclooxygenase-2 expression is increased in frontal cortex of Alzheimer's disease brain. Neuroscience 87: 319–324.
32. RIENDEAU, D., M.D. PERCIVAL, S. BOYCE et al. 1997. Biochemical and pharmacological profile of a tetrasubstituted furanone as a highly selective COX-2 inhibitor. Br. J. Pharmacol. 121: 105–117.

Aβ Modulation: The Next Generation of AD Therapeutics

KEVIN M. FELSENSTEIN[a]

Bristol-Myers Squibb Pharmaceutical Research Institute,
Wallingford, Connecticut 06492, USA

The amyloid β-peptide (Aβ) is the major component of senile plaques in Alzheimer's disease (AD) patients. Aβ is present in the media of cultured cells, plasma, cerebrospinal fluid, and various tissues, including brain, indicating that its production and release are normal physiological events. However, accumulation of the Aβ peptide in the brain, in the form of plaques, is believed to be linked to the pathogenesis of AD. Some forms of AD, mainly early-onset cases, show autosomal dominant inheritance patterns due to the presence of mutated genes, including β-APP, presenilin 1 (PS1), and presenilin 2 (PS2). Additionally, Trisomy 21 individuals, known to contain an extra copy of the β-APP gene and to express higher levels of the β-APP protein, show an increased incidence of plaque and tangle formation paralleling the pathology seen in AD. Aβ is generated from sequential cleavage activities, termed β- and γ-secretase, which liberate the amino and carboxy termini of the Aβ peptide from β-APP, respectively. Approximately, 90% of secreted Aβ peptides are $A\beta_{1-40}$, a relatively soluble form of the peptide, while most of the remaining 10% are $A\beta_{1-42(43)}$. The latter represents species deposited early in the disease that are highly fibrillogenic, which may be essential to the neurotoxic activity *in vitro* and, possibly, *in vivo*. In early onset AD, a higher fraction of the $A\beta_{42x}$ peptide relative to wild-type is secreted, strongly implicating Aβ to the etiology of the disease. Drug discovery efforts targeting the generation of Aβ may result in significantly slowing, stopping, or preventing the disease. Screening efforts have identified compounds that can modulate Aβ production both *in vitro* and *in vivo*. *In vivo* examination of such compounds reveals significant decreases in the concentration of Aβ in the brains of animals within hours after single dose administration. The studies were extended to include plasma and cerebrospinal fluid, where similar decreases were apparent. These efforts have led to the identification of clinical candidates that should form the foundation of the next generation of AD therapeutics. The proprietary nature of the research prevents current details from being published at this time, and the following is meant only to serve as a guide to the rationale behind the potential disease modifying approach.

Alzheimer's disease (AD) is a progressive neurodegenerative disorder marked by loss of memory, cognition, and behavioral stability.[1] AD afflicts 6–10% of the population over age 65 and up to 50% over age 85. It is the leading cause of dementia and the fourth leading cause of death after cardiovascular disease, cancer, and stroke.

[a]Address for correspondence: Kevin Felsenstein, Neuroscience Drug Discovery, Bristol-Myers Squibb Pharmaceutical Research Institute, 5 Research Parkway, Wallingford, CT 06492-7660. Tel.: 92030 677-7671; fax: (203) 677-7569.
e-mail: kevin.felsenstein@bms.com

There is currently no effective treatment for AD. The total net cost related to AD in the U.S. exceeds $100 billion annually. The market for an effective medication is estimated to be between $2 and $8 billion per year in the U.S. The current combined sales of drugs for symptomatic treatment of AD in the seven major markets (U.S., U.K., France, Germany, Japan, Italy, and Spain) exceeds $650 million and is estimated to climb to more than $1.9 billion by 2007. Drug discovery efforts focused on slowing the rate of decline or delaying the onset (5–10 years) of the disease could effectively decrease the incidence of the disease by 50–75% within one generation.[2]

AD does not have a simple etiology; however, it has been associated with certain risk factors including (1) age, (2) family history, and (3) head trauma; other factors include environmental toxins and low level of education. Protective factors include postmenopausal estrogen replacement therapy, long-term use of antiinflammatory drugs, and cigarette smoking.[1,2] Specific neuropathological lesions in the limbic and cerebral cortices include intracellular neurofibrillary tangles consisting of hyperphosphorylated tau and the extracellular deposition of fibrillar aggregates of β-amyloid.[2] Familial, early onset autosomal dominant forms of AD have been linked to missense mutations in the β-amyloid precursor protein (β-APP) and in the presenilin proteins 1 and 2.[3,4] In some patients, late onset forms of AD have been correlated with a specific allele of the apolipoprotein E (apoE) gene, and, more recently, the finding of a mutation in α_2-macroglobulin, which may be linked to at least 30% of the AD population. Despite this heterogeneity, all forms of AD exhibit similar pathological findings.[1,5]

MODULATION OF Aβ AS A THERAPEUTIC TARGET

The rationale for pursuing the modulation of Aβ production as a therapeutic target is as follows:[1–7]

- Amyloid burden in other diseases, e.g., multiple myeloma, type II diabetes mellitus, dialysis arthropathy, and the less common systemic amyloid AA (protein A) and AL (kappa light-chain) amyloidosis, correlates with tissue dysfunction.

- Aβ deposition is relatively specific for AD.

- Aβ deposition is the earliest known pathological evidence of disease

- Aβ deposition is seen in early Down's Syndrome, long before neuronal death or dementia appear.

- Degree of dementia positively correlates with neuritic plaque count.

- Plaque Aβ appears to be neurotoxic.

- Mutations in the β-APP protein cause some rare forms of inherited familial Alzheimer's disease.

- Mutations in other FAD-related genes affect Aβ production both quantitatively and qualitatively.

Genetic analysis provides the best clues for a logical therapeutic approach to AD.[5,6] All mutations, found to date, affect the quantitative or qualitative production of the amyloidogenic Aβ peptide and have given strong support to the "amyloid cascade hypothesis" of AD. Transgenic animals have been developed overexpressing β-APP species bearing familial mutations, which exhibit AD-like histopathology and cognitive deficits. Additionally, Aβ is neurotoxic in several cell systems including cultured neurons. The likely link between Aβ and AD pathology emphasizes the need for a better understanding of the mechanisms of Aβ production and strongly warrants a therapeutic approach at modulating Aβ levels.

PROTEOLYTIC PROCESSING OF β-APP

The release of Aβ is modulated by at least two proteolytic activities referred to as β- and γ-secretase cleaving at the N-terminus (Met-Asp bond) and the C-terminus (residues 40–42 of the Aβ peptide), respectively. In the secretory pathway, there is evidence that β-secretase cleaves first, leading to the secretion of s-APPβ (sβ) and the retention of an 11-kDa membrane-bound carboxy terminal fragment (CTF). The latter is believed to give rise to Aβ, following cleavage by γ-secretase. The γ-secretase is also capable of cleaving the α-secretase-generated 9-kDa CTF giving rise to a non-amyloidogenic 3-kDa secreted fragment (p3). In addition to the α- and β-secretory pathways, a substantial portion of full-length β-APP enters into the endosomal system for Golgi recycling or degradation in the lysosomal system.[1,7]

DIRECTED AND HIGH-THROUGHPUT SCREENING FOR Aβ PRODUCTION INHIBITORS

With Aβ being a product of normal cellular metabolism, transfected cells, stably expressing wild-type and mutant forms of β-APP, can be used to study the mechanisms that regulate its production. Conditioned medium from these cells is assayed by a sandwich ELISA for the quantity of Aβ present and to identify and characterize inhibitors of Aβ production. The primary assay does not distinguish between β- or γ-secretase inhibition or for that matter any other interaction, e.g., presenilin's, that may interfere with Aβ production. Inhibitors are also looked at for their effects on the overall synthesis of β-APP; their effects on secretion of β-APP species; and their effects on intracellular catabolites of β-APP in order to classify them as putative β- or γ-secretase inhibitors. In conjunction with the cell-based ELISA, a cell-free system has been developed that specifically measures a proteolytic activity that detects the γ-secretase cleavage product. This latter assay formed the basis of the biochemistry approach to isolate and identify the proteolytic activity.

BIOLOGY-EVALUATION TIER FOR Aβ PRODUCTION MODULATORS

- Primary Screen: ELISA assay measuring secreted Aβ in culture media produced from β-APP transfected human neuroglioma (H4) cells.

- Secondary Assay(s): Cell-free assays (membrane preparations; detergent extracts; or semipurified/enriched fractions) measuring activities consistent with either β- or γ-secretase. Cell-based assays (transfected cell lines and primary mixed brain cultures) to determine the effect of compounds on overall β-APP metabolism (production, secretion, accumulation, or degradation of C-terminal catabolic products, and production of Aβ isoforms). Additional compound profiling is performed to measure the effects, if any, on overall cellular metabolism and on nonspecific protease inhibitory activity.

- *In vivo* Screen: Lead compounds are screened at a single dose and time point following oral administration utilizing transgenic mice or other small animal species such as guinea pig as a measure of *in-vivo* efficacy, i.e., lowering total Aβ concentrations in the brain. Pharmacokinetic profiling is done in parallel to establish absolute concentrations, brain:plasma ratios, and oral bioavailability. Selected compounds undergo a more rigorous dose response, time course, and chronic administration study; additional pharmacokinetic profiling; examination of plasma and CSF Aβ levels after administration (PO); and drug safety evaluation.

IN VIVO STUDIES

In vivo proof of principle experiments is based on three critical components. The first is a reliable assay to quantitative Aβ in biological samples; the second is an appropriate animal model that either mimics the disease or provides the appropriate endpoint for measuring the effect of compounds on Aβ levels; and the third is the requirement that the compound is orally bioavailable. The final criteria are based on the high probability of this being a long-term, chronically administered drug. Presently, no animal exists that shows all the features of human AD. The creation of models showing elevated levels of Aβ and cognitive deficits allow the investigation of important pathological events that can only be studied in a whole animal model.[8] As of this writing, clinical candidates are currently being carried forward towards the all important first in man studies. The primary goals for the early development are to establish the safety, tolerability, and pharmacokinetic and pharmacodynamic profile and to confirm the putative mechanism of action. Once this is accomplished, proof of principle studies can be initiated to validate the candidates ability to act as a disease modifying agent and to validate the "amyloid cascade" hypothesis of AD.[1–7]

REFERENCES

1. SELKOE, D.J. 1999. Translating cell biology into therapeutic advances in Alzheimer's disease. Nature **399**: A23–A31.
2. GREER, M. & H. MONTEBAN. 1999. A review of quality of life in Alzheimer's disease. Parts 1 and 2: Issues in assessing disease impact and drug effects. Pharmacoeconomics **15**: 641–644.
3. HAASS, C. & B. DE STROOPER. 1999. The presenilins in Alzheimer's disease: proteolysis holds the key. Science **286**: 916–919.
4. WOLFE, M.S., J. DE LOS ANGELES, D.D. MILLER *et al.* 1999. Are presenilins intramembrane-cleaving proteases? Implications for the molecular mechanism of Alzheimer's disease. Biochemistry **38**: 11223–11230.

5. WAGNER, S.L. & B. MUNOZ. 1999. Modulation of amyloid β-protein precursor processing as a means of retarding progression of Alzheimer's disease. JCI **104:** 1329–1332.
6. RACCHI, M. & S. GOVONI. 1999. Rationalizing a pharmacological intervention on the amyloid precursor protein metabolism. Trends Pharmacol. Sci. **20:** 418–423.
7. SINHA, S. & I. LIEBERBURG. 1999. Cellular mechanisms of beta-amyloid production and secretion. Proc. Natl. Acad. Sci. USA **96:** 11049–11053.
8. HSIAO, K., P. CHAPMAN, S. NILSEN et al. 1996. Correlative memory deficits, Abeta elevation, and amyloid plaques in transgenic mice. Science **274:** 99–102.

Prevention and Reduction of AD-type Pathology in PDAPP Mice Immunized with $A\beta_{1-42}$

DORA GAMES,[a] FREDERIQUE BARD, HENRY GRAJEDA,
TERRY GUIDO, KAREN KHAN, FERDIE SORIANO, NICKI VASQUEZ,
NANCY WEHNER, KELLY JOHNSON-WOOD, TED YEDNOCK,
PETER SEUBERT, AND DALE SCHENK

Elan Pharmaceuticals, South San Francisco, California 94080, USA

ABSTRACT: In AD certain brain structures contain a pathological density of $A\beta$ protein deposited into plaques. The effect of genetic mutations found in early onset AD patients was an overproduction of $A\beta_{42}$, strongly suggesting that overproduction of $A\beta_{42}$ is associated with AD. We hypothesized that an immunological response to $A\beta_{42}$ might alter its turnover and metabolism. Young PDAPP transgenic mice were immunized with $A\beta_{1-42}$, which essentially prevented amyloid deposition; astrocytosis was dramatically reduced and there was reduction in $A\beta$-induced inflammatory response as well. $A\beta_{1-42}$ immunization also appeared to arrest the progression of amyloidosis in older PDAPP mice. $A\beta$ immunization appears to increase clearance of amyloid plaques, and may therefore be a novel and effective approach for the treatment of AD.

INTRODUCTION

Alzheimer's disease (AD) is the major cause of dementia and leading cause of death in the elderly. Currently, the estimated U.S. prevalence of AD is 4.6 million patients. Its prevalence will undoubtedly grow with prolonged life expectancy, as the incidence of AD increases with age. The diagnosis of AD requires that, upon postmortem neuropathological exam, certain of the higher cortical and memory-related brain structures contain a pathological density of beta amyloid ($A\beta$) protein deposited into plaques.[1]

Several rare, very aggressive autosomal-dominant familial forms of AD, distinct from the more typical late-onset AD (LOAD), develop a form of the disease similar to LOAD neuropathologically and clinically, except that the age of onset occurs much earlier. Genetic studies in the past decade have uncovered three genes linked to these inherited forms of early onset AD (reviewed in Ref. 2). Perhaps not surprisingly, several different pathogenic mutations in the amyloid precursor protein (APP) gene were identified. Two unrelated genes, the presenilins (PS-1 and PS-2), were also sub-

[a]Address for correspondence: Dora Games, Elan Pharmaceuticals, 800 Gateway Blvd., So. San Francisco, CA 94080. Tel.: (650) 877-7635; fax: (650) 553-7196.
e-mail: dgames@elanpharma.com

sequently identified and dozens of mutations, also pathogenic, established. Careful analysis by several research groups, studying cell culture models, transgenic animals, and patient samples all reached a striking conclusion: every examined disease-linked mutation from the three different genes has a common effect in that $A\beta_{42}$ production is increased (e.g., see Ref. 3). This observation strongly argues that overproduction of $A\beta_{42}$ is associated with AD.

The mutations linked to early onset AD described above represent a fraction (<10%) of AD cases. However, other evidence exists that suggests alteration of $A\beta_{42}$ metabolism is seminal in LOAD. Apolipoprotein E (apoE) has been identified as a risk factor in AD.[4] The allelic variant apoE4 has been shown to increase risk for AD in a dose-dependent manner in numerous studies. In addition, apoE binds $A\beta$ *in vitro* and AD brains with an apoE4 genotype have heavier $A\beta_{42}$ plaque burdens.[5] Perhaps more striking is the observation that brains from a transgenic mouse model of AD show few amyloid deposits if the apoE gene is knocked-out.[6] Although the apoE4 allele is found in less than half of AD cases, $A\beta_{42}$ can be perturbed in other ways, irrespective of genotype. Cerebrospinal fluid (CSF) levels of $A\beta_{42}$ have been shown to be selectively lowered in cohorts of LOAD patients.[7] Given that brain deposition of $A\beta_{42}$ is also unquestionably increasing in these AD patients, this strongly suggests that an alteration of a normal clearance mechanism is happening in the disease. Therefore, a perturbation of $A\beta_{42}$ metabolism is closely linked to AD pathology.

It is also known that in other systemic amyloidogenic diseases, amyloid deposition is typically linked to either abnormal overproduction of the endogenous protein or expression of a genetic variant resulting in production of a particularly amyloidogenic form of the protein (e.g., transthyretin, cystatin C, gelsolin). It has been possible, in certain of these conditions, to show that limiting the production of the amyloidogenic protein leads to its clearance and clinical improvement. In some instances the primary source of production of the amyloidogenic material can be corrected by transplantation. For example, in cases of familial amyloid polyneuropathy due to transthyretin mutation, liver transplantation stops the neurological deterioration and avoids the fatal outcome of the disease by replacing the primary source of synthesis of the mutated amyloidogenic protein. The amyloid deposits regress, and peripheral nerve function frequently improves with this procedure.[8]

The structural and histological similarities of the protein involved in the systemic amyloidoses and AD suggest that a strategy to remove or reduce the pathological amyloid burden brain is a reasonable approach to therapy.

In the following studies we explore a novel therapeutic approach to reduce amyloid burden. We hypothesized that an immunological response to beta amyloid might alter its turnover and metabolism through humoral or cellular responses.

The PDAPP mouse expresses a mutant version of the human amyloid precursor protein (APP) gene (valine at position 717 is mutated to phenylalanine) that is associated with an early-onset and aggressive form of AD inherited in affected families.[9] A platelet-derived growth factor promoter drives the minigene that results in high levels of brain expression of the mutant APP that exceeds the level of the endogenous mouse version of APP by about 4–6 fold. This results in the overproduction of $A\beta$ that deposits plaques in a fashion similar to that found in human AD brains. Importantly, several other of the consequent neurodegenerative changes that occur in AD also develop in PDAPP brains, including the formation of neuritic plaques, astrocytosis, and microgliosis.

To determine whether such an Aβ-specific immune response could potentially prevent or reduce amyloid deposition and the consequential brain pathologies, a group of young, PDAPP transgenic mice were immunized with the specific form of Aβ peptide that initially deposits in amyloid plaques, the 42 amino acid-long Aβ peptide ($A\beta_{1-42}$). We reasoned that an antiamyloid immune response could block the deposition of Aβ or increase its clearance and thus reduce the plaque burden as well as the associated degenerative pathologies in these mice.

In a prophylactic paradigm using young mice with very little or no amyloid deposits, groups of six-week-old, female heterozygous PDAPP transgenic mice were immunized with either 100 μg of amyloid beta-protein (AN1792, $n = 9$), 100 μg of peptides derived from the amyloid plaque-associated protein serum amyloid P component (SAPP; $n = 5$) or phosphate-buffered saline (PBS; $n = 5$). A fourth group received no treatment ($n = 10$). Antigens were emulsified with Freund's adjuvant and delivered by intraperitoneal immunization at a two-week interval for the first two doses and then monthly thereafter for a total of eleven immunizations given over an eleven-month period. At 13 months of age, brains were removed and examined for pathological changes. Computer-assisted quantitative image analysis was performed on immunohistochemically processed brain sections to measure the extent to which the hippocampus was occupied by immunoreactive amyloid deposits (amyloid burden). In addition, the magnitude of dystrophic neuronal pathology associated with neuritic plaques (neuritic dystrophy) and the extent of reactive astrocytosis were determined.

RESULTS

Amyloid Burden

Amyloid deposition was essentially prevented by Aβ immunization. Seven of nine mice immunized with $A\beta_{1-42}$ had no detectable amyloid deposits in their brains. One mouse from this treatment group had a greatly reduced and altered pattern of amyloid deposition, confined to the hippocampus. A single isolated plaque was seen in the final mouse. Quantitative image analyses of the amyloid burden in the hippocampus verified the dramatic reduction achieved in the $A\beta_{1-42}$-treated animals (FIG. 1). The median values of the amyloid burden for the PBS group (2.22%), and for the untreated control group (2.65%) were significantly greater ($p = 0.0005$) than for those immunized with $A\beta_{1-42}$ (0.00%). In contrast, the median value for the SAPP group was 5.74%. Brain tissue from the untreated, control mice contained numerous Aβ amyloid deposits visualized with the Aβ-specific monoclonal antibody 3D6 in the hippocampus, as well as in the retrosplenial cortex. A similar pattern of amyloid deposition was also seen in mice immunized with SAP peptides or PBS. In addition, there was a characteristic involvement of subregions of the brain classically seen in AD, such as the outer molecular layer of the hippocampal dentate gyrus in all three of these control groups.

Neuritic Dystrophy

Brains of those $A\beta_{1-42}$-treated mice that lacked Aβ deposits were also devoid of the dystrophic neurites which compose the neuritic plaques that are typically visual-

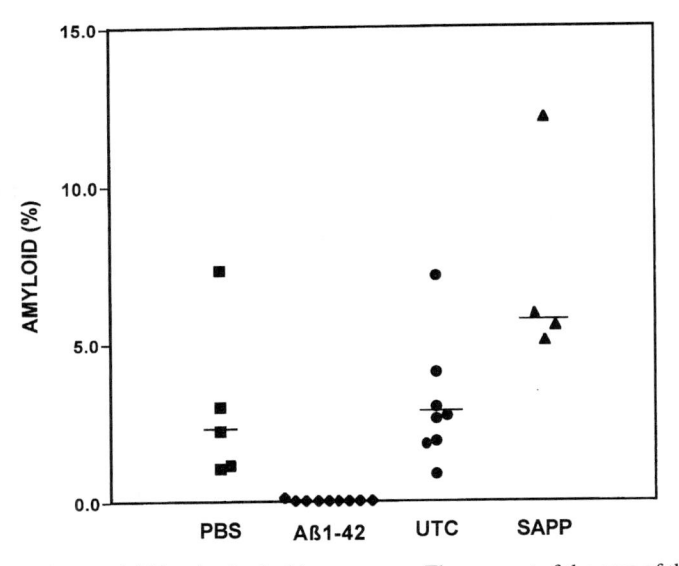

FIGURE 1. Amyloid burden in the hippocampus. The percent of the area of the hippocampal region occupied by amyloid plaques, defined by reactivity with the Aβ-specific mAb 3D6, was determined by computer-assisted quantitative image analysis of immunoreacted brain sections. The values for individual mice are shown sorted by treatment group. The *horizontal line* for each grouping indicates the median value of the distribution. Median values expressed as percentages, are as follows: PBS-immunized (PBS), 2.22; $A\beta_{1-42}$-immunized ($A\beta_{1-42}$), 0.00; untreated control (UTC), 2.65; serum amyloid P component peptide-immunized (SAPP), 5.74. The $A\beta_{1-42}$-treated group has significantly less amyloid than any of the other three groups ($p = 0.001$), which are not significantly different from each other ($p > 0.05$).

ized with the human APP-specific monoclonal antibody 8E5. A small number of dystrophic neurites were present in one $A\beta_{1-42}$-treated mouse, and a single cluster of dystrophic neurites was found in a second treated mouse. Brains from SAPP-injected and the two control groups (PBS-injected and untreated mice) all had numerous neuritic plaques. Quantitative image analyses of the hippocampus, shown in FIGURE 2, demonstrated the virtual elimination of dystrophic neurites in $A\beta_{1-42}$-treated mice (median 0.00%) compared to the PBS recipients (median 0.28%, $p = 0.0005$).

Astrocytosis

Astrocytosis, which is another hallmark of plaque-associated damage, was dramatically reduced in the brains of the entire $A\beta_{1-42}$-injected group. Brains from mice in all other groups contained abundant and clustered glial fibrillary acidic protein (GFAP)-positive astrocytes, a finding typical of Aβ plaque-associated gliosis. A subset of the GFAP-reacted sections were counter-stained with thioflavin S to visualize the Aβ deposits. The GFAP-positive astrocytes colocalized with Aβ plaques in animals receiving SAPP, PBS or no treatment. No such association was found in those $A\beta_{1-42}$-treated mice lacking amyloid plaques, while minimal plaque-

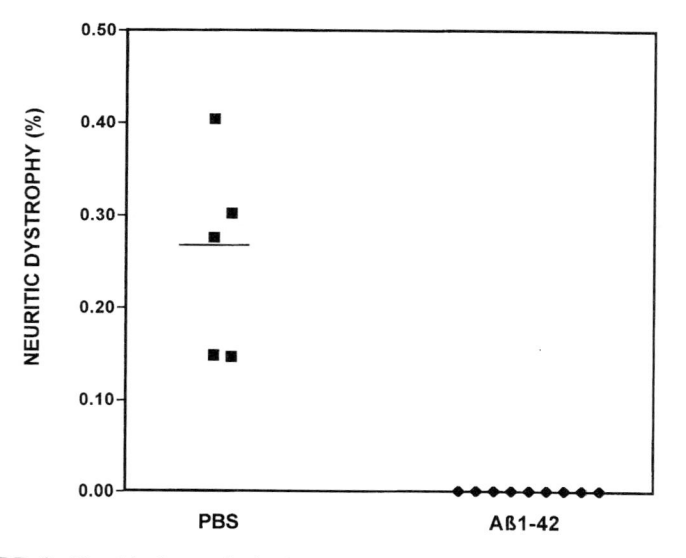

FIGURE 2. Neuritic dystrophy in the hippocampus. The percent of the area of the hippocampal region occupied by dystrophic neurites, defined by their reactivity with the human APP-specific mAb 8E5, was determined by quantitative computer-assisted image analysis of immunoreacted brain sections. The values for individual mice are shown for the $A\beta_{1-42}$-treated group and the PBS-treated control group. The *horizontal line* for each grouping indicates the median value of the distribution. Median values (%) for the PBS- and $A\beta_{1-42}$-treated groups were 0.28 and 0.00, respectively. The difference between groups was significant ($p = 0.0005$).

associated gliosis was identified in the mouse with a greatly reduce amyloid burden from this same group. Again the results of image analyses, shown in FIGURE 3 for the retrosplenial cortex, verified that the reduction in astrocytosis was significant with a median value of 1.55% for those treated with $A\beta_{1-42}$ versus median values greater than 6% for groups immunized with SAP peptides, PBS or unimmunized ($p = 0.0017$).

Microgliosis

Sections of the mouse brains were reacted with a monoclonal antibody specific for MAC-1, a cell surface integrin protein. The resident MAC-1-reactive cell type in the brain is likely to be microglia based on its monocytic lineage and phenotypic morphology. Plaque-associated MAC-1 labeling was lower in the brains of mice treated with $A\beta_{1-42}$ compared to the PBS control group, a finding consistent with the lack of an $A\beta$-induced inflammatory response.

Antibody Responses

Eight of the nine mice immunized with $A\beta_{1-42}$ developed high antibody titers (greater than 10,000) which were maintained throughout the series of injections. The ninth mouse had a lower titer of approximately 1000. Mice immunized with SAPP

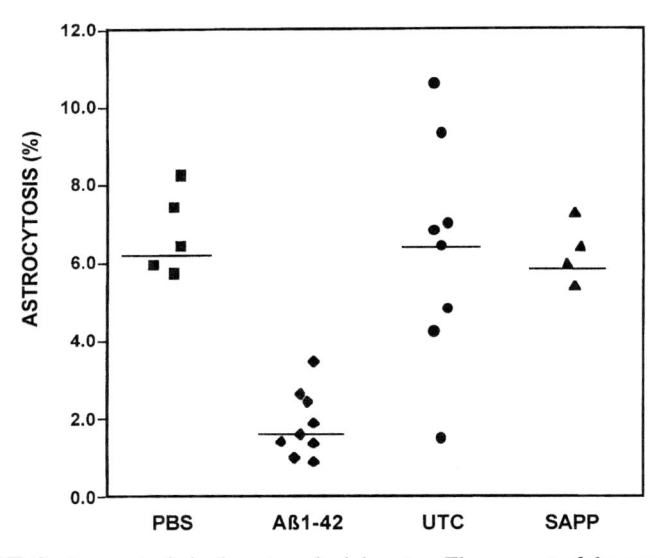

FIGURE 3. Astrocytosis in the retrosplenial cortex. The percent of the area of the cortical region occupied by glial fibrillary acidic protein (GFAP)-positive astrocytes was determined by quantitative computer-assisted image analysis of immunoreacted brain sections. The values for individual mice are shown sorted by treatment group and median group values are indicated by *horizontal lines*. Median percent values for the various groups were as follows: PBS-immunized (PBS), 6.43; $A\beta_{1-42}$-immunized ($A\beta_{1-42}$), 1.56; untreated controls (UTC), 6.625; serum amyloid P component peptides (SAPP), 6.15. The $A\beta_{1-42}$-treated group has significantly less astrocytosis than the other groups ($p = 0.0017$), which are not significantly different from each other.

had much lower titers against SAP ranging from 1000 to 10,000 with the exception of one mouse with a titer greater than 10,000.

Antibody titers to SAP and $A\beta_{1-42}$ were determined for mice that received PBS with adjuvant for a subset of the bleeds, those sera collected at six, ten, and twelve months. The SAP-specific response was negligible at these time points with all titers less than 300. Likewise, the $A\beta_{1-42}$-specific response was also negligible.

The virtual absence of $A\beta$ plaques in the brains of the $A\beta_{1-42}$-treated-mice indicates that the deposition of amyloid was extremely reduced or entirely eliminated. These observations suggest that treatment with $A\beta_{1-42}$ prevented the deposition of $A\beta$ or accelerated its clearance from brain tissue. In addition, the absence of the subsequent degenerative neuronal and reactive inflammatory changes that normally occur with $A\beta$ amyloidosis suggests that the $A\beta_{1-42}$-treated mice never developed the neurodegenerative lesions that typify the progression of AD.

Immunization with SAPP had no impact on either the extent or histopathological appearance of amyloid plaques showing that prevention or clearance of amyloid deposition is not a general response to immunization with plaque-associated proteins.

To evaluate the efficacy of this approach in a setting closer to that anticipated for the clinical treatment of AD, a second study was designed to begin the $A\beta$ immunizations when amyloid plaques are already present in the brains of the PDAPP mice and during a period when the rate of amyloid deposition accelerates to achieve levels comparable to that of established AD. A central question addressed in this study was whether immunization with Aβ could arrest the progression of amyloidosis under these conditions.

For this study, approximately eleven-month-old PDAPP transgenic mice ($n = 24$) were immunized repeatedly with $Aβ_{1-42}$ combined with adjuvant. As a negative control, a parallel group of 24 transgenic littermates was immunized with PBS combined with adjuvant. One-half of each group was sacrificed at 15 months of age, after four months of treatment totaling six immunizations, and the remaining animals were sacrificed at 18 months of age, following seven months of treatment and a total of nine immunizations. Groups of untreated PDAPP mice, aged 12, 15, and 18 months, were also included for certain of the comparisons to the immunized groups. At these time points, brains were removed to quantitatively assess, by immunohistochemical analysis, the amyloid burden, neuritic dystrophy, astrocytosis, and microgliosis.

RESULTS

$Aβ_{1-42}$ Effects on Amyloid Burden

Quantitative image analysis results of $Aβ_{1-42}$ treatment on cortical amyloid burden are shown in FIGURE 4. The median value of cortical amyloid burden was 0.28% in a group of untreated 12-month-old PDAPP mice, representative of the plaque load in experimental mice at the study's initiation. At 18 months, the amyloid burden increased over 17-fold to 4.87% in PBS-treated mice, while $Aβ_{1-42}$-treated mice had a greatly reduced amyloid burden of only 0.01%, notably less than the 12-month untreated and both 15- and 18-month PBS-treated groups. The amyloid burden was significantly reduced in the $Aβ_{1-42}$ at both 15 (96% reduction; $p = 0.003$) and 18 (>99% reduction; $p = 0.0002$) months.

Typically, cortical amyloid deposition in PDAPP mice initiates in the frontal and retrosplenial cortices (RSC) and progresses in a ventral-lateral direction to involve the temporal and entorhinal cortices (EC). Little or no amyloid was found in the EC of 12-month-old mice, the approximate age at which $Aβ_{1-42}$ was first administered. After 4 months of treatment, amyloid deposition was greatly diminished in the RSC, and the progressive involvement of the EC was entirely eliminated by $Aβ_{1-42}$ treatment. The latter observation showed that $Aβ_{1-42}$ completely halted the progression of amyloid that would normally invade the temporal and ventral cortices, as well as arrested or possibly reversed deposition in the RSC.

$Aβ_{1-42}$-associated Cellular and Morphological Changes

In addition to the observation that amyloid deposition was profoundly reduced by $Aβ_{1-42}$, a population of Aβ-positive cells was found in brain regions that typically deposit amyloid. Remarkably, in several brains from the $Aβ_{1-42}$ group, very little or no extracellular cortical amyloid plaques were found. Most of the Aβ immunoreactivity appeared to be contained within cells with large lobular or clumped soma. Phenotypically, these cells resembled activated microglia or monocytes, were immunoreactive with antibodies recognizing ligands expressed by activated monocytes

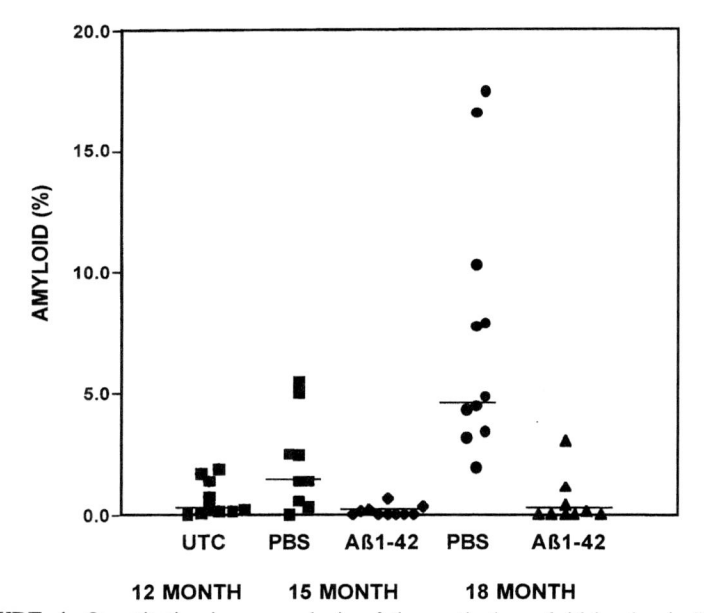

FIGURE 4. Quantitative image analysis of the cortical amyloid burden in PBS- and $A\beta_{1-42}$-treated mice. Amyloid deposition was significantly reduced in the $A\beta_{1-42}$ group compared to the PBS controls at both 15 ($p = 0.003$) and 18 ($p = 0.00002$) months of age. The median value of the amyloid burden for each group is shown by the *horizontal line* on the scatterplot. The median value of the $A\beta_{1-42}$ group compared to the PBS group at 15 and 18 months of age was 0.05% vs. 1.39% and 0.01% vs. 4.87%, respectively. The amyloid burden in a 12-month untreated group, representative of that in the experimental group at the study's initiation, was 0.28%.

and microglia (MHC II and CD11b), and were occasionally associated with the wall or lumen of blood vessels. Comparison of near-adjacent sections labeled with $A\beta$ and MHC II-specific antibodies revealed that similar patterns of cells were recognized by both classes of antibodies. Detailed examination of the $A\beta_{1-42}$-treated brains revealed that the MHC II-positive cells were restricted to the vicinity of the limited amyloid remaining in these animals. Confocal analysis of double-labeled sections confirmed that many MHC II-positive cells contained $A\beta$. Under the fixation conditions employed, the cells were not immunoreactive with antibodies that recognize T cell (CD3, CD3e) or B cell (CD45RA, CD45RB) ligands or leukocyte common antigen (CD45), but were reactive with an antibody recognizing leukosialin (CD43), which cross-reacts with monocytes. No such cells were found in any of the PBS-treated mice.

PDAPP mice invariably develop heavy amyloid deposition in the outer molecular layer of the hippocampal dentate gyrus. The deposition forms a distinct streak within the perforant pathway, consisting of both diffuse and compacted amyloid. The diffuse amyloid was nearly undetectable in the immunized mice. Instead, a number of unusual punctate 3D6-immunoreactive amyloid-positive structures were present, several of which appeared to be amyloid-containing cells.

To determine whether the Aβ-specific antibodies detected in the sera of $Aβ_{1-42}$-treated mice were also associated with deposited brain amyloid, a subset of sections from the $Aβ_{1-42}$- and PBS-treated mice were reacted with an antibody specific for mouse IgG. In contrast to the PBS group, Aβ plaques in $Aβ_{1-42}$-treated brains were coated with endogenous IgG. The difference between the two groups was seen in both the 15- and 18-month groups. Particularly striking was the lack of labeling in the PBS group, despite the presence of a heavy amyloid burden in these mice.

Effects on Neurodegenerative and Gliotic Pathology

Neuritic plaque burden was significantly reduced in the frontal cortex of $Aβ_{1-42}$-treated mice compared to the PBS group at both 15 (84%; $p = 0.03$) and 18 (55%; $p = 0.01$) months of age (FIG. 5). The median value of the neuritic plaque burden increased from 0.32% to 0.49% in the PBS group between 15 and 18 months of age. This contrasted with the greatly reduced development of neuritic plaques in the $Aβ_{1-42}$ group, with neuritic plaque burden median values of 0.05% and 0.22%, at the 15- and 18-month groups, respectively.

Reactive astrocytosis was also significantly reduced in the RSC of $Aβ_{1-42}$-treated mice when compared to the PBS group at both 15 (56%; $p = 0.011$) and 18 (39%; $p = 0.028$) months of age (FIG. 6). Median values of percent astrocytosis in the PBS

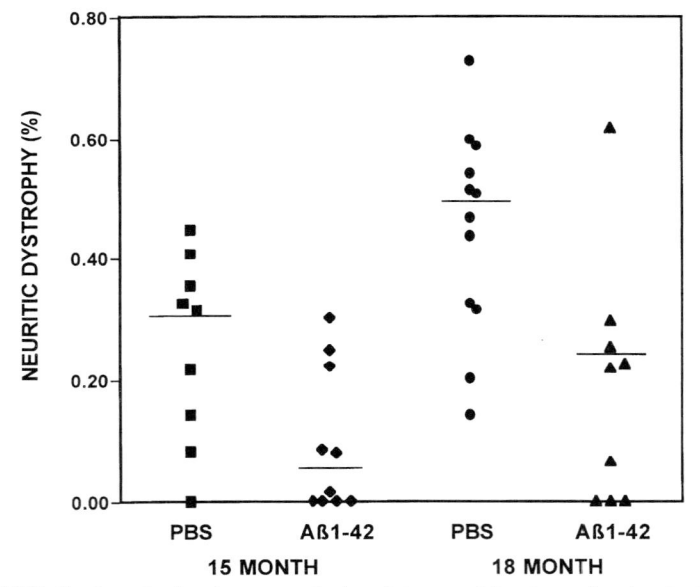

FIGURE 5. Quantitative image analysis of the neuritic plaque burden in PBS- and $Aβ_{1-42}$-treated mice. The percent of the frontal cortex occupied by dystrophic neurites, which compose neuritic plaques, was significantly reduced by $Aβ_{1-42}$ treatment at both 15 ($p = 0.03$) and 18 ($p = 0.01$) months of age. The median value of the neuritic plaque burden for each group is shown by the *horizontal line* on the scatterplot. The median value of the $Aβ_{1-42}$ group compared to the PBS group at 15 and 18 months of age was 0.05% vs. 0.32% and 0.22% vs. 0.49%, respectively.

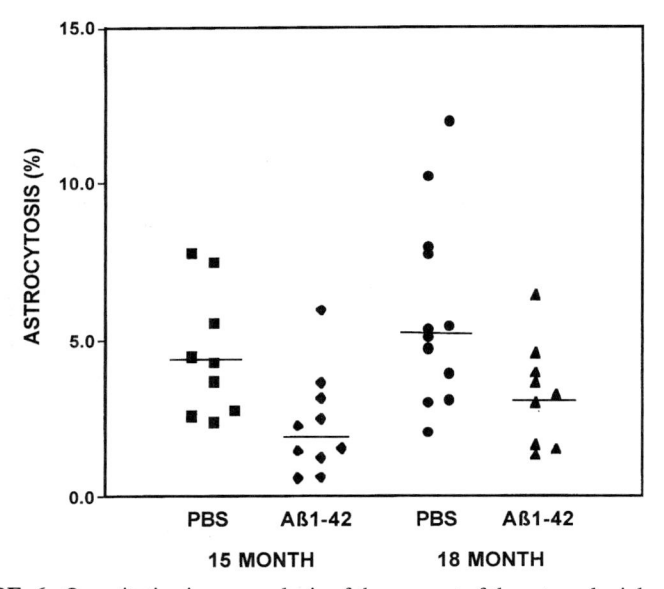

FIGURE 6. Quantitative image analysis of the percent of the retrosplenial cortex occupied by astrocytosis in PBS- and $A\beta_{1-42}$-treated mice. The percent astrocytosis was significantly reduced by $A\beta_{1-42}$ treatment at both 15 ($p = 0.011$) and 18 months ($p = 0.028$) of age. The median value of the percent astrocytosis for each group is shown by the *horizontal line* on the scatterplot. The median value of the $A\beta_{1-42}$ group compared to the PBS group at 15 and 18 months of age was 1.89% vs. 4.26% and 0.20% vs. 5.21%, respectively.

group increased between 15 and 18 months from 4.29% to 5.21%. $A\beta_{1-42}$ suppressed the development of astrocytosis at both time points to 1.89% and 3.2%, respectively.

DISCUSSION AND CONCLUSION

$A\beta_{1-42}$ immunization of young PDAPP mice virtually abolished amyloid plaque formation, while immunization of older, plaque-bearing animals was efficacious in slowing and preventing progressive amyloid deposition and retarding consequential neuropathological changes in the aged brain. In both experiments, immunization with $A\beta_{1-42}$ essentially halted amyloid development in structures that would normally succumb to amyloidosis, a clear example being the complete prevention of amyloid deposition in the entorhinal cortex.

Evidence was seen for what appears to be active, cellular-mediated removal of amyloid in plaque-bearing brain regions in immunized mice. The impression that cells were clearing amyloid plaques was supported by confocal analysis of Aβ-containing microglia. In addition, much of the remaining amyloid assumed a distinct and unusual punctate appearance that lacked diffuse amyloid components and overlapped with the distribution of microglia. Absolute quantification of the plaque-laden cortical area showed no increase in amyloid load. In fact, the involved area at 15 and 18 months of $A\beta_{1-42}$-treated animals tended to be less than the 12-month value of the untreated controls.

The decoration of plaques in $A\beta_{1-42}$-treated animals with endogenous IgGs suggests a mechanism by which monocytic cells could be recruited into the CNS to clear amyloid plaques. The association of $A\beta$- and MHC II-positive cells with blood vessels further supports the existence of an active trafficking mechanism.

The lower extent of neuritic plaque formation and astrogliosis in $A\beta_{1-42}$-treated animals is another indication of a favorable outcome associated with $A\beta$ immunization. A strong implication from these observations is that $A\beta$ immunization increases clearance of amyloid plaques from the brain, and significantly prevents a host of consequential pathologies. The overall positive effects of this treatment on neuropathology suggest that an immune-mediated approach to limiting amyloidosis may be a novel, effective therapeutic approach for the treatment of AD.

REFERENCES

1. MCKHANN, G., D. DRACHMAN, M. FOLSTEIN et al. 1984. Clinical diagnosis of Alzheimer's disease: report of the NINCDS-ADRDA Work Group under the auspices of the Department of Health and Human Services Task Force on Alzheimer's Disease. Neurology **34:** 939–944.
2. SELKOE, D.J. 1996. Cell biology of the β-amyloid precursor protein and the genetics of Alzheimer's disease. Cold Spring Harbor Symp. Quant. Biol. **61:** 587–596.
3. SCHEUNER, D., C. ECKMAN, M. JENSEN et al. 1996. Secreted amyloid β-protein similar to that in the senile plaques of Alzheimer's disease is increased in vivo by the presenilin 1 and 2 and APP mutations linked to familial Alzheimer's disease. Nat. Med. **2:** 864–870.
4. STRITTMATTER, W.J., A.M. SAUNDERS, D. SCHMECHEL et al. 1993. Apolipoprotein E: high avidity binding to β-amyloid and increased frequency of type 4 allele in late-onset familial Alzheimer's disease. Proc. Natl. Acad. Sci. USA **90:** 1977–1981.
5. REBECK, G.W., J.S. REITER, D.K. STRICKLAND & B.T. HYMAN. 1997. Apolipoprotein E in sporadic Alzheimer's disease: allelic variation and receptor interactions. Neuron **11:** 575–580.
6. BALES, K.B., T. VERINA, R.C. DODEL et al. Lack of apolipoprotein E dramatically reduces amyloid β-peptide deposition. Nat. Genet. **17:** 263–264.
7. GALASKO, D., L. CHANG, R. MOTTER et al. 1998. High cerebrospinal fluid tau and low amyloid β 42 levels in the clinical diagnosis of Alzheimer's disease and relation to apolipoprotein E genotype. Arch. Neurol. **55:** 937–945.
8. BERGETHON, P.R., T.D. SABIN, D. LEWIS et al. 1996. Improvement in the polyneuropathy associated with familial amyloid polyneuropathy after liver transplantation. Neurology **47:** 944–951.
9. GAMES, D., D. ADAMS, R. ALESSANDRINI et al. 1995. Alzheimer-type neuropathology in transgenic mcie overexpressing V717F beta-amyoid precursor protein. Nature (London) **373:** 523–527.

Treatment with the Selective Muscarinic Agonist Talsaclidine Decreases Cerebrospinal Fluid Levels of Total Amyloid β-Peptide in Patients with Alzheimer's Disease

C. HOCK,[a,h] A. MADDALENA,[a] I. HEUSER,[b] D. NABER,[c] W. OERTEL,[d]
H. VON DER KAMMER,[e] M. WIENRICH,[f] A. RASCHIG,[f] M. DENG,[g]
J.H. GROWDON,[g] AND R.M. NITSCH[a]

[a]*Department of Psychiatry Research, University of Zürich, Switzerland*

[b]*Central Institute of Mental Health, Mannheim, Germany*

[c]*Department of Psychiatry, University of Hamburg, Hamburg, Germany*

[d]*Department of Neurology, University of Marburg, Marburg, Germany*

[e]*Center for Molecular Neurobiology, University of Hamburg, Hamburg, Germany*

[f]*Boehringer Ingelheim Co., Germany, and*

[g]*Department of Neurology, Massachusetts General Hospital,
Boston, Massachusetts, USA*

ABSTRACT: Brain amyloid load in Alzheimer's disease (AD) is, at least in genetic forms, associated with overproduction of amyloid β-peptides (Aβ). Thus, lowering Aβ production is a central therapeutic target in AD and may be achieved by modulating such key enzymes of amyloid precursor protein (APP) processing as β-, γ-, and α-secretase activities. Talsaclidine is a selective muscarinic M1 agonist that stimulates the nonamyloidogenic α-secretase pathway in model systems. Talsaclidine was administered double-blind, placebo-controlled, and randomized to 24 AD patients and cerebrospinal fluid (CSF) levels of total Aβ were quantitated before and after 4 weeks of drug treatment. We observed that talsaclidine decreases CSF levels of Aβ significantly over time within the treatment group ($n = 20$) by a median of 16% as well as compared to placebo ($n = 4$) by a median of 27%. We conclude that treatment with selective M1 agonists may reduce Aβ production and may thus be further evaluated as a potential amyloid-lowering therapy of AD.

INTRODUCTION

Brain amyloid deposits in Alzheimer's disease (AD) are composed of aggregated amyloid β-peptides (Aβ) derived from proteolytic cleavage of the amyloid precursor protein (APP).[1] Aβ comprises a group of approximately 4-kD peptides, the predom-

[h]Address for correspondence: Dr. Christoph Hock, Department of Psychiatry Research, University of Zürich, Lenggstrasse 31, CH-8029 Zürich 8, Switzerland. Tel.: +41-1-384-2271; fax: +41-1-384-2275.

e-mail: chock@bli.unizh.ch

inant forms of which, $A\beta_{40}$ and $A\beta_{42}$, are 40 and 42 amino acid residues in length.[2,3] $A\beta_{40}$ and $A\beta_{42}$ are products of at least two protease activities termed β- and γ-secretase that cleave at the N- and C-termini, respectively, of the $A\beta$ domain within APP.[1] In contrast, activation of α-secretase cleaves APP within the $A\beta$ domain and results in the production of nonamyloidogenic fragments including the nontoxic and probably neurotrophic secreted APP (APPsα). Theoretically, brain amyloid load may be lowered by reduction of $A\beta$ production, aggregation, or toxicity, or by removing amyloid from brain. Lowering $A\beta$ production may be achieved by either decreasing β- or γ-secretase, and, alternatively, by increasing α-secretase activities. APP processing via the nonamyloidogenic α-secretase pathway can be stimulated by cell surface receptors including muscarinic M1, serotonergic 5-HT 2_b and 2_c, and metabotropic glutamate mGlu R1α receptors, and several neuropeptides.[4–6] Talsaclidine is a selective muscarinic M1 agonist.[7,8] Talsaclidine increased the release of APPs and decreased levels of total $A\beta$ in such model systems as transfected HEK295 cells, transfected human U373 astrocytoma cells, and neuroblastoma cells as well as in hippocampal slices from rat brain. We administered talsaclidine as well as placebo to 24 patients with a clinical diagnosis of probable AD and assayed for cerebrospinal fluid (CSF) levels of total $A\beta$ before and after 4 weeks of drug treatment. We hypothesized that treatment with talsaclidine decreases CSF levels of $A\beta$.

SUBJECTS AND METHODS

Subjects

Diagnosis of probable AD was made according to the National Institute of Neurological and Communicative Disorders and Stroke–Alzheimer's Disease and Related Disorders Association (NINCDS-ADRDA) criteria.[9] All patients were community-dwelling, and were referred to the psychogeriatric research ward from general practitoners, neurologists, and psychiatrists for diagnostic purposes and screening for clinical trials. Patients were carefully examined and received a thorough clinical work-up. Psychometric testing included the Mini Mental State (MMS)[10] as a global screening instrument for dementia. There were 24 participants in the study. Among the inclusion criteria was age <85, MMS between 12 and 26, and absence of relevant systemic disorders.

Medication

Talsaclidine was given t.i.d in a constant dosage to the patients in four panels. Panel 1: 2.5/5 mg (corresponds to talsaclidine fumarate 1.5/2.9 mg), Panel 2: 10/20 mg (5.9/11.8 mg), Panel 3: 40/60 mg (23.5/35.3 mg), Panel 4: 80 mg (b.i.d./t.i.d.) (48.0 mg) within a multicenter trial. The ability of talsaclidine to elicit muscarinic responses was investigated in various *in vitro* and *in vivo* models.[7]

Protocol

AD patients were free of psychotropic medication prior to treatment with talsaclidine, except for hypnotics such as oxazepam, zolpidem, zopiclone, and

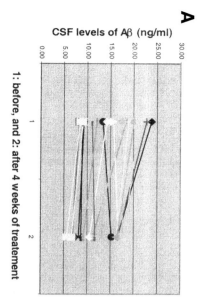

A

CSF levels of Aβ (ng/ml)

1: before, and 2: after 4 weeks of treatment

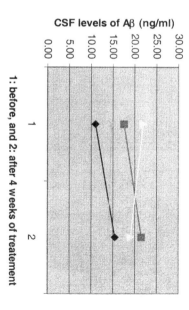

B

CSF levels of Aβ (ng/ml)

1: before, and 2: after 4 weeks of treatement

FIGURE 1. CSF levels of Aβ during treatment with talsaclidine. CSF levels of Aβ **(a)** decrease during treatment with talsaclidine but **(b)** do not change during treatment with placebo.

chloral hydrate when patients were pretreated with such substances. Informed consent was taken from each patient and their caregivers before the investigation. The study was approved by the local ethics committee. All procedures were in accordance with the Helsinki Declaration of 1975, as revised in 1983. Within one week of dementia testing, and before treatment with talsaclidine, CSF was obtained by lumbar puncture according to conventional techniques. CSF samples were frozen on dry ice immediately upon withdrawal at the bedside in 0.5-ml aliquots and stored at −85°C until biochemical analyses. A second lumbar puncture was performed after four weeks of treatment with talsaclidine, and the CSF obtained was processed identically to the first lumbar puncture. Total Aβ was measured by ELISA using the mAb 6E10 and 22c4.

STATISTICAL ANALYSES

Statistical analyses of data were done by two-tailed t-tests for dependent and as independent samples.

RESULTS

CSF levels of Aβ at baseline ranged from 8.19 to 23.89 ng/ml ($n = 24$). Mean Aβ concentrations were 15.05 ± 4.93 ng/ml (mean ± SD). After four weeks of treatment with talsaclidine, the mean CSF levels of Aβ decreased from 14.79 ± 5.06 ng/ml to 12.41 ± 4.04 ng/ml ($n = 20$) ($p <0.01$, paired samples t-test) (FIG. 1a). We observed no change in CSF levels of Aβ during treatment with placebo (16.32 ± 4.63 to 17.50 ± 3.43 ng/ml, $n = 4$) (FIG. 1b).

We observed that talsaclidine decreases CSF levels of Aβ significantly over time within the treatment group ($n = 20$) by a median of 16% ($p <0.01$, paired samples t-test) as well as compared to placebo ($n = 4$) by a median of 27% ($p <0.01$, independent samples t-test).

DISCUSSION

We demonstrate here that treatment with the selective muscarinic M1 agonist talsaclidine, in contrast to placebo, lowered CSF levels of total Aβ in patients with AD. This finding extends results from cell culture and brain slice models where stimulation of M1 receptors was shown to stimulate nonamyloidogenic APP processing.[4–6] Thus, treatment with M1 agonists may constitute a reasonable therapeutic strategy to lower brain amyloid load in humans.

Activation of the α-secretase pathway by cholinergic agents seems to depend on selectivity for muscarinic receptor subtypes. Stimulation of M2 receptors does not affect APP processing,[4] or blocks the M1 effect when stimulated simultaneously.[11]

Although CSF levels of Aβ may reflect to some extent the brain amyloid burden, several confounding factors have to be considered. These include CSF flow dynamics and exchange rates, further processing and modification of APP derivatives in CSF, and nonneuronal sources of APP derivatives.

$A\beta_{42}$ peptide is the major component of amyloid in plaques, while $A\beta_{40}$ is the major amyloid form in the cerebral microvasculature.[12] However, the majority of $A\beta$ in the CSF is $A\beta_{40}$, whereas $A\beta_{42}$ peptides make up less than 10%. CSF levels of total $A\beta$ and $A\beta_{40}$ were reported to be normal in AD as compared to controls[13–15] or slightly decreased.[16] CSF levels of $A\beta_{42(43)}$ were shown to be decreased in AD as compared to control groups,[17–21] whereas ratios of $A\beta_{42}/A\beta_{40}$ are significantly increased in genetic cases of AD.[22,23] Recently, Almkvist *et al.*[24] reported, that CSF levels of $A\beta_{42}$ may increase preclinically in nonaffected PS1 H163T mutation carriers, along with a subsequent decline over time, ending up finally in decreased levels of soluble $A\beta_{42}$ peptides in affected carriers. Thus, $A\beta_{42}$ may increase preclinically in CSF, and then decrease over time. A longitudinal study on CSF levels of $A\beta$ peptides reported by Kanai *et al.*[25] showed an increase of the $A\beta_{40}/A\beta_{42(43)}$ ratio at stages that may correspond to the conversion phase of mild cognitive impairment to clinically obvious AD, suggesting that CSF levels of $A\beta_{42(43)}$ may decrease and $A\beta_{40}/A\beta_{42(43)}$ ratios may increase at early stages in sporadic AD. Thus, CSF levels of $A\beta$ peptides are dependent on the stage of the disease and on the presence of genetic risk factors.

In addition to the potential value as markers of disease risk or progression, CSF levels of $A\beta$ may be used as a surrogate markers to monitor effects of specific therapies aimed to reduce brain amyloid deposition by lowering $A\beta$ production. Such therapies may be realized by either decreasing β- or γ-secretase, or by increasing α-secretase activities. Shifting APP processing to the nonamyloidogenic pathways should be accompanied by increased levels of APPsα and decreased levels of $A\beta$ peptides in the brain, and subsequently, in CSF. The present study indicates that CSF levels of total $A\beta$ change under a therapy designed to alter APP processing. Therefore, monitoring CSF levels of $A\beta$ may be a useful tool to evaluate new amyloid-lowering therapeutic strategies based on altering secretase activities. Possibly, this applies also for other therapeutic strategies such as clearing amyloid from brain, e.g., by means of immunization against $A\beta$ peptides.[26] Likely, such therapies will lead to increased CSF levels of $A\beta$ peptides.

In summary, treatment with the selective M1 agonist talsaclidine reduced CSF levels of total $A\beta$ in patients with AD. We conclude that monitoring CSF levels of $A\beta$ may constitute a valuable to tool to evaluate the mechanism of action of amyloid-lowering drugs in patients with AD.

ACKNOWLEDGMENTS

The study protocol was added to a multicenter trial sponsored by Boehringer Ingelheim Pharma, Germany. Among the centers were dementia research units at the Universities of Basel, Mannheim, Hamburg, Munich, Marburg, and Tübingen, as well as dementia care centers in Hannover, St.Malo, and Draveil.

REFERENCES

1. PRICE, D.L., R.E. TANZI, D.R. BORCHELT & S.S. SISODIA. 1998. Alzheimer's disease: genetic studies and transgenic models. Annu. Rev. Genet. **32:** 461–493.

2. SHOJI, M., T.E. GOLDE, J. GHISO *et al.* 1992. Production of the Alzheimer amyloid β-protein by normal proteolytic processing. Science **258:** 126–129.

3. VIGO-PELFREY, C., D. LEE, P. KEIM *et al.* 1993. Characterization of amyloid peptide from human cerebrospinal fluid. J. Neurochem. **61:** 1965–1968.

4. NITSCH, R.M., B.E. SLACK, R.J. WURTMAN & J.H. GROWDON. 1992. Release of Alzheimer amyloid precursor derivatives stimulated by activation of muscarinic acetylcholine receptors. Science **258:** 304–310.

5. NITSCH, R.M. & J.H. GROWDON. 1994. Role of neurotransmission in the regulation of amyloid β-protein precursor processing. Biochem. Pharmacol. **47:** 1275–1284.

6. NITSCH, R.M., C. KIM & J.H. GROWDON. 1997. Metabotropic glutamate receptor subtype mGluR1a stimulates the secretion of the amyloid beta protein precursor ectodomain. J. Neurochem. **69:** 704–712.

7. ENSINGER, H.A., H.N. DOODS, A.R. IMMEL-SEHR *et al.* 1993. WAL 2014: a muscarinic agonist with preferential neuron-stimulating properties. Life. Sci. **52:** 473–480.

8. GROWDON, J.H. 1997. Muscarinic agonists in Alzheimer's disease. Life Sci. **60:** 993–998.

9. MCKHANN, G., D. DRACHMAN, M. FOLSTEIN *et al.* 1984. Clinical diagnosis of Alzheimer's disease: report of the NINCDS-ADRDA Work Group under the auspices of Department of Health and Human Services Task Force on Alzheimer's Disease. Neurology **34:** 939–944.

10. FOLSTEIN, M.F., S.E. FOLSTEIN & P.R. MCHUGH. 1975. Mini Mental State: a practical method for grading the cognitive state of patients for the clinician. J. Psychiatry Res. **12:** 189–198.

11. FARBER, S.A., R.M. NITSCH, J.G. SCHULTZ & R.J. WURTMAN. 1995. Regulated secretion of the β-amyloid precursor protein in rat brain. J. Neurosci. **15:** 7442–7450.

12. ALONZO, N.C., B.T. HYMAN, G.W. REBECK & S.M. GREENBERG. 1998. Progression of cerebral amyloid angiopathy: accumulation of amyloid β-40 in affected vessels. J. Neuropathol. Exp. Neurol. **57:** 353–359.

13. PIRTTILA, T., K.S. KIM, P.D. MEHTA *et al.* 1994. Soluble amyloid beta-protein in the cerebrospinal fluid from patients with Alzheimer's disease, vascular dementia and controls. J. Neurol. Sci. **127**(1): 90–95.

14. NITSCH, R.M., G.W. REBECK, M. DENG *et al.* 1995. Cerebrospinal fluid levels of amyloid β-protein in Alzheimer's disease: inverse correlation with severity of dementia and effect of apolipoprotein E genotype. Ann. Neurol. **37:** 512–518.

15. HOCK, C., S. GOLOMBOWSKI, F. MULLER-SPAHN *et al.* 1998. Cerebrospinal fluid levels of amyloid precursor protein and amyloid beta-peptide in Alzheimer's disease and major depression: inverse correlation with dementia severity. Eur. Neurol. **39:** 111–118.

16. SOUTHWICK, P.C., S.K. YAMAGATA, C.L. ECHOLS *et al.* 1996. Assessment of amyloid beta-protein in cerebrospinal fluid as an aid in the diagnosis of Alzheimer's disease. J. Neurochem. **66:** 259–265.

17. MOTTER, R., C. VIGO-PELFREY, D. KHOLODENKO *et al.* 1995. Reduction of β-amyloid peptide42 in the cerebrospinal fluid of patients with Alzheimer's disease. Ann. Neurol. **38:** 643–648.

18. IDA, N., T. HARTMANN, J. PANTEL *et al.* 1996. Analysis of heterogenous βA4 peptides in human cerebrospinal fluid and blood by a newly developed sensitive Western blot assay. J. Biol. Chem. **271:** 22908–22914.

19. TAMAOKA, A., N. SAWAMURA, T. FUKUSHIMA *et al.* 1997. Amyloid beta protein42(43) in cerebrospinal fluid of patients with Alzheimer's disease. J. Neurol. Sci. **148:** 41–45.

20. GALASKO, D., L. CHANG, R. MOTTER *et al.* 1998. High cerebrospinal fluid tau and low amyloid beta42 levels in the clinical diagnosis of Alzheimer disease and relation to apolipoprotein E genotype. Arch. Neurol. **55:** 937–945.

21. SHOJI, M., E. MATSUBARA, M. KANAI *et al.* 1998. Combination assay of CSF tau, A beta 1–40 and A beta 1–42(43) as a biochemical marker of Alzheimer's disease. J. Neurol. Sci. **158:** 134–140.

22. SUZUKI, N., T.T. CHEUNG, X.D. CAI *et al.* 1994. An increased percentage of long amyloid beta protein secreted by familial amyloid beta protein precursor (beta APP(717)) mutants. Science **264:** 1336–1340.

23. SCHEUNER, D., C. ECKMAN, M. JENSEN *et al.* 1996. Secreted amyloid β-protein similar to that in senile plaques of Alzheimer's disease is increasd *in vivo* by the presenilin 1

and 2 and APP mutations linked to familial Alzheimer's disease. Nature Med. **2:** 864–870.

24. ALMKVIST, O., M. JENSEN, H. BASUN *et al.* 1998. Low levels of $A\beta_{42}$ in cerebrospinal fluid are related to cognitive dysfunction in carriers of the APP 670/671 and PS1 163 gene mutations. Neurobiol. Aging **19**(4S): 161.

25. KANAI, M., E. MATSUBARA, K. ISOE *et al.* 1998. Longitudinal study of cerebrospinal fluid levels of tau, A beta1–40, and A beta1–42(43) in Alzheimer's disease: a study in Japan. Ann. Neurol. **44:** 17–26.

26. SCHENK, D., R. BARBOUR, W. DUNN *et al.* 1999 Immunization with amyloid-beta attenuates Alzheimer-disease-like pathology in the PDAPP mouse. Nature **400:** 173–177.

Metal Chelation as a Potential Therapy for Alzheimer's Disease

MATH P. CUAJUNGCO,[a] KYLE Y. FAGÉT,[a] XUDONG HUANG,[a]
RUDOLPH E. TANZI,[b] AND ASHLEY I. BUSH[a,c]

[a]Laboratory for Oxidation Biology, Massachusetts General Hospital, and
Department of Psychiatry, Harvard Medical School,
Boston, Massachusetts 02115, USA

[b]Genetics and Aging Unit, Massachusetts General Hospital,
Charlestown, Massachusetts 02129, USA

ABSTRACT: Alzheimer's disease is a rapidly worsening public health problem. The current lack of effective treatments for Alzheimer's disease makes it imperative to find new pharmacotherapies. At present, the treatment of symptoms includes use of acetylcholinesterase inhibitors, which enhance acetylcholine levels and improve cognitive functioning. Current reports provide evidence that the pathogenesis of Alzheimer's disease is linked to the characteristic neocortical amyloid-β deposition, which may be mediated by abnormal metal interaction with Aβ as well as metal-mediated oxidative stress. In light of these observations, we have considered the development of drugs that target abnormal metal accumulation and its adverse consequences, as well as prevention or reversal of amyloid-β plaque formation. This paper reviews recent observations on the possible etiologic role of Aβ deposition, its redox activity, and its interaction with transition metals that are enriched in the neocortex. We discuss the effects of metal chelators on these processes, list existing drugs with chelating properties, and explore the promise of this approach as a basis for medicinal chemistry in the development of novel Alzheimer's disease therapeutics.

INTRODUCTION

Alzheimer's disease (AD) is a progressive neurodegenerative disorder characterized by extracellular deposits of amyloid-β protein (Aβ), the main component of neuritic or senile and diffuse plaques.[1] Pathogenic mutations of the APP gene close to or within the Aβ domain are linked to forms of familial AD (FAD).[2] Inheritance of mutations on chromosome 14 (presenilin-1),[3] or chromosome 1 (presenilin-2)[4] produces the more aggressive form of the disease (early-onset age of 25–45 years). Moreover, apolipoprotein-E (apoE) ε4 allele on chromosome 19 has been identified

[c]Address for correspondence: Dr. Ashley Bush, Director, Laboratory for Oxidation Biology, Genetics & Aging Unit MGH, 13th Street Bldg. 149, Charlestown, MA 02129. Tel.: (617) 726-8244; fax: (617) 724-9610.
e-mail: BUSH@helix.mgh.harvard.edu

as a risk factor for late-onset AD.[5] More recently, a genetic deletion of the α_2-macroglobulin (A2M) gene on chromosome 12 was discovered to be another risk factor for AD.[6]

Although the effects of the genetic lesions that cause FAD are to elevate $A\beta_{1-42}$ levels,[7] the mere presence of $A\beta_{1-42}$ cannot initiate amyloid deposition since the peptide is a normal component of healthy CSF.[8] If elevated cortical $A\beta$ concentrations were solely responsible for the initiation of amyloid, it would be difficult to explain why the amyloid deposits are focal (related to synapses and the cerebrovascular lamina media) and not uniform in their distribution. Importantly, overexpression of $A\beta_{1-42}$ from birth, which occurs in genetic forms of AD (FAD and Down's syndrome), does not induce amyloid deposition in childhood.[9] In these cases, $A\beta$ deposition still occurs in an age-dependent, albeit accelerated manner. Also, we have found the total levels of $A\beta$ measured in postmortem brain tissue from AD cases are increased to the same extent in both brain regions that form abundant amyloid (e.g., hippocampus) compared to tissues that do not form amyloid (such as cerebellum).[10] From these observations, it seems unlikely that $A\beta$ overproduction alone initiates $A\beta$ deposition, and thus, it is more likely that there are neurochemical factors, altered as a stochastic consequence of aging, that initiate $A\beta$ deposition in sporadic AD and FAD. The plaque deposits of $A\beta$ appear then to be a morphological variation of $A\beta$ accumulation caused by neurochemical interactions that are specific to the neocortex. The availability of high concentrations of Cu(II) and Zn(II) is a specific feature of neocortical tissue that could explain the condensation of $A\beta$ as plaque. Here, we review current evidence for abnormal metal interactions in AD and discuss the potential therapeutic effect of metal chelators against AD pathology.

CEREBRAL ZINC, COPPER AND IRON LEVELS IN AD

There is an emerging consensus in the literature to indicate that the homeostases of zinc, copper, and iron are significantly altered in the AD brain tissue (reviewed in Refs. 11,12). For example, abnormal levels of zinc, copper, or iron have been found in several subcortical regions such as the hippocampus, amygdala, and olfactory bulb, as well as the neocortex.[11,12] A recent well-controlled study using microparticle-induced X ray emission (PIXE) analysis of the cortical and accessory basal nuclei of the amygdala indicated that zinc, copper, and iron accumulate in the neuropil and plaques of the AD brain where their concentrations are 3–5-fold increased compared to age-matched controls (TABLE 1). In fact, the concentrations of these metal ions, particularly the redox active Cu and Fe (implicated in free radical reactions)[13] are normally concentrated in those regions of the brain most affected by AD pathology. Evidence for abnormal Cu homeostasis in AD includes a 2.2-fold increase in the concentration of CSF Cu,[14] and an accompanying increase in ceruloplasmin in the brain and CSF of AD patients.[15] Similarly, there is an extensive literature describing abnormal levels of Fe and Fe-binding proteins in AD.[16] It has been demonstrated that the Fe found within the amyloid deposits of human brains and in amyloid-bearing APP transgenic mice brains is redox-active.[17]

TABLE 1. Micro-PIXE analysis of metal ion concentrations in Alzheimer's disease plaque and neuropil

	Zinc μg/g (μM)[a]	Copper μg/g (μM)*	Iron μg/g (μM)*
Senile plaque	69 (1055)	25 (393)	53 (940)
AD neuropil	51 (786)	19 (304)	39 (695)
Control neuropil	23 (346)	4 (69)	19 (338)

[a]Adapted from Ref. 18. For purposes of comparison we have converted the published values into molar concentrations assuming a sample density of 1 g/cm^3.

BIOMETALS AND RISK FACTORS FOR ALZHEIMER'S DISEASE

The metal binding proteins, A2M[19] and apoE,[20] are typically found in senile plaques.[21] A2M mediates Aβ degradation via its low density-related lipoprotein (LRP) receptor.[22] A2M binding with Aβ, which is enhanced by the presence of zinc, precludes Aβ fibrillogenesis and reduces its associated neurotoxicity.[23] Meanwhile, of the three apoE isoforms, the ε4 isoform has been found to be the least effective in inhibiting Cu(II)- and Zn(II)-induced precipitation of Aβ,[20] a finding compatible with the apoE ε4 allele being an independent risk factor for AD.[5] It is interesting to note that AD patients carrying the apoE ε4 allele have been found to have elevated serum zinc and copper levels, providing an association between abnormal metal metabolism and apoE risk for AD.[24] Both iron and copper have been shown to enhance the toxicity of Aβ in cultures,[25,26] and copper toxicity is enhanced by nontoxic concentrations of Aβ via Aβ-mediated glutathione depletion.[27]

APP AND Aβ ARE METAL-BINDING PROTEINS

Investigating the role of brain biometals as a potential target for therapeutic remedies in AD stemmed from a series of *in vitro* studies that found that synthetic Aβ and purified APP exhibited several physicochemical interactions with Zn(II), Cu(II), and to a lesser extent, Fe(III), at low micromolar and submicromolar concentrations of the metal ions.[28–34] Hence, disruption in the homeostasis of these metals could possibly contribute to abnormal metal-Aβ interactions in AD.

Specific and saturable binding sites for zinc (APP 181–200; $K_a = 750$ nM)[28] and copper (APP 135–155; $K_d = 10$ nM)[35] were identified within the cysteine-rich region on the ectodomain of APP 695. These sites have homology in all known members of the APP superfamily.[31] This indicates that zinc and copper interaction with the protein may play an important, evolutionary conserved role in APP function and metabolism.

While Zn(II) binding to APP is believed to have a structural role, APP can reduce Cu(II) to Cu(I), which results in oxidation of Cys-144 and Cys-155 and a corresponding intramolecular disulfide bridge formation.[36] The resulting APP-Cu(I) complex is prone to redox reactions that result in site-specific APP fragmentation.[37] The Cys-144 residue of APP was determined to be necessary for this chemical reaction.[38]

Aβ_{1-40} specifically and saturably binds zinc, manifesting high-affinity binding (K_d = 107 nM) with a 1:1 (zinc:Aβ) stoichiometry, and low-affinity binding (K_d = 5.2 μM) with a 2:1 stoichiometry.[29] This binding is histidine-mediated, since it is abolished by acidic pH, and by chemical blocking of the histidine residues.[34] More importantly, His-13 is believed to be an important residue in zinc-mediated Aβ assembly.[39] The zinc binding site was mapped to a stretch of contiguous residues between positions 6–28 of the Aβ sequence. Occupation of the zinc binding site, which straddles the lysine 16 position of α-secretase site, inhibits α-secretase type (tryptic) cleavage and so may influence the generation of Aβ from APP, and may increase the biological half-life of Aβ by protecting the peptide from proteolytic attack.[30] Zinc concentrations above 300 nM rapidly precipitate synthetic human Aβ_{1-40}.[29,32,33] Interestingly, zinc may also preserve the α-helical conformation of Aβ_{1-40}, which may explain why precipitation of Aβ by Zn(II) is reversible, and that Zn(II)-assembled Aβ can be resolubilized by chelation.[33]

Aβ is also precipitated by Cu(II) in a reaction that is potentiated by mildly acidic (pH 6.6) conditions. The stoichiometry of Cu:Aβ increases from zero when Aβ is soluble to 1.0–2.5 when Aβ is aggregated by Cu(II).[34,40] Aβ_{1-40} has higher-affinity (log K_{app} 10) and lower-affinity (log K_{app} 7.0) binding sites for Cu, but the affinity of Cu for Aβ_{1-42} is greater for both sites (log K_{app} 17.3 and log K_{app} 8.0, respectively).[40] The high-affinity Cu(II) binding site on Aβ_{1-42} is of such high affinity that it is very likely to be occupied *in vivo*. However, under mildly acidic conditions (pH 6.8), the affinity of Aβ_{1-40} and Aβ_{1-42} for Zn(II), but not Cu(II) decreases at the lower-affinity binding sites.[40]

Unlike Zn(II), both Cu(II) and Fe(III) induce greater Aβ aggregation under mildly acidic conditions (e.g., pH 6.8–7.0).[32,34] However, Aβ binds equimolar amounts of Cu(II) and Zn(II) at pH 7.4, while Cu(II) displaces Zn(II) from Zn(II):Aβ aggregates under acidic conditions (pH 6.6).[40] Aβ_{1-42} markedly aggregates in the presence of trace amounts (<0.1 μM) of Cu(II).

OXIDATIVE MECHANISMS OF Aβ NEUROTOXICITY

Both Aβ deposition in the neocortex, and oxidative stress, are considered closely related to the pathogenesis of AD. The deposition of Aβ in the neocortex of APP transgenic mice overexpressing Aβ is accompanied by some neuropathological features of AD such as neuronal loss,[41] and signs of oxidative damage[42] suggesting that the neurotoxic events of AD are seminally related to Aβ accumulation. Many studies have now confirmed that Aβ is neurotoxic in cell culture[43] and *in vivo*.[44] Therefore, prevention of Aβ deposition could be a therapeutic target in AD.

Focus on the pathogenic relevance of oxidative stress in AD was stimulated by the report that treatment of AD subjects with the antioxidant vitamin E delays decline in independent functioning.[45] Metabolic signs of oxidative stress such as oxygen radical-mediated damage of brain proteins, lipids, and nucleic acids, as well as systemic signs of oxidative stress and the response of antioxidant systems have all been observed in AD.[46,47] The biochemical relationship between $A\beta$ deposition in AD and oxidative stress is complex, and the mechanisms underlying the association between oxidation and amyloid deposition are not well understood.

Synthetic $A\beta$ peptides exert toxicity through mechanisms that involve the generation of cellular hydrogen peroxide (H_2O_2).[48] The observed cytotoxicity is abolished by $O_2^{-\bullet}/H_2O_2$ scavengers.[49] Taken together, the chemical nature of oxidation stress in AD indicates that H_2O_2 levels may be elevated in the AD brain. While Zn(II) is redox-inert, we recently reported that the binding of trace concentrations of redox-active metals Cu(II) and Fe(III) to $A\beta$ engenders the cell-free catalytic production of H_2O_2 from O_2 via metal reduction.[50] The redox activities of $A\beta$ species are greatest for $A\beta_{42} > A\beta_{40} >> $rat $A\beta_{40}$, a chemical relationship that corresponds to the participation of the respective peptide in amyloid pathology, as well as the peptide's H_2O_2-mediated toxicity in cell culture.[26] It is interesting to note that the $A\beta$ peptide has a selective vulnerability to Cu-mediated OH• attack that oxidizes the peptide, emulating the chemical changes seen in the $A\beta$ extracted from AD brain (Atwood *et al.* submitted).

METAL COMPLEXING PROPERTIES OF CHELATING AGENTS: AN OVERVIEW

The term chelator originated from the Greek word "chele," which means "crab's claw."[51,52] This term defines the complexes formed by a ligand (a molecule with at least two donor groups or coordination number) with their substrates (ions) such that a "ring" system is established. The process of creating such a ring structure is well correlated with the formation of a more stable complex.[52] Denticity (from the word "dens," meaning tooth) is used to describe the number of available donor groups of a chelating agent to bind metal ions.[52] For example, bidentate refers to two donor groups, tridentate to three, quinquidentate to five, and so forth. Some chelators are able to form multidentate complexes, while others can only attain a monodentate or bidentate chelate rings. For multidentate ligands, the dissociation constant (K_d; a constant that reflects the intrinsic strength of metal-ligand binding) can vary markedly for different species.[51] Some chelators have the ability to directly permeate cell membranes prior to or upon binding metal ions (e.g., see Ref. 53). Other chelators become membrane permeable after esterification, or by acquiring a nonpolar state following metal complexation.[51] In addition, some chelators are ionophores since their chelating sites have limited flexibility and thus would prefer cations that fit easily into their molecular structure.[52] Ionophores may selectively enhance the permeability of metal ions in lipid membranes of cells as in the case of calcium ionophore A23187 (calcimycin), which facilitates entry of calcium ions into cells.[54] Similarly, pyrithione is a zinc chelator that neutralizes zinc neurotoxicity, but also has an ionophoric property.[53] Hence chelators may act to either deprive biological systems of metal ions, or may have the opposite effect of promoting metal uptake into cells.

EFFECTS OF METAL CHELATORS
ON Aβ PATHOPHYSIOLOGY

Inhibition of the Redox Activity and Aggregation of Aβ

FAD-linked mutations of APP, presenilin-1 and presenilin-2, increase both Aβ amyloid burden and $A\beta_{1-42}$ production, underscoring the role that the longer Aβ species plays in AD pathogenesis.[7] Hence, much effort has focused on the mechanisms of $A\beta_{1-42}$-mediated fibrillogenesis. A landmark *in vitro* study in this area was that of Jarrett *et al.*[55] who reported that $A\beta_{1-40}$, which is kinetically stable at 20 μM in solution for nine days, is destabilized over that interval by "seeding" with 2 μM $A\beta_{1-42}$ fibrils. This work has been considerably augmented and has lead to a theory of nucleation-dependence or "seeding" of amyloidogenic peptides in several neurodegenerative diseases. We extended the work of Jarrett *et al.*[55] and found that addition of Zn(II), Cu(II), and Fe(III) enhanced $A\beta_{1-42}$-initiated seeding of $A\beta_{1-40}$ (Huang *et al.* submitted). However, we measured the concentrations of these metal ions that contaminate the incubation buffer and found levels to be 0.1–0.5 μM, great enough to precipitate Aβ. Therefore, we tested the effects of chelators upon this classic nucleation reaction, and found that polyamincarboxylic acid compounds like diethylene tetraamine pentaacetic acid (DTPA), and cyclohexane diamine tetraacetic acid (CDTA), both high-affinity Cu(II) and Zn(II) chelators, abolished the seeding reaction. Furthermore, NMR spectroscopy proved that these compounds do not interact directly with the peptide. These findings indicate that metal ions are essential for the initiation of nucleation-dependent fibrillogenesis.

We have shown that Aβ reduces Cu and Fe, and that Aβ can generate H_2O_2 through a metal-dependent reaction.[50] We thus tested the possibility that metal chelators could interfere with the redox activity of Aβ. We observed that BP and DTPA abolished (at a 200-fold molar excess) the H_2O_2 generated by Aβ (10 μM) interacting with Fe(III)-citrate (1 μM).[50] We repeated this experiment using a 200-molar excess of desferrioxamine (DFO, a high-affinity Fe[III] chelator), and found that DFO was ineffective in preventing H_2O_2 formation unlike BP and DTPA.[56] These results suggest that the ability of a compound to inhibit Aβ:metal-mediated redox activity is not simply a product of its affinity, but that other factors such as stereochemistry of the metal binding site, play important roles.

Resolubization of Aβ Plaques **in Vitro** *and in Postmortem Human and APP Transgenic Mouse Brain Tissue*

We have shown *in vitro* that zinc-induced[33] or copper-induced[34] precipitation of Aβ peptide is a chelation-reversible event. Interestingly, zinc-precipitated Aβ is denser and less easily resolubilized than copper-induced precipitates.[20] Indeed, Aβ is resolubilized and extracted from postmortem AD and non-AD control brains using metal chelators.[57] High-affinity Cu/Fe/Zn chelators such as N,N,N′,N′-tetrakis-(2-pyridylmethyl)-ethylenediamine (TPEN) and bathocuproine disulfonic acid (BC), markedly enhanced the resolubilization of Aβ deposits from postmortem AD and non-AD brain samples.[57] The observed increase in extractable Aβ correlated with significant depletion in zinc (30%) and to a lesser extent, copper, in each of the AD cases examined ($n = 10$) when compared with PBS-alone treated tissue.[57] The ability

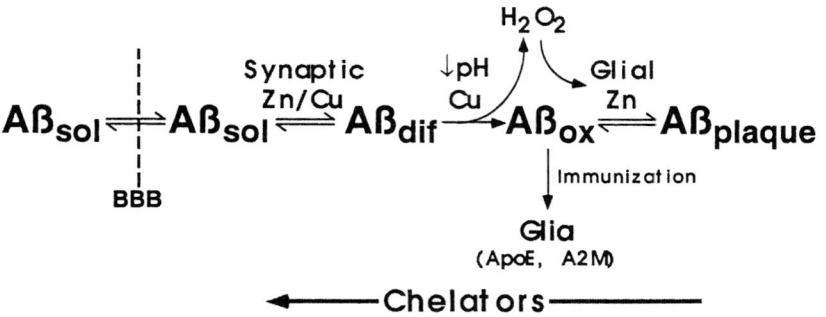

FIGURE 1. A model for the role of metal/Aβ interaction in AD. Aβ is a normal soluble constituent of biological fluids including plasma and brain interstitial fluids (Aβ$_{sol}$). During epochs of metabolic stress (e.g., head injury, hypoxia, etc.), the uptake of zinc and copper via energy-dependent uptake mechanisms after they are released into the synapse is inhibited. This raises the concentration of zinc and copper in the synaptic vicinity, precipitating Aβ at that site as diffuse amyloid deposits on histology (Aβ$_{dif}$). These deposits would ordinarily resolve as the metabolic stress diminishes and the interstitial zinc and copper concentrations decrease to normal again. If on the other hand, the concentration of Cu(II) remains high then Cu(II) may displace Zn(II) from Aβ (especially under acidotic conditions)[34] abnormally generating H$_2$O$_2$ and oxidizing Aβ (carbonyl modification). Soluble oxidized forms of Aβ (Aβ$_{ox}$) are protease resistant,[64] and therefore abnormally long-lived in the cortical interstitium where they drive up the H$_2$O$_2$ levels even more, taxing the cellular scavenging mechanisms (e.g., glutathione), and contributing to neurotoxicity.[25–27] The elevated H$_2$O$_2$, being freely permeable, crosses the membrane of the neighboring glia and reacts with metallothionein, causing the liberation of the metallothionein-held pool of Zn(II).[11,65] The Zn(II) liberated into the interstitium by the glia precipitates the oxidized forms of Aβ into plaque deposits that, as a result, have very high (~1 mM) levels of Zn(II)[18,66,67] but no longer produce H$_2$O$_2$ so that plaque deposits become sites of decreased oxidative damage to neighboring tissue.

The plaque contains oxidized protease-resistant Aβ that is cemented together by Zn(II), which induces even further resistance to proteolysis,[30] so generating a deposit that defies clearance until disaggregated by a chelator.[57,58] Treatment with a compound that complexes both Zn(II) and Cu(II) promotes the dissolution of Aβ plaque and diffuse deposits[57,58] while simultaneously shutting down H$_2$O$_2$ production,[26,50] and facilitating the clearance of damaged forms of Aβ by the glia. Damaged/oxidized forms of Aβ may be antigenically foreign, and cleared by activated glia, perhaps explaining how immunization of transgenic animals with synthetic Aβ may work to clear Aβ by promoting glial recognition of oxidized Aβ forms.[68]

Synaptic zinc is more likely than copper to be responsible for the initial precipitation of Aβ as diffuse deposits, because: (a) Zn(II) induces the precipitation of Aβ far more extensively at pH 7.4 *in vitro* than does Cu(II);[30,34] (b) the concentration of synaptic Zn(II) reached during neurotransmission is 10–20-fold higher than that reached by Cu(II);[69,70] and (c) the distribution of vesicular (synaptically released) Zn(II) in the brain corresponds to the sites of the brain that are most prone to amyloid pathology—the cerebral cortex, and not the subcortical gray matter or the cerebellum.[69]

of a chelator to extract Aβ depended upon the presence of Mg(II) and Ca(II), hence the chelating compound needed must be more selective for Zn(II) and Cu(II), than Ca(II) and Mg(II). Higher concentrations of Cu/Zn chelator caused a paradoxical decrease in the amount of Aβ released, because the sequestration of Ca/Mg from the sample became substantial. This work was further extended on APP transgenic

"Hsiao" mouse brain samples using either triethylenetetraamine (TETA; a high-affinity Cu[II] chelator) or bicinchoninic acid (BCA; a Cu[I]-selective chelator) giving similar results to that of the human study.[58]

The Chelating Class of Molecule as a Pharmacological Possibility in AD

Presently, the only AD therapeutic agents approved by the FDA are acetylcholine esterase (AChE) inhibitors (e.g., donepezil), which enhance cholinergic neurotransmission by hindering the breakdown of acetylcholine. This approach, while providing modest clinical gains, is not believed to retard the progression of the underlying disease. Hence, there is a need to find a suitable drug that attacks the disease at its pathogenesis.

We have reviewed findings which suggest that metal complexing agents may have therapeutic benefits in AD. In the last few years, chelation therapy has become increasingly promoted as a therapy for AD, both by individual medical practitioners and by lay groups and even at internet web sites. However, the growing practice of intravenous infusions of EDTA is based upon largely unscientific interpretations of the neurochemical problems in AD, and can lead to systemic metal ion depletion.

One previous clinical trial of the chelator compound DFO was reported to significantly arrest the progression of the disease.[59] Although the DFO trial was thought to target Al(III), it is possible that the beneficial effect of the treatment was due to chelation of Fe(III), Cu(II), and Zn(II). Indeed, the authors reported verbally (International Conference on Alzheimer's Disease, Padua, 1992) that postmortem metal analysis on brain tissue of study-subjects indicated that although aluminum levels were lower than placebo controls, zinc and iron levels were also decreased in the brains of DFO-treated subjects. This is because, like all chelators, DFO has only a relative selectivity for aluminum, and will also complex with zinc, copper, and iron.[60] Although the results of Crapper-McLachlan and colleagues[59] have not yet been reproduced, further consideration of the removal of zinc, copper, and iron from brain Aβ collections as a therapeutic maneuver seems warranted (FIG. 1). DFO is a charged molecule that does not easily penetrate the blood-brain barrier and is easily degraded after it is administered.[52] Further clinical research into the effects of DFO may have been met with diminished enthusiasm, since the administration of DFO is associated with discouraging difficulties including the nonspecific problems of systemic metal ion depletion (e.g., anemia), and the problem of administration of a twice-daily, painful intramuscular injection.

We propose that the metal binding sites on Aβ may provide an appropriate drug target for rational drug design. Although the 3-D structure of Aβ is unknown, our data indicate that the redox active metal binding site on the protein is subject to steric principles, and therefore small compounds with great specificity for this site may be developed. The principles of pharmacotherapeutic molecule complexing a metal-binding site on a protein target is actually well developed in pharmacology. Several well-known antibiotic, anticonvulsive, antitumor, and antiinflammatory drugs (TABLE 2) exert their pharmacological action by interacting with the Cu-, Zn-, or Fe-active site of their target protein. Disulfiram, for example, blocks enzyme activity by chelating the zinc-catalytic site of alcohol dehydrogenase.[61] Nonsteroidal antiinflammatory drugs (NSAIDs) such as aspirin, diflunisal, ibuprofen, naproxen sodium, indomethacin, *d*-penicillamine, etc., block the heme-iron catalytic site on

TABLE 2. A list of drugs that possess chelating properties

Usage	Drug name	Metal Chelate	Reference
Antiinflammatory; Aanalgesic	Aspirin, indometha-cin, *d*-penicil-lamine, ibuprofen	copper, iron, zinc	62,71–73
Antibiotic; antitumor; sedative	Bleomycin, etham-butol, thalidomide	copper, iron, zinc	74-76
Antioxidant; dietary supplement	α-lipoic acid	zinc, copper, manganese	77
Anticonvulsant	Valproate sodium, phenytoin	copper, selenium, zinc	78,79
Alcohol abuse	Tetraethyl thiuram disulfide or diethyl dithiocarbamate (disulfiram/ antabuse)	copper, zinc	53

cyclooxygenase/arachidonic acid pathway.[62] Intriguingly, the use of these drugs has also been reported to reduce the epidemiological risk for AD,[63] but their therapeutic value is still uncertain (see also Progress Report on Alzheimer's Disease, NIA/NIH publication).

CONCLUDING REMARKS

Our current findings indicate that an ideal therapeutic drug to dissolve Aβ amyloid would involve a compound that is relatively selective for Cu(I), Zn(II), and possibly Fe(III), but does not sequester Mg(II) or Ca(II), and that coordinates metal ions in the cerebral amyloid mass but not systemically. Charged species cannot diffuse through biological membranes and thus are confined to the tissue compartment where they were administered. Electrically neutral and nonpolar molecules are ideal chelators, since they are best absorbed across the gastrointestinal tract and achieve a broad distribution throughout various tissues. Finally, tissue and target selectivity of the chelator-drug is essential in order to prevent other biologically important metal ions from becoming systemically depleted during therapy.

REFERENCES

1. GLENNER, G.G. & C. WONG. 1984. Alzheimer's disease: initial report of the purification and characterization of a novel cerebrovascular amyloid protein. Biochem. Biophys. Res. Commun. **120:** 885–890.
2. CHARTIER-HARLIN, M.C., F. CRAWFORD & H. HOULDEN. 1991. Early-onset Alzheimer's disease caused by mutations at codon 717 of the β-amyloid precursor protein gene. Nature **353:** 844–846.
3. SHERRINGTON, R., E.I. ROGAEV, Y. LIANG *et al.* 1995. Cloning of a gene bearing missense mutations in early-onset familial Alzheimer's disease. Nature **375:** 755–760.

4. LEVY-LAHAD, E., E.M. WIJSMAN, E. NEMENS *et al.* 1995. A familial Alzheimer's disease locus on chromosome 1. Science **269:** 970–973.
5. SAUNDERS, A.M., W.J. STRITTMATTER, D. SCHMECHEL *et al.* 1993. Association of apolipoprotein E allele ε4 with late-onset familial and sporadic Alzheimer's disease. Neurology **43:** 1467–1472.
6. BLACKER, D., M.A. WILCOX, N.M. LAIRD *et al.* 1998. Alpha-2 macroglobulin is genetically associated with Alzheimer's disease. Nat. Genet. **19:** 357–360.
7. SCHEUNER, D., C. ECKMAN, M. JENSEN *et al.* 1996. Secreted amyloid β-protein similar to that in the senile plaques of Alzheimer's disease is increased *in vivo* by the presenilin 1 and 2 and APP mutations linked to familial Alzheimer's disease. Nat. Med. **2:** 864–870.
8. TAMAOKA, A., N. SAWAMURA, T. FUKUSHIMA *et al.* 1997. Amyloid beta protein 42(43) in cerebrospinal fluid of patients with Alzheimer's disease. J. Neurol. Sci. **148:** 41–45.
9. LEMERE, C.A., J.K. BLUSZTAJN, H. YAMAGUCHI *et al.* 1996. Sequence of deposition of heterogeneous amyloid beta-peptides and apoE in Down syndrome: implications for initial events in amyloid plaque formation. Neurobiol. Dis. **3:** 16–32.
10. McLEAN, C., R.A. CHERNY, F. FRASER *et al.* 1999. Soluble pool of Aβ amyloid as a determinant of severity of neurodegeneration in Alzheimer's disease. Ann. Neurol. **46:** 860–866.
11. CUAJUNGCO, M.P. & G.J. LEES. 1997. Zinc metabolism in the brain: relevance to human neurodegenerative disorders. Neurobiol. Dis. **4:** 137–169.
12. ATWOOD, C.S., X. HUANG, R.D. MOIR *et al.* 1999. Role of free radicals and metal ions in the pathogenesis of Alzheimer's disease. Metal Ions Biol. Syst. **36:** 309–364.
13. HALLIWELL, B. & J.M.C. GUTTERIDGE. 1984. Oxygen toxicity, oxygen radicals, transition metals and disease. Biochem. J. **219:** 1–14.
14. BASUN, H., L.G. FORSSELL, L. WETTERBERG & B. WINBLAD. 1991. Metals and trace elements in plasma and cerebrospinal fluid in normal aging and Alzheimer's disease. J Neural. Transm. Park. Dis. Dement. Sect. **3:** 231–258.
15. LOEFFLER, D.A., P.A. LEWITT, P.L. JUNEAU *et al.* 1996. Increased regional brain concentrations of ceruloplasmin in neurodegenerative disorders. Brain Res. **738:** 265–274.
16. ROBINSON, S.R., D.F. NOONE, J. KRIL & G.M. HALLIDAY. 1995. Most amyloid plaques contain ferritin-rich cells. Alzheimer's Res. **1:** 191–196.
17. SMITH, M.A., P.L.R. HARRIS, L.M. SAYRE & G. PERRY. 1997. Iron accumulation in Alzheimer's disease is a source of redox-generated free radicals. Proc. Natl. Acad. Sci. USA **94:** 9866–9868.
18. LOVELL, M.A., J.D. ROBERTSON, W.J. TEESDALE *et al.* 1998. Copper, iron and zinc in Alzheimer's disease senile plaques. J. Neurol. Sci. **158:** 47–52.
19. MIYATA, M. & J.D. SMITH. 1996. Apolipoprotein E allele-specific antioxidant activity and effects on cytotoxicity by oxidative insults and beta-amyloid peptides. Nat. Genet. **14:** 55–61.
20. MOIR, R.D., C.S. ATWOOD, D.M. ROMANO *et al.* 1999. Differential effects of apolipoprotein E isoforms on metal-induced aggregation of Aβ using physiological concentrations. Biochemistry **38:** 4595–4603.
21. REBECK, G.W., S.D. HARR, D.K. STRICKLAND & B.T. HYMAN. 1995. Multiple, diverse senile plaque-associated proteins are ligands of an apolipoprotein E receptor, the α_2-macroglobulin receptor/low-density lipoprotein receptor-related protein. Ann. Neurol. **37:** 211–217.
22. QIU, W.Q., W. BORTH, Z. YE *et al.* 1996. Degradation of amyloid β-protein by a serine protease-α_2-macroglobulin complex. J. Biol. Chem. **271:** 8443–8451.
23. DU, Y., K.R. BALES, R.C. DODEL *et al.* 1998. α_2-Macroglobulin attenuates β-amyloid peptide 1–40 fibril formation and associated neurotoxicity in cultured fetal rat cortical neurons. J. Neurochem. **70:** 1182–1188.
24. GONZÁLEZ, C., T. MARTÍN, J. CACHO *et al.* 1999. Serum zinc, copper, insulin and lipids in Alzheimer's disease epsilon 4 apolipoprotein E allele carriers. Eur. J. Clin. Invest. **29:** 637–642.
25. SCHUBERT, D. & M. CHEVION. 1995. The role of iron in beta amyloid toxicity. Biochem. Biophys. Res. Commun. **216:** 702–707.

26. HUANG, X., M.P. CUAJUNGCO, C.S. ATWOOD *et al.* 1999. Cu(II) potentiation of Alzheimer's Aβ neurotoxicity: correlation with cell-free hydrogen peroxide production and metal reduction. J. Biol. Chem. **274:** 37111–37116.
27. WHITE, A.R., A.I. BUSH, K. BEYREUTHER *et al.* 1999. Exacerbation of copper toxicity in primary neuronal cultures depleted of cellular glutathione. J. Neurochem. **72:** 2092–2098.
28. BUSH, A.I., G. MULTHAUP, R.D. MOIR *et al.* 1993. A novel zinc(II) binding site modulates the function of the βA4 amyloid protein precursor of Alzheimer's disease. J. Biol. Chem. **268:** 16109–16112.
29. BUSH, A.I., W.H. PETTINGELL, G. MULTHAUP *et al.* 1994. Rapid induction of Alzheimer Aβ amyloid formation by zinc. Science **265:** 1464–1467.
30. BUSH, A.I., W.H. PETTINGELL, M.D. PARADIS & R.E. TANZI. 1994. Modulation of Aβ adhesiveness and secretase site cleavage by zinc. J. Biol. Chem. **269:** 12152–12158.
31. BUSH, A.I., W.H. PETTINGELL, M.D. PARADIS *et al.* 1994. The amyloid β-protein precursor and its mammalian homologues: evidence for a zinc-modulated heparin-binding superfamily. J. Biol. Chem. **269:** 26618–26621.
32. BUSH, A.I., R.D. MOIR, K.M. ROSENKRANZ & R.E. TANZI. 1995. Zinc and Alzheimer's disease. Science **268:** 1921–1923.
33. HUANG, X, C.S. ATWOOD, R.D. MOIR *et al.* 1997. Zinc-induced Alzheimer's Aβ$_{1-40}$ aggregation is mediated by conformational factors. J. Biol. Chem. **272:** 26464–26470.
34. ATWOOD, C.S., R.D. MOIR, X. HUANG *et al.* 1998. Dramatic aggregation of Alzheimer Aβ by Cu(II) is induced by conditions representing physiological acidosis. J. Biol. Chem. **273:** 12817–12826.
35. HESSE, L., D. BEHER, C.L. MASTERS & G. MULTHAUP. 1994. The beta A4 amyloid precursor protein binding to copper. FEBS Lett. **349:** 109–116.
36. MULTHAUP, G., A. SCHLICKSUPP, L. HESSE *et al.* 1996. The amyloid precursor protein of Alzheimer's disease in the reduction of copper(II) to copper(I). Science **271:** 1406–1409.
37. MULTHAUP, G., T. RUPPERT, A. SCHLICKSUPP *et al.* 1998. Copper-binding amyloid precursor protein undergoes a site-specific fragmentation in the reduction of hydrogen peroxide. Biochemistry **37:** 7224–7230.
38. RUIZ, F.H., M. GONZÁLEZ, M. BODINI 1999. Cysteine 144 is a key residue in the copper reduction by the beta-amyloid precursor protein. J. Neurochem. **73:** 1288–1292.
39. LIU, S.T., G. HOWLETT & C.J. BARROW. 1999. Histidine-13 is a crucial residue in the zinc ion-induced aggregation of the A beta peptide of Alzheimer's disease. Biochemistry **38:** 9373–9378.
40. ATWOOD, C.S., R.C. SCARPA, X. HUANG *et al.* 2000. Characterization of copper interactions with Alzheimer Aβ peptides: identification of an attomolar affinity copper binding site on Aβ$_{1-42}$. J. Neurochem. **75:** 1219–1233.
41. STURCHLER-PIERRAT, C., D. ABRAMOWSKI, M. DUKE *et al.* 1997. Two amyloid precursor protein transgenic mouse models with Alzheimer disease-like pathology. Proc. Natl. Acad. Sci. USA **94:** 13287–13292.
42. SMITH, M.A., K. HIRAI, K. HSIAO *et al.* 1998. Amyloid-beta deposition in Alzheimer transgenic mice is associated with oxidative stress. J. Neurochem. **70:** 2212–2215.
43. YANKNER, B.A., L.K. DUFFY & D.A. KIRSCHNER. 1990. Neurotrophic and neurotoxic effects of amyloid β protein: reversal by tachykinin neuropeptides. Science **250:** 279–282.
44. EMRE, M., C. GEULA, B.J. RANSIL & M.M. MESULAM. 1992. The acute neurotoxicity and effects upon cholinergic axons of intracerebrally injected beta-amyloid in the rat brain. Neurobiol. Aging **13:** 553–559.
45. SANO, M., C. ERNESTO, R.G. THOMAS *et al.* 1997. A controlled trial of selegiline, alpha-tocopherol, or both as treatment for Alzheimer's disease. The Alzheimer's Disease Cooperative Study. N. Engl. J. Med. **336:** 1216–1222.
46. MECOCCI, P., U. MACGARVEY & M.F. BEAL. 1994. Oxidative damage to mitochondrial DNA is increased in Alzheimer's disease. Ann. Neurol. **36:** 747–751.
47. SMITH, M.A., P.L. RICHEY, S. TANEDA *et al.* 1994. Advanced Maillard reaction end products, free radicals, and protein oxidation in Alzheimer's disease. Ann. N.Y. Acad. Sci. **738:** 447–454.

48. BEHL, C., J.B. DAVIS, R. LESLEY & D. SCHUBERT. 1994. Hydrogen peroxide mediates amyloid β protein toxicity. Cell **77**: 817–827.
49. BRUCE, A.J., B. MALFROY & M. BAUDRY. 1996. β-Amyloid toxicity in organotypic hippocampal cultures: protection by Euk-8, a synthetic catalytic free radical scavenger. Proc Natl. Acad. Sci. USA **93**: 2312–2316.
50. HUANG, X., C.S. ATWOOD, M.A. HARTSHORN *et al.* 1999. The Aβ peptide of Alzheimer's disease directly produces hydrogen peroxide through metal ion reduction. Biochemistry **38**: 7609–76016.
51. MELLOR, D.P. 1964. Historical background and fundamental concepts. *In* Chelating Agents and Metal Chelates. F.P. Dwyer & D.P. Mellor, Eds.: 1–50. Academic Press. New York.
52. MAY, P.M. & R.A. BULMAN. 1983. The present status of chelating agents in medicine. Prog. Med. Chem. **20**: 225–336.
53. CUAJUNGCO, M.P. & G.J. LEES. 1998. Diverse effects of metal chelating agents on the neuronal cytotoxicity of zinc in the hippocampus. Brain Res. **799**: 97–107.
54. BLAU, L., R.B. STERN & R. BITTMAN. 1984. The stoichiometry of A23187- and X537A-mediated calcium ion transport across lipid bilayers. Biochim. Biophys. Acta **778**: 219–223.
55. JARRETT, J.T., E.P. BERGER & P.T LANSBURY, JR. 1993. The carboxy terminus of the β amyloid protein is critical for the seeding of amyloid formation: implications for the pathogenesis of Alzheimer's disease. Biochemistry **32**: 4693–4697.
56. BUSH, A.I., X. HUANG & D.P. FAIRLIE. 1999. The possible origin of free radicals from amyloid β peptides in Alzheimer's disease. Neurobiol. Aging **268**: 335–337.
57. CHERNY, R.A., J.T. LEGG, C.A. MCLEAN, *et al.* 1999. Aqueous dissolution of Alzheimer's disease Aβ amyloid deposits by biometal depletion. J. Biol. Chem. **274**: 23223–23228.
58. GRAY, D.N., R.A. CHERNY, C.L. MASTERS *et al.* 1998. Resolubilization of Alzheimer and APP transgenic beta amyloid plaque by copper chelators [abstract]. Soc. Neurosci. Abstr. **24**: 722.
59. CRAPPER-MCLACHLAN, D.R., A.J. DALTON, T.P.A. KRUCK *et al.* 1991. Intramuscular desferrioxamine in patients with Alzheimer's disease. Lancet **337**: 1304–1308.
60. HIDER, R.C. & A.D. HALL. 1991. Clinically useful chelators of tripositive elements. Prog. Med. Chem. **28**: 41–173.
61. LANGELAND, B.T. & J.S. MCKINLEY-MCKEE. 1996. The effects of disulfiram on equine hepatic alcohol dehydrogenase and its efficiency against alcoholism: vinegar effect. Alcohol Alcohol. **31**: 75–80.
62. RAO, G.H. & J.G. WHITE. 1985. Comparative pharmacology of cyclooxygenase inhibitors on platelet function. Prostaglandins Leukotrienes Med. **18**: 119–131.
63. MCGEER, P.L., M. SCHULZER & E.G. MCGEER. 1996. Arthritis and anti-inflammatory agents as possible protective factors for Alzheimer's disease: a review of 17 epidemiologic studies. Neurology **47**: 425–432.
64. STADTMAN, E.R. 1992. Protein oxidation and aging. Science **257**: 1220–1224.
65. CUAJUNGCO, M.P. & G.J. LEES. 1997. Zinc and Alzheimer's disease: is there a direct link? Brain Res. Rev. **23**: 219–236.
66. LEE, J.-Y., I. MOOK-JUNG & J.-Y. KOH. 1999. Histochemically reactive zinc in plaques of the Swedish mutant beta-amyloid precursor protein transgenic mice. J. Neurosci. **19**(RC10): 1–5.
67. SUH, S.W., K.B. JENSEN, M.S. JENSEN *et al.* 1999. Histological evidence implicating zinc in Alzheimer's disease. Brain Res. **852**: 274–278.
68. SCHENK, D., R. BARBOUR, W. DUNN, *et al.* 1999. Immunization with amyloid-beta attenuates Alzheimer-disease-like pathology in the PDAPP mouse. Nature **400**: 173–177.
69. FREDERICKSON, C.J. 1989. Neurobiology of zinc and zinc-containing neurons. Int. Rev. Neurobiol. **31**: 145–328.
70. HARTTER, D.E. & A. BARNEA. 1988. Brain tissue accumulates 67copper by two ligand-dependent saturable processes. J. Biol. Chem. **263**: 799–805.
71. RUSSANOV, E.M., D.E. DIMITROVA, E.A. IVANCHEVA & M.D. KIRKOVA. 1986. The effects of aspirin, indomethacin and their copper complexes on phospholipase activity and on lipid peroxidation in rat liver microsomes. Acta Physiol. Pharmacol. Bulg. **12**: 36–43.

72. PETERSON, D.A., J.M. GERRARD, G.H. RAO & J.G. WHITE. 1979. Inhibition of ferrous ion induced oxidation of arachidonic acid by indomethacin. Prostaglandins Med. **2:** 97–108.
73. PERRET, D. 1981. The metabolism and pharmacology of *d*-penicillamine in man. J. Rheumatol. (Suppl.) **7:** 41–50.
74. DORR, R.T. 1992. Bleomycin pharmacology: mechanism of action and resistance, and clinical pharmacokinetics. Semin. Oncol. **19**(Suppl. 5)**:** 3–8.
75. SHESKIN, J., R. GORODETZKY, E. LOEWINGER & A. WEINREB. 1981. *In vivo* measurements of iron, copper and zinc in the skin of prurigo nodularis patients treated with thalidomide. Dermatologica **162:** 86–90.
76. WEISMANN, K. 1986. Chelating drugs and zinc. Dan. Med. Bull. **33:** 208–211.
77. PACKER, L., E.H. WITT & H.J. TRITSCHLER. 1995. Alpha-lipoic acid as a biological antioxidant. Free Radical Biol. Med. **19:** 227–250.
78. HURD, R.W., H.A. VAN RINSVELT, B.J. WILDER *et al.* 1984. Selenium, zinc, and copper changes with valproic acid: possible relation to drug side effects. Neurology **34:** 1393–1395.
79. PALM, R. & G. HALLMANS. 1982. Zinc and copper metabolism in phenytoin therapy. Epilepsia **23:** 453–461.

Regulation of Gene Expression by Muscarinic Acetylcholine Receptors

A Comprehensive Approach for the Identification of Regulated Genes

HEINZ VON DER KAMMER,[a,d] MANUEL MAYHAUS,[a] CLAUDIA ALBRECHT,[a] BARBARA ANDRESEN,[a] JAROSLAV KLAUDINY,[b] CÜNEYT DEMIRALAY,[a] AND ROGER M. NITSCH[a,c]

[a]Center for Molecular Neurobiology, University of Hamburg, Martinistr. 51, 20246 Hamburg, Germany

[b]Institute of Chemistry, Slovak Academy of Sciences, Dubravska cesta 9, 84238 Bratislava, Slovak Republic

[c]Department of Psychiatry Research, University of Zürich, August-Forel-Str. 1, 8008 Zürich, Switzerland

Muscarinic acetylcholine receptors (mAChRs) are members of a superfamily of G-protein-coupled cell surface receptors.[1,2] In brain, m1 and m3 mAChRs are present on somatodendritic plasma membranes of large pyramidal neurons throughout the cortex and the hippocampus, as well as on small cholinergic interneurons in the striatum. In contrast, m2 and m4 mAChRs are predominantly localized to presynaptic terminals and the axons of the large basal forebrain projection neurons that innervate cortical and hippocampal cholinergic target cells. Cellular responses of mAChRs include the activation of neurite outgrowth, the fine-tuning of membrane potentials, and the regulation of mitogenic growth responses in cells that are not terminally differentiated.[3] mAChRs are involved in long-term potentiation and synaptic plasticity[4] alterations in neuronal structure and function that have been proposed to be associated with rapid and transient transcription of activity-dependent genes.[5–7] mAChRs are also involved in the activity-dependent regulation of α-secretase processing of the β-amyloid precursor protein,[8–10] associated by reduced generation of β-amyloid peptides, the principal component of amyloid plaques in Alzheimer's disease brains.[11–13] Alzheimer brains show progressive loss of cholinergic innervation from the basal forebrain to the cerebral cortex, hippocampus, and amygdala.[14–16] These changes of the cholinergic system correlate with cognitive decline;[17] therefore, different therapeutic strategies for Alzheimer's disease were developed that enhance cholinergic function including the use of cholinomimetic drugs like m1 mAChR agonists.[18,19]

In order to identify genes that are regulated by mAChRs, we developed an mRNA differential display (DD) approach, which yielded highly consistent results.[20] A set

[d]Address correspondence to: Dr. Heinz von der Kammer, Center for Molecular Neurobiology, University of Hamburg, Martinistr. 5, D-20246 Hamburg, Germany. Tel.: +49-40-42803-6273; fax: +49-42803-6598.

e-mail: kammer@plexus.uke.uni-hamburg.de

of 64 distinct random primers was specifically designed to approach a statistically comprehensive analysis of all mRNA species in a defined cell population. A partial screen analyzing mRNAs generated in response to 1 h of m1 mAChR stimulation revealed 10 distinct immediate-early genes: Egr-1, Egr-2, Egr-3, NGFi-B, ETR101, c-jun, jun-D, Gos-3, and hCyr61, as well as the previously unknown gene Gig-2. A more detailed study of the mAChR-coupled regulation of the Egr family showed that mAChRs can regulate Egr-1, Egr-2, Egr-3, and Egr-4 at the level of transcription, as well as functional protein synthesis.[21] The ability of different mAChR subtypes to stimulate Egr-1 expression suggests that similar genes are controlled by acetylcholine both in pre- and postsynaptic neuronal populations. Our studies showed binding to, and activation of, EGR-promoter sequences followed by the synthesis of functional protein as a result of mAChR stimulation.[21] EGR-1 increases the promoter activity and gene expression of acetylcholinesterase (AChE), a serine hydrolase that catalyzes the breakdown of acetylcholine. m1 mAChR activation specifically increases AChE gene promoter activity,[21] and leads to a significant induction of AChE mRNA expression.[22] Moreover, *in vivo* experiments using adult rats that were treated with the cholinergic immunotoxin 192 IgG-saporin revealed a dramatic decrease of AChE activity in cortex, hippocampus, and in the cholinergic cell bodies in the medial septum.[23] AChE transcription may be involved in a receptor-coupled feedback mechanism by which increases in cholinergic transmission are limited by up-regulated AChE expression and accelerated breakdown of acetylcholine at the cholinergic synapses.

In our study several new genes were identified to be induced by activation of m1 mAChRs. hCyr61, an immediate-early gene that is a member of the CCN gene family of Ctgf, Cyr61, and nov that encodes secretory signaling factors,[24] was induced within 15 min.[20] Binding to heparin-containing components of the extracellular matrix, Cyr61 promotes cell growth, adhesion, proliferation, chemotaxis, and migration.[25,26] As a ligand of the integrin $a_v\beta_3$, Cyr61 induces angiogenesis, neovascularization, and tumor growth.[27] In addition, Gig-2 (for G-protein-coupled receptor induced gene 2), a previously unknown gene, was found to be upregulated by m1 mAChR within 40 min of stimulation. Receptor stimulation also triggered Gig-2 expression in the presence of cycloheximide, indicating that Gig-2 is an immediate-early gene. In *in vivo* experiments, the muscarinic agonist pilocarpine strongly induced both hCyr61 and Gig-2 expression in neurons of several, but different, layers of the brain cortex, the hippocampal CA1 region, and the putamen. In preliminary studies in order to analyze gene expression in m1 cells 3 h after stimulation with carbachol, we identified two other new genes that are induced by mAChRs: Gig-3 and Gig-4.[22] Like AChE, some of these genes may be target genes that are under the control of the above immediate-early genes.

Together, our data show that muscarinic receptors induce a complex and sustained pattern of expression of genes that may be involved in the regulation of cholinergic transmission, as well as in the control of cellular functions in postsynaptic cholinergic target cells. The biological functions of early effector genes including Cyr61, CTGF, and Gig-2 may be directly involved in such cellular responses as growth, adhesion, and plasticity; transcription factors induce a set of target genes that encode late effector proteins including AChE, LM04, Gig-3, and Gig-4. Together, both early- and late-effector proteins may act together mediating such activity-dependent long-term cellular responses as neurite growth, synaptic plasticity, LTP, and memory and learning. Drugs designed to activate mAChRs including AChE inhibitors and m1-agonists currently tested in clinical trials for the treatment of Alzheimer's disease may be expected to stimulate transcription of Egr genes along with EGR-dependent target genes.

REFERENCES

1. BONNER, T.I. 1989. New subtypes of muscarinic acetylcholine receptors. Trends Pharmacol. Sci. (Suppl.) 11–15.
2. WESS, J. 1993. Molecular basis of muscarinic acetylcholine receptor function. Trends Pharmacol. Sci. **14:** 308–314.
3. CONKLIN, B.R., M.R. BRANN, N.J. BUCKLEY, A.L. MA, T.I. BONNER & J. AXELROD. 1988. Stimulation of arachidonic acid release and inhibition of mitogenesis by cloned genes for muscarinic receptor subtypes stably expressed in A9 L cells. Proc. Natl. Acad. Sci. USA **85:** 8698–8702.
4. DI CHIARA, G., M. MORELLI & S. CONSOLO. 1994. Modulatory functions of neurotransmitters in the striatum: ACh/dopamine/NMDA interactions. Trends Neurosci. **17:** 228–233.
5. MORGAN, J.I. & T. CURRAN. 1991. Stimulus-transcription coupling in the nervous system: involvement of the inducible proto-oncogenes fos and jun. Annu. Rev. Neurosci. **14:** 421–451.
6. ABRAHAM, W.C., S.E. MASON, J. DEMMER, *et al.* 1993. Correlations between immediate early gene induction and the persistence of long-term potentiation. Neuroscience **56:** 717–727.
7. HUERTA, P.T. & J.E. LISMAN. 1993. Heightened synaptic plasticity of hippocampal CA1 neurons during a cholinergically induced rhythmic state. Nature **364:** 723–725.
8. NITSCH, R.M., B.E. SLACK, R.J. WURTMAN & J.H. GROWDON. 1992. Release of Alzheimer amyloid precursor derivatives stimulated by activation of muscarinic acetylcholine receptors. Science **258:** 304–307.
9. NITSCH, R.M., S.A. FARBER, J.H. GROWDON & R.J. WURTMAN. 1993. Release of amyloid beta-protein precursor derivatives by electrical depolarization of rat hippocampal slices. Proc. Natl. Acad. Sci. USA **90:** 5191–5193.
10. FARBER, S.A., R.M. NITSCH, J.G. SCHULZ & R.J. WURTMAN. 1995. Regulated secretion of beta-amyloid precursor protein in rat brain. J. Neurosci. **15:** 7442–7451.
11. LEE, R.K.K., R.J. WURTMAN, A.J. COX & R.M. NITSCH. 1995. Amyloid precursor protein processing is stimulated by metabotropic glutamate receptors. Proc. Natl. Acad. Sci. USA **92:** 8083–8087.
12. NITSCH, R.M., M. DENG, J.H. GROWDON & R.J. WURTMAN. 1996. Serotonin 5-HT2a and 5-HT2c receptors stimulate amyloid precursor protein ectodomain secretion. J. Biol. Chem. **271:** 4188–4194.
13. NITSCH, R.M., A. DENG, R.J. WURTMAN & J.H. GROWDON. 1997. Metabotropic glutamate receptor subtype mGluR1alpha stimulates the secretion of the amyloid. J. Neurochem. **69:** 704–712.
14. COYLE, J.T., D.L. PRICE & M.R. DELONG. 1983. Alzheimer's disease: a disorder of cortical cholinergic innervation. Science **219:** 1184–1190.
15. PEARSON, R.C.A., M.M. ESIRI, R.W. HIORNS, G.K. WLCOCK & T.P.S. POWELL. 1985. Anatomical correlates of the distribution of the pathological changes in the neocortex in Alzheimer disease. Proc. Natl. Acad. Sci. USA **82:** 4531–4533.
16. SAMUEL, W., R.D. TERRY, R. DETERESA, N. BUTTERS & E. MASLIAH. 1994. Clinical correlates of cortical and nucleus basalis pathology in Alzheimer dementia. Arch. Neurol. **51:** 772–778.
17. TERRY, R.D. & R. KATZMAN. 1983. Senile dementia of the Alzheimer type. Ann. Neurol. **14:** 497–506.

18. LEVEY, A.I. 1996. Muscarinic acetylcholine receptor expression in memory circuits: implications for treatment of Alzheimer disease. Proc. Natl. Acad. Sci. USA **93:** 13541–13546.
19. LADNER, C.J. & J.M. LEE. 1998. Pharmacological drug treatment of Alzheimer disease: the cholinergic hypothesis revisited. J. Neuropathol. Exp. Neurol. **57:** 719–731.
20. VON DER KAMMER, H., C. ALBRECHT, M. MAYHAUS, B. HOFFMANN, G. STANKE & R.M. NITSCH. 1999. Identification of genes regulated by muscarinic acetylcholine receptors: application of an improved and statistically comprehensive mRNA differential display technique. Nucleic Acids Res. **27:** 2211–2218.
21. VON DER KAMMER, H., M. MAYHAUS, C. ALBRECHT, J. ENDERICH, M. WEGNER & R.M. NITSCH. 1998. Muscarinic acetylcholine receptors activate expression of the EGR gene family of transcription. J. Biol. Chem. **273:** 14538–14544.
22. VON DER KAMMER, H., C. DEMIRALAY, B. HOFFMANN, C. ALBRECHT, M. MAYHAUS & R.M. NITSCH. 2000. Biochem. Soc. Trans. In press.
23. NITSCH, R.M., S. ROSSNER, C. ALBRECHT, et al.. 1998. Muscarinic acetylcholine receptors activate the acetylcholinesterase gene promoter. J. Physiol. (Paris) **92:** 257–264.
24. BORK, P. 1993. The modular architecture of a new family of growth regulators related to connective tissue growth factor. FEBS Lett. **327:** 125–130.
25. KIREEVA, M.L., B.V. LATINKIC, T.V. KOLESNIKOVA, et al.. 1997. Cyr61 and Fisp12 are both ECM-associated signaling molecules: activities, metabolism, and localization during development. Exp. Cell Res. **233:** 63–77.
26. KIREEVA, M.L., F. MO, G.P. YANG & L.F. LAU. 1996. Cyr61, a product of a growth factor-inducible immediate-early gene, promotes cell proliferation, migration, and adhesion. Mol. Cell. Biol. **16:** 1326–1334.
27. BABIC, A.M., M.L. KIREEVA, T.V. KOLESNIKOVA & L.F. LAU. 1998. CYR61, a product of a growth factor-inducible immediate early gene, promotes angiogenesis and tumor growth. Proc. Natl. Acad. Sci. USA **95:** 6355–6360.

Cholinergic Modulation of Amyloid Processing and Dementia in Animal Models of Alzheimer's Disease

O. ISACSON[a] AND L. LIN

Neuroregeneration Laboratories, McLean Hospital/Harvard Medical School, Belmont, Massachusetts 02478, USA

INTRODUCTION

Alzheimer's disease (AD) regional cerebral pathology is partially characterized by diffuse and dense-core amyloid deposition, neurofibrillary tangles, and loss of afferent cortical input from subcortical cholinergic and monoaminergic neurons. The potential interactions between these separate neuropathological findings in the evolution of AD dementia and brain damage have not been fully elucidated. For example, correlations of dementia with postmortem amyloid plaques and neurofibrillary tangles are generally unreliable, unless strictly defined to stage of disease or anatomical subregions. Evidence of cerebrocortical and hippocampal dysfunction (such as atrophy or metabolic dysfunction), possibly resulting from neuronal damage and the loss of afferent synaptic control, are considered a better correlate with signs of dementia. The severe loss of cholinergic function in AD[1] and the profound effect on memory function of the CNS cholinergic system[2–4] suggest that cognitive deficits in AD may be due in part to that specific pathology. More recent *in vivo* observations imply that neuronal degeneration of the cholinergic system and amyloid pathology may be interrelated.[5–7] Loss of cholinergic input to the neocortex and hippocampus increases amyloid precursor protein (APP) levels and reduces nonamyloidogeneic processing of APP. Linking these systems are studies showing how Aβ can interfere with cholinergic neurotransmission, implying Aβ not only in plaque formation, but also in cholinergic dysfunction. Interactions between the cholinergic system and Aβ-related systems may therefore be central to AD pathogenesis. These data also imply that drugs or cell repair designed to enhance cholinergic synaptic function, ACh synthesis, release, receptor-activations, or increase the effects of ACh neurotransmission may inhibit AD pathology by reducing the Aβ burden as well as improving cognitive function.

[a]Address for correspondence: O. Isacson, Neuroregeneration Laboratories, McLean Hospital/ Harvard Medical School, 115 Mill St., Belmont, MA 02478. Tel.: (617) 855-3283; fax: (617) 855-3284.

e-mail: isacson@helix.mgh.harvard.edu

AMYLOID PRECURSOR PROTEIN AND
CHOLINERGIC FUNCTION

APP is an abundant glycoprotein with a long N-terminal domain, a single membrane spanning unit, and a minor cytoplasmic C-terminal tail.[2,9] Aβ is generated by the proteolytic cleavage of APP[10] and released under normal conditions in brain,[11,12] indicating that Aβ may have physiological functions. Inhibition of ACh release by Aβ has been shown in the frontal cortex and hippocampus.[13] Demonstrations that Aβ can reduce choline levels of neurons by either enhancing leakage of choline or decreasing choline uptake[13,14] indicate that Aβ can interfere with normal cholinergic neurotransmission. Further data show that Aβ depresses cholinergic physiological activity by reducing muscarinic M1 receptor coupling to G protein.[15] This effect on the muscarinic M1 receptor would be amyloidogenic.[10,16] Intriguingly, in addition to its infamous Aβ generation, APP itself may in its cleaved secreted form have significant neurobiological functions and regulate neurotransmission by trophic or pharmacological actions. The nonamyloidogenic processing pathway, termed the α-secretase pathway, principally acts on cell surfaces and within the trans-Golgi network.[17] If APP cleavage occurs at both the N-terminus (β-secretase) and C-terminus (γ-secretase) of the Aβ domain, an Aβ peptide is produced; and if secreted in sufficient concentrations, it will aggregate to form amyloid.[11,12,17–19] Alternatively, APP can also be reinternalized from the cell surface into the acidic endosomal-lysosomal compartment and processed to yield multiple C-terminal derivatives, some of which contain intact Aβ sequences that are potentially amyloidogenic.[17–19] The enzymes involved in the APP processing pathways have not been conclusively identified, although presenilin 1 appears to be the γ-secretase.[20]

Several studies have demonstrated that APP processing is under the control of G-protein linked receptors, for example, cholinergic, serotoninergic, and glutamatergic receptor.[21–23] Binding to these receptors can accelerate APPs secretion and reduce Aβ formation.[21–23] Of interest, muscarinic ACh receptors appear to have a potential role in the regulation of APP processing. Nitsch et al.[16] first demonstrated that agonist stimulation of muscarinic receptors by carbachol enhances APPs release in cells selectively expressing M1 and M3 receptor subtypes. In contrast, APPs release in cells made to express M2 or M4 and wild-type cells was not modified on balance by muscarinic activation, indicating that regulation of APP processing is receptor subtype specific.[23] Activation of the M1 receptor with carbachol reduces Aβ secretion,[24] and M1 selective receptor activation increased APPs release, while the nonselective muscarinic agents did not modify APP processing.[25] When M2 antagonist was added to the cell preparations, the nonselective agonist behaved as selective M1 agonists, implicating an inhibitory action of the M2 receptor on M1 receptor-enhanced APP processing.[26] These findings are consistent with the view that only selective activation of the M1 subtype can result in increased nonamyloidogenic processing of APP. Since M1 and M3 receptors are linked to protein kinase C, whereas stimulation of M2 and M4 receptors inhibit adenylate cyclase,[10] this could explain the differences seen, given that activation of protein kinase C promotes APPs secretion,[24,27,28] which in turn can be blocked by PKC inhibitors.[22,29] APP secretion proceeds in the absence of either cytoplasmic or extracellular phosphorylation.[28] PKC activation may therefore lead to phosphorylation and activation of additional kinases, potentially involved in APP processing.[30] While these *in vitro* cell culture studies proposed a reasonable scheme for cholinergic control of APP processing, *in vivo* studies in animals confirming these effects have been lacking.

In a series of *in vivo* lesion studies of cholinergic synaptic loss and cognitive function, we administered a muscarinic receptor agonist (RS86) to rats (normal, aged, and those with severe basal forebrain cholinergic deficits induced by 192 IgG-saporin). The levels of the cell-associated APP in neocortex, hippocampus, and striatum, as well as APPs in CSF, were determined by Western blots. The treatment with muscarinic receptor agonist reduced APP levels in neocortex and hippocampus, and elevated APPs in CSF.[7] These effects on APP processing by the muscarinic agonist treatment were found in normal and aged rats and those with cholinergic denervation.

CAN CHOLINERGIC DEFICITS CONTRIBUTE TO BOTH AMYLOID PATHOLOGY AND COGNITIVE DYSFUNCTION?

Rats with excitotoxic lesions of the basal forebrain cholinergic system show increased APP mRNA and APP synthesis in cerebral cortex.[31] Fimbria-fornix lesions also cause significant accumulation of APP in the hippocampus.[32] More recently, it was demonstrated that selective neuronal loss of cholinergic neurons expressing the low-affinity NGF receptor (p75) in the basal forebrain produced increased APP immunoreactivity in cholinoceptive layers of the frontal cortex and hippocampus.[5,6] Similar investigations showed that the secreted form of APP (APPs) was reduced while levels of full-length APP increased significantly.[33] Such findings strongly support the idea that APP levels or processing may be under the control of the basal forebrain cholinergic system, presumably mediated through M1 muscarinic receptors on cholinoceptive target cells.[33,34] Nonetheless, other types of cell damage and loss of neurotransmission (for example, serotonin and norepinephrine[31]) also cause APP expression, and cognitive problems, suggesting that APP could be a rather generalized response to CNS damage or disrupted neurotransmitter function that would increase amyloid-load and brain dysfunction.

Multiple copies of the APP gene probably causes Down's syndrome, having a progressive development of AD-like brain degeneration and loss of brain function.[35] APP and derivatives may be directly involved in brain functions serving learning and memory. Aβ infused into the cerebral ventricles in rats[36] and mice[37] disrupted learning and memory. A concomitant decreased cholinergic activity was seen in frontal cortex and hippocampus.[36] Data exist showing that transgenic mice overexpressing isoforms of human APP will eventually display reduced learning and memory.[38–41] Notably, cognitive deficits are also seen in mice overexpressing the normal C-terminal 104 amino acid of APP, which contains the Aβ sequence.[41] Mice with both mutant APP and presenilin 1 transgenes have less spontaneous alternations in a two-armed maze, without signs of amyloid deposition.[42] These genetic manipulations in mice suggest a potential role of elevated membrane bound APP or released Aβ in cognitive dysfunction. In contrast, the secreted form of APP (APPs) can improve memory performance in animal experiments and block the confusion caused by scopolamine.[43] A peptide-fragment of the APPs caused cognitive improvement and increased the number of presynaptic terminals in the cerebral cortex of rats.[44] We discovered that increased APP levels in cerebral cortex correlated with cognitive deficits observed in a water maze in 192 IgG-saporin lesioned rats.[7] Impaired glucose utilization in hippocampus was registered in APP transgenic mice with behavioral deficits,[40] which resemble the impairment in glucose uptake and CNS-specific glucose transporters found in AD brain.[45,46] Decreased glucose uptake can suppress the production of ATP and increased neuronal vulnerability to excitotoxicity,[47] which may contribute to degenerative process and cognitive deficits seen in AD. We have also found marked reductions in glucose utilization (Browne et al., unpublished observations) in a number of regions including cortex and hippocampus in 192 IgG-saporin lesioned rats with selective cholinergic loss and behavioral deficits suggesting a role of impaired cellular energy systems in altered APP processing and cognitive deficits in AD.

ACKNOWLEDGMENT

This work was supported in part by a donation from the Irving and Betty Brudnick Research Fund at McLean Hospital.

REFERENCES

1. REISINE, T.D., H.I. YAMAMURA, E.D. BIRD et al. 1978. Pre- and postsynaptic neurochemical alterations in Alzheimer's disease. Brain Res. 159: 477–481.
2. COLLERTON, D. 1986. Cholinergic function and intellectual decline in Alzheimer's disease. Neuroscience 19: 1–28.
3. COYLE, J.D., D.L. PRICE & M.R. DELONG. 1983. Alzheimer's disease: a disorder of cortical cholinergic innervation. Science 219: 1184–1190.
4. BARTUS, R.T., R.L. DEAN III, B. BEER & A.S. LIPPA. 1982. The cholinergic hypothesis of geriatric memory dysfunction. Science 217: 408–417.
5. LEANZA, G. 1998. Chronic elevation of amyloid precursor protein expression in the neocortex and hippocapmus of rats with selective cholinergic lesions. Neurosci. Lett. 257: 53–56.
6. LIN, L., C. LEBLANC, T. DEACON & O. ISACSON. 1998. Chronic cognitive decifits and amyloid precursor protein elevation after immunotoxin lesions of the basal forebrain cholinergic system. Neuroreport 9: 547–552.
7. LIN, L., A. GEORGIEVSKA, A. MATTSSON & O. ISACSON. 1999. Cognitive changes and modified processing of amyloid precursor protein in the cortical and hippocampal system after cholinergic synapse loss and muscarinic receptor activation. Proc. Natl. Acad. Sci. USA 96: 12108–12113.
8. SELKOE, D.J. 1994. Normal and abnormal biology of the β-amyloid precursor protein. Annu. Rev. Neurosci. 17: 489–517.
9. KANG, J., H.-G. LEMAIRE, A. UNTERBECK et al. 1987. The precursor of Alzheimer's disease amlyoid A4 protein resembles a cell-surface receptor. Nature 325: 733–736.
10. NITSCH, R.M. & J.H. GROWDON. 1994. Role of neurotransmission in the regulation of amyloid beta-protein precursor processing. Biochem. Pharmacol. 47: 1275–1284.
11. HAASS, C., M.G. SCHLOSSMACHER, A.Y. HUNG et al. 1992. Amyloid bete-peptide is produced by cultured cells during normal metabolism. Nature 359: 322–325.
12. SHOJI, M., T.E. GOLDE, J. GHISO et al. 1992. Production of the Alzheimer amyloid β protein by normal proteolytic processing. Science 258: 126–327.
13. KAR, S., A. ISSA, D. SETO et al. 1998. Amyloid beta-peptide inhibits high-affinity choline uptake and acetylcholine release in rat hippocampal slices. J. Neurochem. 70: 2179–2187.

14. GALDZICKI, Z. 1994. β-Amyliod increases choline conductance of PC12 cells: possible mechanism of toxicity in Alzheimer's disease. Brain Res. **646:** 332–336.
15. KELLY, J.F., K. FURUKAWA, S.W. BARGER *et al.* 1996. Amyloid β-peptide disrupts carbachol-induced muscarinic cholinergic signal transduction in cortical neurons. Proc. Natl. Acad. Sci. USA **93:** 6753–6758.
16. NITSCH, R.M., B.E. SLACK, R.J. WURTMAN & J.H. GROWDON. 1992. Release of Alzheimer amyloid precursor derivatives stimulated by activation of muscarinic acetylcholine receptors. Science **258:** 304–310.
17. HAASS, C., A. HUNG, M. SCHLOSSMACHER *et al.* 1993. Beta-amyloid peptide and a 3-kDa fragment are derived by distinct cellular mechanism. J. Biol. Chem. **268:** 3021–3024.
18. GOLDE, T., S. ESTUS, L. YOUNKIN *et al.* 1992. Processing of the amyloid precursor protein to potentially amyloidgenic derivatives. Science **255:** 728–730.
19. ESTUS, S., T. GOLDE, T. KINISHITE *et al.* 1992. Potentially amyloidgenic, carboxyl-terminal derivatives of the amyloid protein precursor. Science **255:** 726–728.
20. WOLFE, M., W. XIA, B. OSTASZEWSKI *et al.* 1999. Two transmembrane aspartates in presenilin-1 required for presenilin endoproteolysis and γ-secretase activity. Nature **398:** 513–517.
21. LEE, R., R. WURTMAN, A. COX & R. NITSCH. 1995. Amyloid precursor protein processing is stimulated by metabotropic glutamate receptors. Proc. Natl. Acad. Sci. USA **92:** 8083–8087.
22. NITSCH, R.M., M. DENG, J.H. GROWDON & R.J. WURTMAN. 1996. Serotonin 5-HT2a and 5-HT2c receptors stimulate amyloid precursor protein ectodomain secretion. J. Biol. Chem. **271:** 4188–4194.
23. NITSCH, R.M., S.A. FARBER, J.H. GROWDON & R.J. WURTMAN. 1993. Release of amyloid β-protein precursor derivatives by electrical depolarization of rat hippocamal slices. Proc. Natl. Acad. Sci. USA **90:** 5191–5193.
24. HUNG, A.Y., C. HAASS, R.M. NITSCH *et al.* 1993. Activation of protein kinase C inhibits cellular production of the amyloid β-protein. J. Biol. Chem. **268:** 22959–22962.
25. MULLER, D.M., K. MENDLA, S.A. FARBER & R.M. NITSCH. 1997. Muscarinic M1 receptor agonists increase the secretion of the amyloid precursor protein ectodomain. Life Sci. **60:** 985–998.
26. FARBER, S., R. NITSH, J. SCHULZ & R. WURTMAN. 1995. Regulated secretion of β-amyloid precursor protein in rat brain. J. Neurosci. **15:** 7442–7451.
27. CAPORASO, G.L., S.E. GANDY, J.D. BUXBAUM *et al.* 1992. Protein phosphorylation regulates secretion of Alzheimer-beta/A4 amyloid precursor protein. Proc. Natl. Acad. Sci. USA **89:** 3055–3059.
28. GABUZDA, D., J. BUSCIGLIO & B.A. YANKNER. 1993. Inhibition of β-amyloid production by activation of protein kinase C. J. Neurochem. **61:** 2326–2329.
29. SLACK, B.E., J. BREU, M.A. PETRYNIAK *et al.* 1995. Tyrosine phosphorylation-dependent stimulation of amyloid beta precursor protein secretion by the M3 muscarinic acetylcholine receptor. J. Biol. Chem. **270:** 8337–8344.
30. HUNG, A.Y. & D.J. SELKOE. 1994. Selective ectodomain phosphorylation and regulated cleavage of β-amyloid precursor protein. EMBO J. **13:** 534–542.
31. WALLACE, W., S.T. AHLERS, J. GOTLIB *et al.* 1993. Amyloid precursor protein in the cerebral cortex is rapidly and persistently induced by loss of subcortical innervation. Proc. Natl. Acad. Sci. USA **90:** 8712–8716.
32. BEESON, J.G., E.R. SHELTON, H.W. CHAN & F.H. GAGE. 1994. Age and damage induced changes in amyloid protein precursor immunohistochemistry in the rat brain. J. Comp. Neurol. **342:** 69–77.
33. ROSSNER, S., U. UEBERHAM, J. YU *et al.* 1997. *In vivo* regulation of amyloid precursor protein secretion in rat neocortex by cholinergic activity. Eur. J. Neurosci. **9:** 2125–2134.
34. ROSSNER, S. 1997. Cholinergic immunolesions by 192-saporin: a useful tool to stimulate pathogenic aspects of Alzheimer's disease. Int. J. Dev. Neurosci. **15:** 837–850.
35. RUMBLE, B., R. RETALLACK, C. HILBICH *et al.* 1989. Amyloid A4 protein and its precursor in Down's syndrome and Alzheimer's disease. N. Engl. J. Med. **320:** 1446–1452.
36. NABESHIMA, T. & A. NITTA. 1994. Memory impairment and neuronal dysfunction induced by beta-amyloid protein in rats. Tohoku J. Exp. Med. **174:** 241–249.

37. MAURICE, T., B.P. LOCKHART & A. PRIVAT. 1996. Amnesia induced in mice by centrally administered β-amyloid peptides involves cholinergic dysfunction. Brain Res. **706:** 181–193.
38. MORAN, P.M., L.S. HIGGINS, B. CORDELL & P.C. MOSER. 1995. Aged-related learning deficits in transgenic mice expressing the 751-amino acid isoform of human β-amyloid precursor protein. Proc. Natl. Acad. Sci. USA **92:** 5341–5345.
39. HSIAO, K., P. CHAPMAN, S. NILSEN *et al.* 1996. Correlative memory deficits, Aβ elevation, and amyloid plaques in transgenic mice. Science **272:** 99–102.
40. HSIAO, K.K., D.R. BORCHELT, K. OLSON *et al.* 1995. Aged-related CNS disorder and early death in transgenic FVB/N overexpressing Alzheimer amyloid precursor protein. Neuron **15:** 1203–1218.
41. NALBANTOGLU, J., G. TIRADO-SANTIAGO, A. LAHSAINI *et al.* 1997. Impaired learning and LTP in mice expressing the carboxy terminus of the Alzheimer amyloid precursor protein. Nature **387:** 500–505.
42. HOLCOMB, L., M.N. GORDON, E. MCGOWAN *et al.* 1998. Accelerated Alzheimer's-type phenotype in transgenic mice carrying both mutant amyloid precursor protein and presenilin 1 transgenes. Nat. Med. **4:** 97–100.
43. MEZIANE, H., J.-C. DODART, C. MATHIS *et al.* 1998. Memory-enhancing effects of secreted forms of the β-amyloid precursor protein in normal and amnestic mice. Proc. Natl. Acad. Sci. USA **95:** 12683–12688.
44. ROCH, J., E. MASLIAH, A. ROCH-LEVECQ *et al.* 1994. Increase of synaptic density and memory retention by a peptide representing the trophic domain of the amyloid beta/A4 protein precursor. Proc. Natl. Acad. Sci. USA **91:** 7450–7454.
45. SIMS, N. 1990. Altered glucose metabolism in Alzheimer's disease. Ann. Neurol. **27:** 691–693.
46. SIMPSON, I.A., K.R. CHUNDU, T. DAVIES-HILL *et al.* 1994. Decreased concentrations of GLUT1 and GLUT3 glucose transporters in the brains of patients with Alzheimer's disease. Ann. Neurol. **35:** 546–551.
47. NOVELLI, A., J. REILLY, P. LYSKA & R. HENNEBERRY. 1988. Glutamate becomes neurotoxic via the *N*-methy-D-aspartate receptor when intracellular enery levels are reduced. Brain Res **451:** 205–212.

M1 Muscarinic Agonists as Potential Disease-Modifying Agents in Alzheimer's Disease

Rationale and Perspectives

A. FISHER,[a,b] D.M. MICHAELSON,[c] R. BRANDEIS,[a] R. HARING,[a] S. CHAPMAN,[a] AND Z. PITTEL[a]

[a]Israel Institute for Biological Research, Ness-Ziona, Israel

[c]Tel Aviv University, Ramat Aviv, Israel

ABSTRACT: A cholinergic hypofunction in Alzheimer's disease (AD) may lead to formation of β-amyloids that might impair the coupling of M1 muscarinic ACh receptors (mAChRs) with G proteins. This disruption in coupling can lead to decreased signal transduction, to a reduction in levels of trophic amyloid precursor proteins (APPs), and to generation of more β-amyloids that can also suppress ACh synthesis and release, aggravating further the cholinergic deficiency. These "vicious cycles," a presynaptic and a postsynaptic one, may be inhibited, in principle, by M1 selective agonists. Such properties can be detected in the functionally selective M1 agonists from the AF series [e.g., project drugs, AF102B, AF150(S)]. These M1 agonists promote the nonamyloidogenic APP processing pathways and decrease tau protein phosphorylation. The effects on tau proteins suggest a link between M1 mAChR-mediated signal transduction system(s) and the neuronal cytoskeleton via regulation of phosphorylation of tau microtubule-associated protein. This may indicate a dual role for M1 agonists: as inhibitors of two "vicious cycles," one induced by β-amyloids, and the other due to overactivation of certain kinases (e.g., glycogen synthase kinase-3, GSK-3) or downregulation of phosphatases, respectively. Prolonged administration of AF150(S) in apolipoprotein E-knockout mice restored cognitive impairments, cholinergic hypofunction, and tau hyperphosphorylation, and unveiled a high-affinity binding site to M1 mAChRs. Except M1 agonists, there are no reports of compounds having such combined effects, for example, amelioration of cognition dysfunction and beneficial modulation of APPs together with tau phosphorylation. This unique property of M1 agonists to alter different aspects of AD pathogenesis could represent the most remarkable, yet unexplored, clinical value of such compounds.

INTRODUCTION

The rationale behind development of M1-selective muscarinic agonists in Alzheimer's disease (AD) rests upon two themes: the cholinergic hypothesis of memory and learning (symptomatic treatment), and the potential of such compounds to be disease-modifying agents via muscarinic regulation of amyloid metabolism and tau phosphorylation (for a review, see Ref. 1).

[b]Address for correspondence: Dr. Abraham Fisher, Israel Institute for Biological Research, P.O. Box 19, Ness-Ziona 74100, Israel. Tel: + (972)-8-381-603; fax: + (972)-8-381-615.
e-mail: fisher_a@netvision.net.il

M1-type muscarinic receptors (mAChRs) have an important role in cognitive processing, are relatively unchanged in AD, and therefore may serve as a target for an antidementia drug treatment. M1 agonists may offer a significant advantage in treating AD because they might allow the continuation of symptomatic treatment of cognitive decline when the already-approved cholinesterase inhibitors (AChE-Is) no longer work. However, some muscarinic agonists showed disappointing results in phase III studies in AD patients. Most of these agonists lacked M1 selectivity *in vivo* and/or had several major clinical limitations, sufficient to raise serious questions as to why these compounds reached the stage of clinical testing at all.[1] The proper M1 muscarinic agonists have not yet been tested in comprehensive clinical trials in AD.

RESULTS AND DISCUSSION

There is now justified hope that M1 agonists could provide limited causal therapy. Thus a relationship among the formation of Aβ peptide and amyloid plaques, tau phosphorylation, and the loss of cholinergic function in AD brains was reported (for a review, see Ref. 1).

M1 Agonists and β-Amyloid Processing

Cholinergic stimulation of M1 mAChRs can increase cleavage of amyloid precursor proteins (APPs) in the middle of its β-amyloid region.[1,2] This cleavage produces the secreted, nonamyloidogenic APPs (α-APPs), preventing the formation of Aβ peptide. M1 agonists may be of value in preventing amyloid formation by selectively promoting the "α-secretase" processing pathway in AD. It can be deduced that M1 selective agonists may alter APP processing in cortex and hippocampus where M1 mAChRs are abundant. TABLE 1 summarizes results obtained *in vivo* in a number of laboratories, including ours, on the relation between the cholinergic system and Aβ.[4–7] The following conclusions can be drawn: (a) A chronic cholinergic hypofunction induced by either the cholinotoxin AF64A (rats: 3 nmole/side, icv, 7 and 30 days postinjection; unpublished data) or the immunotoxin 192 IgG-saporin produces a decrease in α-APPs that indicates a reduction in α-secretase activity;[5–7] (b) in rabbits, where the sequence of $\beta A_{(1-42)}$ is similar to humans, a chronic cholinergic hypofunction elevates βA;[6] (c) activation of protein kinase C (PKC) in transgenic (Tg) mice that produces elevated human βA^4 or direct activation of mAChR (mostly of M1 type) in 192 IgG-saporin lesioned rats[7] reduces $\beta A_{(1-42)}$ and attenuates the 192 IgG-saporin effects on APP, respectively.

M1 mAChR Dephosphorylation of Tau Proteins

Tau microtubule-associated protein is neuronal specific, and its expression is necessary for neurite outgrowth. Hyperphosphorylated tau proteins constitute the principal fibrous component of the neurofibrillary tangle pathology in AD. Stimulation of M1 decreased tau phosphorylation.[8] This was shown in studies *in vitro* (cell cultures)[8–10] and *in vivo* [in apolipoprotein E (ApoE)-deficient mice][11] (TABLE 2 and below). The effects on tau proteins suggest a link between M1 mAChR-mediated signal transduction system(s) and the neuronal cytoskeleton via regulation of phos-

TABLE 1. The relationship between cholinergic hypofunction and APP processing *in vivo*

Study	α-APPs	β-amyloids
Swedish FAD (APP670/671 mutation)[3]	α-APPs (CSF) is reduced and correlates with cognitive impairment	$\beta A_{(1-42)}$ is elevated
Tg mice (Swedish FAD) $\pm$ PKC activation[4]	PKC-activation leads to α-APPs— no change; β-APPs reduction	$\beta A_{(1-42)}$ is elevated PKC-activation leads to $\beta A_{(1-42)}$ reduction
AF64A-treated rats (icv)	HP: α-APPs is reduced APP-M[a] is elevated	Not tested
192 IgG saporin-lesioned rats[5]	CT:[b] α-APPs is reduced APP-M is elevated	Not reported
192 IgG saporin-lesioned rabbits[6]	Not reported	CT: $\beta A_{(1-42)}$ and $\beta A_{(1-40)}$ 8- and 2.5-fold increase
192 IgG saporin-lesioned rats; $\pm$ RS-86 (limited electivity for M1 mAChR)[7]	−RS86	APP-M is elevated (CT, H[c])	α-APPs is reduced (CSF)	Not reported Elevated APP-M correlates with cognitive impairment
	+RS86	APP-M is reduced (CT, H)	α-APPs is elevated (CSF)	

[a]APP-M, membrane-bound APP; [b]CT, cortex; [c]HP, hippocampus.

TABLE 2. Evidence for the claim that M1 agonists can decrease tau hyperphosphorylation

Experiment	Summary
PC12M1 cell cultures $\pm$ AF102B, carbachol[8]	Stimulation of M1 mAChR decreased tau phosphorylation
CHO-M1AChR co-transfected with tau and GSK3β $\pm$ carbachol, xanomeline, SB202026[9,10]	Muscarinic agonists reduce tau phosphorylation through PKC activation and via GSK-3 inhibition. Carbachol induces a decrease in tau phosphorylation and an increase in the formation of microtubule bundles.
Primary cortical cell cultures $\pm$ carbachol[9,10]	Carbachol induces a decrease in tau phosphorylation.
ApoE-deficient mice versus control[11]	Tau proteins in ApoE-deficient mice contain a hyperphosphorylated "hot spot" domain, localized N-terminally to the microtubule-binding domain.
ApoE-deficient mice and control $\pm$ AF150(S) (0.5 mg/kg, p.o., 5 days/week for three weeks), respectively[11]	Tau epitopes that reside in the hyperphosphorylated hot spot are dephosphorylated by AF150(S), but unaffected in controls. Tau epitopes that flank the hot spot domain are dephosphorylated by AF150(S) in both groups. Epitopes located at the N and C terminal of tau are unaffected by AF150(S) in both groups.

phorylation of tau microtubule-associated protein. Moreover it may indicate a dual role for M1 agonists, as inhibitors of "vicious cycles" induced by β-amyloids and overactivation of certain kinases (e.g., GSK3) and/or downregulation of phosphatases, respectively.[12]

Studies in ApoE-deficient Mice

ApoE-deficient mice have memory deficits, synaptic loss of basal forebrain cholinergic projections, and hyperphosphorylation of distinct epitopes of the microtubule-associated protein tau (TABLE 2). These impairments are restored by subchronic treatment with AF150(S) (0.5 mg/kg, po 5 days/week for three weeks).[11] These findings suggest that ApoE deficiency results in hyperphosphorylation of a distinct tau domain whose excess phosphorylation can be reduced by M1 muscarinic treatment. A linkage can be proposed between the muscarinic signal transduction system(s) and the neuronal cytoskeleton via regulation of phosphorylation of tau microtubule-associated protein. It can be speculated that activation of M1 mAChRs might provide a novel treatment strategy for AD by modifying tau processing in the brain.[11] AF150(S) completely abolished working memory impairments in this model in a Morris Water Maze test. Furthermore, this cognitive improvement in ApoE-deficient mice was associated with a parallel restoration to control values of reduced ChAT and AChE and elevated M1 mAChR brain levels, respectively.[13] Interestingly, under similar experimental conditions, rivastigmine, an AChE-Is effective in AD, restored only cognitive impairments, but not AChE levels.[13] In both control and ApoE-deficient mice the prolonged treatment with AF150(S) revealed a two-site displacement curve of tritiated pirenzepine using AF150(S) as the competing ligand [K_H = 0.1 ± 0.1 μM (37%) and K_L = 15.3 ± 6 μM]. This indicates that the compound behaves as an efficacious M1 agonist *in vivo*, without producing tolerance following long-term treatment. Interestingly, control and ApoE-deficient mice that received a saline treatment exhibited a single-site binding curve for AF150(S) [K_L = 4.6 ± 0.6 μM]. From these and other studies (not shown), it can be speculated that no tolerance is expected to occur in AD patients when treated with partial M1 agonists [e.g., AF150(S)].

Studies in Other Animal Models

Some of the M1 agonists, including the AF series, were tested in a variety of animal models. AF102B and AF150(S) restored memory and learning deficits in a variety of animal models, which mimic cholinergic deficits reported in AD, without producing adverse central and peripheral side effects at effective doses and showing a relatively wide safety margin (> 200- to 500-fold).[1]

CONCLUSIONS AND PERSPECTIVES

Because Aβ is a natural constituent of body fluids, it is not known how inhibition of its formation would affect normal function. Inhibition of β/γ-secretases would lead to accumulation of APP or its Aβ-containing fragments if the inactivated α-secretase remains unmodified. These fragments can be potentially neurotoxic.

Therefore, attempts to reduce Aβ in AD should target the α-secretase. In this context, the ability of M1 agonists to stimulate APP secretion and Aβ reduction (via activation of α-secretase) might lead to a relatively direct route of Aβ reduction.

Disappointing results with some of the tested agonists should not discourage development of more selective M1 agonists. There are now experimental data to claim that M1 agonists may have not only a palliative effect (on cognition and behavior in AD) but also slow the progression of AD by altering the mechanisms responsible for disposal of Aβ and of tau phosphorylation/dephosphorylation. Except for M1 agonists, there are no reports on compounds with combined effects, for example, amelioration of cognition and modulation of Aβ and tau phosphorylation. This unique property of M1 agonists could represent the most remarkable value of such compounds. The compound with the least adverse effects profile and a high selectivity for M1 mAChR, both *in vitro* and *in vivo*, should be selected to evaluate the therapeutic potential of M1 agonists designed to influence the onset, progression, and prevalence of various target populations at risk for developing AD. Clinical trials with selective M1 agonists on Aβ levels in CSF taken from AD patients will be reported in the near future. Such studies, if positive, may indicate that M1 agonists have an important role also in affecting amyloid processing in AD patients. M1-selective agonists will thus allow testing the M1 mAChR-mediated effects on amyloids and tau in AD patients more directly than with other tools. All these findings may strengthen the cholinergic hypothesis in Alzheimer's disease.

REFERENCES

1. FISHER, A. 1999. Muscarinic receptor agonists in Alzheimer's disease. More than just symptomatic treatment. CNS Drugs **12**: 197–214.
2. NITSCH, R.N., B.E. SLACK, R.J. WURTMAN *et al.* 1992. Release of Alzheimer amyloid precursor derivatives stimulated by activation of muscarinic acetylcholine receptors. Science **58**: 304–307.
3. ALMKVIST, O., H. BASUN, S.L. WAGNER *et al.* 1997. Cerebrospinal fluid levels of α-secretase-cleaved soluble amyloid precursor protein mirror cognition in Swedish family with Alzheimer disease and a gene mutation. Arch. Neurol. **54**: 641–644.
4. SAVAGE, M.J,. S.P. TRUSKO, D.S. HOWALAND *et al.* 1998. Turnover of amyloid beta-protein in mouse brain and acute reduction of its level by phorbol ester. J. Neurosci. **185**: 1743–1752.
5. ROSSNER, S., U. UEBERHAM, J. YU *et al.* 1997. *In vivo* regulation of amyloid precursor protein secretion in rat neocortex by cholinergic activity. Eur. J. Neurosci. **9**: 2125–2134.
6. POTTER, P.E., T.G. BEACH, D.G. WALKER *et al.* 1999. Immunotoxin-induced cortical cholinergic denervation leads to vascular beta-amyloid deposition: a model of cerebral amyloid angiopathy. Soc. Neurosci. Abstr. **25**: 519.11.
7. LIN, L., B. GEORGIEVSKA, A. MATTSSON *et al.* 1999. Cognitive changes and modified processing of amyloid precursor protein in the cortical and hippocampal system after cholinergic synapse loss and muscarinic receptor activation. Proc. Natl. Acad. Sci. USA **96**: 12108–12113.
8. SADOT, E., D. GURWITZ, J. BARG *et al.* 1996. Activation of M1-muscarinic acetylcholine receptor regulates tau phosphorylation in transfected PC12 cells. J. Neurochem. **66**: 877–880.
9. FORLENZA, O., J. SPINK, O. OLESON *et al.* 1998. Muscarinic agonists reduce tau phosphorylation in transfected cells and in neurons. Neurobiol. Aging **19**: S218.
10. FORLENZA, O. & W.F. GATTAZ. 1998. Rev. Psiq. Clin. **25**: 114–117.

11. GENIS, I., A. FISHER & D.M. MICHAELSON. 1999. Site-specific dephosphorylation of tau in apolipoprotein E–deficient and control mice by M1 muscarinic agonist treatment. J. Neurochem. **12:** 206–213.
12. FISHER, A., R. BRANDEIS, S. CHAPMAN *et al.* 1998. M1 muscarinic agonist treatment reverses cognitive and cholinergic impairments of apolipoprotein E–deficient mice. J. Neurochem. **70:** 1991–1997.
13. CHAPMAN, S., A. FISHER, M. WEINSTOCK *et al.* 1998. The effects of the acetylcholinesterase inhibitor ENA713 and the M1 agonist AF150(S) on apolipoprotein E deficient mice. J. Physiol. (Paris) **92:** 299–303.

Cholinesterase Inhibitors Stabilize Alzheimer's Disease

EZIO GIACOBINI[a]

Department of Geriatrics, University Hospitals of Geneva,
University of Geneva Medical School, Geneva, Switzerland

ABSTRACT: During the last decade, a systematic effort to develop a pharmacological treatment for Alzheimer disease (AD) has resulted into three drugs being registered for the first time in the USA and Europe for this specific indication. All three are cholinesterase inhibitors (ChEI). The major therapeutic effect of ChEI on AD patients is to maintain cognitive function at a constant level during a six-month to one-year period of treatment, as compared to placebo. Additional drug effects might slow cognitive deterioration and improve behavioral and daily living conditions. Comparison of clinical effects of six ChEI demonstrates a rather similar magnitude of improvement in cognitive measures. For some drugs, this may represent an upper limit, whereas for other it may still be possible to further increase the benefit. In order to maximize and prolong positive drug effects, it is important to start early and adjust dosage during the treatment. Recent studies show that in many patients the stabilization effect produced by ChEI can be prolonged for as long as a 24-month period. In order to explain the stabilizing effect of ChEI, a mechanism other than AChE inhibition, based on β-amyloid metabolism, is postulated.

CHOLINESTERASE INHIBITORS STABILIZE COGNITIVE SYMPTOMS OF ALZHEIMER'S DISEASE

Cholinesterase inhibitors presently in clinical trials in Japan, the USA, and Europe include approximately 10 drugs, most of which have already advanced to clinical phase III and IV; three [(tacrine, rivastigmine (ENA 713), and donepezil (E2020)] are registered in the USA and/or in Europe. Another two ChEI (metrifonate and galanthamine) are pending registration. TABLE 1[1–18] compares the effects of eight ChEI on the ADAS-cog test using ITT (intention to treat) criteria. The duration of these controlled trials varied between 12 and 30 weeks (mostly 24 weeks), and the total number of tested patients was 8,864. At least 1,200 additional patients have been tested since the publication of these reports, bringing the total number to above 10,000. Based on the results of these studies, eight ChEI tested under similar criteria on patients of similar age, education, and degree of disease severity, originating from 26 countries, produced statistically significant improvements using rating scales of standardized and validated measures of both cognitive and noncognitive function. The first observation is a similarity in magnitude of cognitive effect for all eight

[a]Address for correspondence: Ezio Giacobini, University Hospitals of Geneva, Department of Geriatrics, University of Geneva, Medical School, CH-1226 Thonex, Geneva, Switzerland. Tel.: +41-22-305 -6522; fax: +41-22-305-6515.
e-mail: Ezio.Giacobini@hcuge.ch

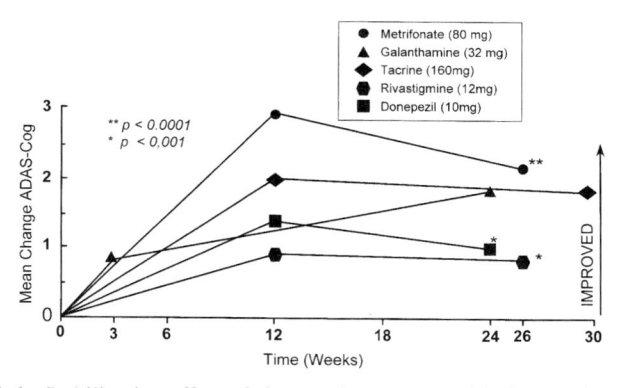

FIGURE 1. Stabilization effect of six-month treatment with five cholinesterase inhibitors. The patients change little cognitively from baseline during this period. (Modified from Giacobini[20].)

drugs when expressed as a difference between drug- and placebo-treated patients (TABLE 1).[1-18] Maximal differences in ADAS-cog (for eight drugs, at all doses) between drug-treated and placebo-treated patients averaged approximately 4.0 points (range 2.9–6.8). The highest difference of 6.8 points was seen for the MSF (methane sulphonyl-fluoride) 16-week study in a small number of patients. In the same study, for five drugs, an average difference in 1–2 ADAS-cog points above baseline was seen at the end of the study (range 0.5–2.2)[19,20] (FIG. 1). As seen in TABLE 1, the difference in cognitive effect between low and high dose is not constantly dose-dependent but seems to vary depending on the therapeutic window of that particular drug. Similarity in cognitive effect suggests a ceiling value average of approximately 5–6 ADAS-cog points for patients at the mild-to-moderate stages (MMSE 23-15) of the disease. The results suggest that some drugs (such as metrifonate) may have not been tested at their full capacity. Stratification analysis shows that for several drugs some patients demonstrate rates of improvement higher than 5, and up to 11 ADAS-cog points. Therefore, higher doses of some ChEI could increase the difference from the placebo. Similarity in clinical effects is also supported by the close values obtained on clinical global scales, such CIBIC-plus (interview-based impression of change-plus), representing an average of 0.4 points for tacrine, ENA 713, and metrifonate after 24 weeks of treatment.[19,20] For tacrine, the high percentage of dropouts and frequency of side effects suggest a practical limit in ChE inhibition as well as in drug effect. For other ChEI (e.g., metrifonate and donepezil), in spite of high AChE inhibition (70–80%), severity of side effects does not seem to represent a limiting factor. In general, the percentage of improved patients varies from about 25% (donepezil, high dose) to about 50% (tacrine, high dose), with an average of 34%.[19,20] These figures indicate that at least one-third of treated patients show a significant positive response (responders). Approximately 20% of patients do not improve (nonresponders) at the given dosage. It is plausible to think that the percent of responders could be increased from the present 35% to 50% by using higher doses of those ChEI that produce less severe side effects at higher dosages. The relationship between AChE (erythrocytes) or BuChE (plasma) inhibition (or drug concen-

TABLE 1. Comparison of the effect of eight cholinesterase inhibitors on ADAS-cog test (ITT)[a]

References	Drugs (No. of Patients)	Doses (mg/Day)	Duration of Study (Weeks)	Treatment Difference from Placebo[b]	Baseline[c]	Improved patients (%)	Dropout (%)	Side Effects (%)
Farlow et al.[1] Knapp et al.[2]	tacrine (THA) (1131)	120-160	30	4.0-5.3	0.8-2.8	30-50	55-73	40-58
Canal et al.[3] Imbimbo et al.[4]	eptastigmine (491)	45	25	4.7	1.8	30	12	35
Rogers & Friedhoff[5] Rogers et al.[6] Doody et al.[7] Burns et al.[8]	donepezil (E2020) (1452)	5-10	24	2.8-4.6	0.7-1	40-58	5-13	6-13
Anand et al.[9] Rossler et al.[10] Spencer &Noble[11]	rivastigmine (ENA 713) (2831)	6-12	24	1.9-4.9	0.7-1.2	25-37	15-36	15-28
Becker et al.[12] Morris et al.[13]	metrifonate (2440)	25-75	12-26	2.8-3.1	-0.75-0.5	35	2-21	2-12
Raskind et al.[14] Farlow et al.[15]		60-80	26	3.9	2.2	40	15	7
Wilkinson et al.[16]	galanthamine (289)	30	12	3.3	1.8	—	33	—
Moss et al.[17]	MSF[d] (15)	10-13	16	6.8	3.4	80	0	—
Thal et al.[18]	physostigmine (475)	30-36	24	2.9	1.8	29-24	26.61	70-80

[a]NOTE: ADAS-cog = AD Assessment Scale-cognitive subscale. ITT, intention to treat. Total number of patients: 8864.
[b]Study end point vs. placebo.
[c]Study end point vs. baseline.
[d]MSF, methane sulphonyl-flouride 3 times/week. Physostigmine, controlled release.

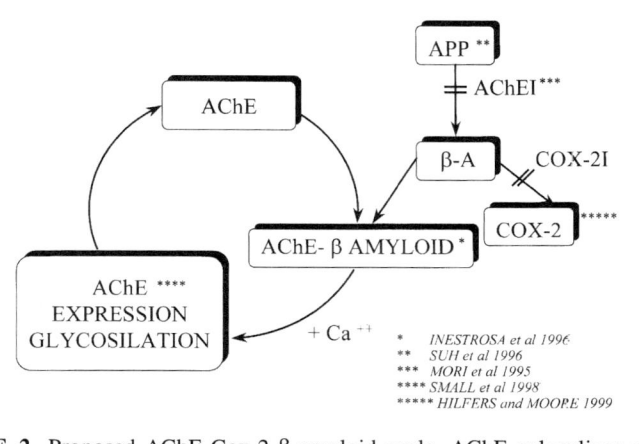

FIGURE 2. Proposed AChE-Cox-2 β-amyloid cycle. AChE colocalizes with β-amyloid and accelerates β-amyloid formation and deposition in AD brain. β-amyloid increases both AChE and Cox-2 expression in brain. Inhibition of AChE activity, inhibiting APP (amyloid precursor protein) release, reduces β-amyloid deposition and indirectly β-amyloid-enhanced Cox-2 expression. This mechanism could contribute to the patient's long-term cognitive improvement.

tration) and cognitive effect shows that different compounds display different levels of optimal ChE inhibition, ranging from a low of 30% to a high of 70%.[19,20] Data available after six months for six ChEI suggest that patients treated with the active compound change little cognitively from baseline from the beginning of the trial to the end of the trial.[19,20] As an example, in a USA study with ENA 713, patients administered placebo for 26 weeks deteriorated over four points on the ADAS-cog compared to only 0.3 points in patients given 6–12 mg/day of the drug. The same trend is true for the metrifonate-treated patients. Stabilization of cognitive deterioration could indicate either a primary, protective, and structural effect, or a more long-lasting improvement of cholinergic synaptic function (as reflected by the cognitive improvement measured by ADAS-cog). The slow return to the deterioration line after washout also suggests additional effects due to a secondary still-unknown effect of the compound.[21–22] The mechanism postulated by us is based on the AChE-β amyloid cycle shown in FIGURE 2.[21–26] Based on this hypothesis, ChEI may differ from one another not only with respect to the magnitude but also to the duration of the clinical effect.

LONG-LASTING STABILIZATION EFFECT OF ChEI

Recent data from 12- to 24-month open trials and one randomized placebo-controlled trial suggest that optimization and maintenance of clinical effects for one year or more is a feasible goal in many patients. Clinical studies lasting for periods longer than one year (up to 4.5 years) are listed in TABLE 2.[25–29] The data indicate that benefit differences can be maintained in a number of patients for up to 12–24 months for five different inhibitors (donepezil, tacrine, metrifonate, rivastigmine,

TABLE 2. Long-term efficacy of five cholinesterase inhibitors in patients with Alzheimer's disease

References	Drug	No. of Pts.[a]	Max Treatment Duration/ Yrs	Test	Benefit Difference
Rogers & Friedhoff[27]	donepezil	1600	2	ADAS-COG	positive
Mohs et al.[32]	donepezil	431[b]	1	ADFAC-CDR	positive
Winblad et al.[31]	donepezil	286[b]	1	GBS-MMSE	positive
Jelic et al.[28]	tacrine	25	1	MMSE-EEG	positive
Farlow et al.[15]	metrifonate	605	3	ADAS-COG., MMSE	positive
Anand et al.[29]	rivastigmine	2149	2	ADAS-COG, MMSE, CIB IC+, GDS	positive
Rainer &Mucke[30]	galanthamine	44	3	ADAS-cog	positive

[a]Total number of patients: 3540.
[b]Prospective, placebo controlled, double blind.

and galanthamine). With regard to global improvement in the ADAS-cog score, this may be a 15- to 20-point gain, representing an 18- to 24-month difference. The long-term stabilizing effects of ChEI are also suggested by the fact that if drug treatment is discontinued the clinical effect does not halt abruptly (such as could be expected from a symptomatic effect), but continues for several weeks following cessation of AChE inhibition. A newly demonstrated feature of ChEI and of muscarinic agonists is their ability to enhance the release of nonamyloidogenic-soluble derivatives of amyloid precursor protein (APPs) *in vitro* and *in vivo* and possibly to slow down formation of amyloidogenic compounds in brain[21,22] (FIG. 2). Controlled clinical trials monitoring CSF levels of biological markers (A-beta-42 and phosphorylated tau), combined with multiple MRI volumetric determinations of specific hippocampal regions extending to 24 months, should be able to show whether or not the demonstrated pharmacological effect of AChEI on APP metabolism[21] (FIG. 2) exerts an antideterioration and protective effect.

Based on recent data, present and future potential uses for AChEI are in (1) preclinical–presymptomatic stages in at-risk individuals with minimal cognitive impairment (MCI, CDR O); (2) early AD patients with manifested symptoms (CDR 0.5–1), presently representing the most frequently treated group; and (3) late AD (CDR 1.5–2) patients with behavioral symptoms (either alone or, in the future, in combination with muscarinic or nicotinic agonists). Combinations of ChEI with estrogens, antioxidants, or antiinflammatory agents might also represent future alternatives to ChEI monotreatment. The effect of these drugs is based on mechanisms different from the ones postulated for ChEI. Improved clinical knowledge and diagnosis may provide novel indications for expanding the use of ChEI to other areas of dementia, such as cerebrovascular disease (multiple infarct dementia), Lewy body disease, parkinsonism, frontal–temporal lobe disorder, and Down syndrome. Clinical trials are in progress for some of these disorders.

REFERENCES

1. FARLOW, M., S.I. GRACON, L.A. HERSHEY et al. 1992. Controlled trial of tacrine in Alzheimer's disease. J. Am. Med. Assoc. **268:** 2523–2529.
2. KNAPP, M.J., D.S. KNOPMAN & P.R.A. SOLOMON. 1994. 30 week randomized controlled trial of high-dose tacrine in patients with Alzheimer's disease J. Am. Med. Assoc. **271:** 985–991.
3. CANAL, I. & B.P. IMBIMBO. 1996. Clinical trials and therapeutics: relationship between pharmacodynamic activity and cognitive effects of eptastigmine in patients with Alzheimer's disease. Clin. Pharmacol. Therap. **15:** 49–59.
4. IMBIMBO, B.P., P. MARTELLI, W.M. TROETEL et al. 1999. Efficacy and safety of eptastigmine for the treatment of patients with Alzheimer's disease. Neurology **52:** 700–708.
5. ROGERS, S. L. & T. FRIEDHOFF. 1996. The efficacy and safety of donepezil in patients with Alzheimer's disease: results of a US multicentre, randomized, double-blind, placebo-controlled trial. Dementia **7:** 293–230.
6. ROGERS, S.L., M.R. FARLOW, S.R. DOODY et al. 1998. A 24 week, double blind placebo controlled trial of donepezil in patients with AD. Neurology **50:** 136–145.
7. DOODY, R.S. 1998. Treatment of Alzheimer's disease. Neurologist **3:** 279–289 (Abstr. 880), S 209.
8. BURNS, A., M. ROSSOR, J. HECKER et al. 1999. The effects of donepezil in Alzheimer's Disease—results from a multinational trial. Dementia **10:** 237–244.
9. ANAND, R., R.D. HARTMAN & P.E. HAYES. 1996. An overview of the development of SDZ ENA 713, a brain selective cholinesterase inhibitor disease. In Alzheimer Disease: From Molecular Biology to Therapy. R. Becker & E. Giacobini, Eds.: 239–243. Birkhäuser. Boston, MA.
10. ROSSLER, M., R. ANAND, A. CICIN-SIAN et al. 1999. Efficacy and safety of rivastigmine in patients with Alzheimer's disease: international randomized controlled trial. Br. Med. J. **318:** 633–658.
11. SPENCER, M.C. & S. NOBLE. 1998. Rivastigmine. a review of its use in Alzheimer's Disease. Drugs & Aging **1** (Suppl. 5): 391–411.
12. BECKER, R., J.A. COLLIVER, S.J. MARKWELL et al. 1996. Double-blind, placebo-controlled study of metrifonate, an acetylcholinesterase inhibitor for Alzheimer disease. Alzheimer Dis. Assoc. Discord. **1:** 124–131.
13. MORRIS, J., P. CYRUS, J. ORAZEM et al. 1998. Metrifonate benefits cognitive, behavioral, and global function in patients with Alzheimer's disease. Neurology **50:** 1222–1230.
14. RASKIND, M., P. CYRUS, B. RUZICKA & B.I. GULANSKI. 1999. The effects of Metrifonate on the cognitive, behavioral and functional performance of Alzheimer's disease patients. J. Clin. Psychol. **60:** 318–325.
15. FARLOW, M.R, P.A. CYRUS & B. GULANSKI. 1998. Metrifonate improves the cognitive deficits of Alzheimer's disease patients in a dose-related manner. Am. Geriatr. Soc. Meeting Seattle, Abstr. A15.
16. WILKINSON, D. 1997. Galanthamine hydrobromide—results of a group study. Eighth Congress Int. Psychoger. Jerusalem. Abstr. 7025.
17. MOSS, D.E., P. BERLANGA, M.M. HAGAN et al. 1999. Methanesulphonyl fluoride (MSF). Alzheimer Dis. Assoc. Discord. **13:** 20–25.
18. THAL, L.J., J.M. FERGUSON, J. MINTZER et al. 1999. Randomized trial of controlled release physostigmine. Neurology **52:** 1146–1152.
19. GIACOBINI, E. 1998. Cholinesterase inhibitors for Alzheimer's disease therapy, from tacrine to future applications. Neurochem. Int. **32:** 413–419.
20. GIACOBINI, E. 2000. Cholinesterase and cholinesterase inhibitors. From molecular biology to therapy. Chapter 12. Martin Dunitz Publishers. London.
21. MORI, F., C.C. LAI, F. FUSI & E. GIACOBINI. 1995. Cholinesterase inhibitors increase secretion of APPs in barin cortex. Neuroreport **6:** 633–636.

22. GIACOBINI, E. 1996. Cholinesterase inhibitors do more than inhibit cholinesterase. *In* Alzheimer Disease: From Molecular Biology to Therapy. R. Becker & E. Giacobini, Eds.: 187–204. Birkhäuser. Boston, MA.

23. INESTROSA, N., A. ALVAREZ, C.A. PEREZ *et al.* 1996. Acetylcholinesterase accelerates assembly of amyloid-beta-peptides into Alzheimer's fibrils: possible role of the peripheral site of the enzyme. Neuron **16:** 881–891.

24. SUH, Y.-H., Y.H. CHONG, S.-H. KIM *et al.* 1996. Molecular physiology, biochemistry, and pharmacology of Alzheimer's amyloid precursor protein (APP). Ann. N.Y. Acad. Sci. **786:** 169–183.

25. SMALL, D.H., G. SBERNA, Q.X. LI *et al.* The beta-amyloid protein influence on acethylcholinesterase expression, assembly and glycosylation. Sixth Int. Conf. on Alzheimer's Disease and Related Disorders. Amsterdam.

26. HILFERS, M.A. & S.A. MOORE. 1999. Amyloid-beta peptide induces cyclooxygenase-2 expression and activity in brain-derived cells. Soc. Neurosci. **25** (Abstr. 450.1) p. 1105.

27. ROGERS, S. & L. FRIEDHOFF. 1998. Long-term efficacy and safety of donepezil in the treatment of Alzheimer's disease. Eur. Neuropsychopharmacol. **8:** 67–75.

28. JELIC, V., K. AMBERLA, O. ALMKVIST *et al.* 1998. Long-term tacrine treatment slows the increase of theta power in the EEG of mild Alzheimer patients compared to untreated controls. Fifth Int. Geneva/Springfield Symposium on Advances in Alzheimer Therapy. Geneva. Abstr. 147.

29. ANAND, R., R. HARTMAN, J. MESSINA *et al.* 1998. Long-term treatment with rivastigmine continue to provide benefits for up to one year. Fifth Int. Geneva/Springfield Symposium on Advances in Alzheimer Therapy. Geneva. Abstr. 18.

30. RAINER, M. & H.A.M. MUCKE. 1999. Long-term cognitive benefit from galanthamine in Alzheimer's disease. Int. J. Geriatr. Psychiatry **1:** 197–201.

31. WINBLAD, B., K. ENGEDAL, H. SOININEN *et al.* 1999. Donepezil enhances global function, cognition and activities of daily living compared with placebo one year. 12th Congr. ECNP. Abstr. 30. London.

32. MOHS, R., R. DOODY, J. MORRIS *et al.* 1999. Donepezil preserves functional status in Alzheimer's disease patients. Eur. Neuropsychol. Suppl 5, Abstr. S328.

Nasal Aβ Treatment Induces Anti-Aβ Antibody Production and Decreases Cerebral Amyloid Burden in PD-APP Mice

C.A. LEMERE,[a,c] R. MARON,[a] E.T. SPOONER,[a] T.J. GRENFELL,[a] C. MORI,[a] R. DESAI,[a] W.W. HANCOCK,[b] H.L. WEINER,[a] AND D.J. SELKOE[a]

[c]*Department of Neurology, Harvard Medical School and Center for Neurologic Diseases, Brigham and Women's Hospital, Boston, Massachusetts 02115, USA*

[b]*Department of Pathology, Harvard Medical School and LeukoSite, Inc., Cambridge, Massachusetts 02142, USA*

Amyloid accumulation[1] and accompanying inflammation—including both the activation of glial cells[2] and the accrual of inflammatory proteins, such as complement,[3,4] cytokines,[5] and acute phase proteins[6–8]—play key roles in the pathogenesis of Alzheimer's disease (AD).[9] Mucosal administration of proteins implicated in a disease can decrease organ-specific inflammatory processes in a number of animal models of autoimmune disorders, including those affecting the nervous system, principally by inducing antiinflammatory IL-4/IL-10 (Th2) and TGFβ immune responses in mucosal lymphoid tissue that then act systemically.[10] For example, oral or nasal administration of myelin basic protein (MBP)[11–13] or the acetylcholine receptor[14,15] can suppress experimental autoimmune encephalomyelitis (EAE) and experimental myasthenia gravis, respectively.

In an effort to reduce the inflammation associated with Aβ deposition via mucosal tolerance, we tested the effects of nasal or oral administration of Aβ$_{1-40}$ peptide and a control protein, myelin basic protein (MBP), by treating 52 PD-APP transgenic mice, an animal model with certain key features of AD,[16–18] on a weekly basis for seven months (ages 5 to 12 months). Doses were chosen based on preliminary nasal and oral studies in nontransgenic mice. Treatment groups included (1) untreated ($n = 7$); (2) MBP oral, 500 μg ($n = 5$); (3) MBP nasal, 50 μg ($n = 6$); (4) Aβ oral, 10 μg ($n = 9$); (5) Aβ oral, 100 μg ($n = 9$); (6) Aβ nasal, 5 μg ($n = 7$); and (7) Aβ nasal, 25 μg ($n = 9$). During the first week, mice were fed five times or nasally treated three times on consecutive days. Thereafter, mice were fed or nasally treated each week for seven months and then sacrificed. The brain from each mouse was removed and divided in half along the sagittal midline. One hemisphere was formalin fixed and embedded in paraffin for immunohistochemical analysis. Of the contralateral hemispheres, half were snap frozen for biochemical analysis; the other half were embedded sagittally in OCT and snap frozen for cryosectioning and immunohistochemistry.

[c]Address for correspondence: Cynthia A. Lemere, Center for Neurologic Diseases, Harvard Institutes of Medicine 622, 77 Avenue Louis Pasteur, Boston, MA 02115-5716. Tel.: (617) 525-5214; fax: (617) 525-5252.
e-mail: lemere@cnd.bwh.harvard.edu

As previously described for PD-APP transgenic mice,[16–18] moderate variability in the amount of Aβ deposition was observed in the mice, even in the untreated group. Computerized image analysis was performed to quantitate the amount of Aβ deposition in each brain. The three control groups showed no significant differences in mean Aβ burden from each other (untreated = 3.31 ± 2.35; oral MBP = 5.78 ± 2.97; and nasal MBP = 3.87 ± 4.86). In view of this lack of effect of MBP treatment, the large Aβ variation among individual mice, and the limited number of mice available to us for this study, we compared each of the four Aβ treatment groups to the mice in the three control groups. A substantial (60%) and significant ($p < 0.037$; two-tailed Mann-Whitney U test) reduction was revealed in the percent area occupied by Aβ immunoreactivity (IR) in hippocampus in mice treated nasally with 25 μg Aβ ($1.72 ± 1.39$, $n = 9$), as compared with controls ($4.18 ± 3.47$, $n = 18$). The mice treated nasally with 5 μg of Aβ also showed a reduction in Aβ burden, but their mean levels did not differ significantly from the controls. The mean Aβ plaque burden in the mice treated orally with Aβ did not differ significantly from control groups.

This reduction in Aβ plaque burden in mice treated nasally with 25 μg Aβ was paralleled by a significant decrease in $Aβ_{X–42}$ levels in brain homogenates, as detected by Aβ ELISA. The mean levels of $Aβ_{X–42}$ (pmol/g) among the three control groups of mice (untreated: 453 ± 96; oral MBP: 887 ± 584; nasal/MBP: 535 ± 460) showed no statistical difference from each other. Brains of the nasal Aβ 25 μg–treated mice contained a mean of 282 ± 187 pmol/g of $Aβ_{X–42}$, representing a 52% decrease ($p < 0.033$; repeated measures ANOVA) when compared to a mean of 592 ± 383 pmol/g for the control mice. When the mean $Aβ_{X–42}$ level of the nasal Aβ 25 μg–mice (282 ± 187 pmol/g) was compared to that (453 ± 96) of the untreated mice alone, a significant decrease of 38% ($p < 0.044$) was observed. As in the case of Aβ imaging, $Aβ_{X–42}$ ELISA revealed no significant changes in brain Aβ levels in either of the oral Aβ treatment groups (oral Aβ, 10 μg: 763 ± 566; oral Aβ, 100 μg: 661 ± 477), compared to the controls (592 ± 383). A small decrease in the far less abundant $Aβ_{X–40}$ species was observed in the nasal Aβ 25 μg mice (mean: 16 ± 10 pmol/g) versus control mice (mean: 24 ± 12 pmol/g), but the difference was not significant.

The decrease in Aβ deposition observed in the mice treated chronically with nasal Aβ 25 μg was accompanied by corresponding decreases in microglial activation, reactive astrocytosis, accrual of complement, and neuritic dystrophy. However, even within this group, the level of plaque-associated inflammation corresponded with Aβ plaque burden: mice with moderate levels of Aβ deposition had moderate numbers of activated microglia, reactive astrocytes, dystrophic neurites, and complement; those with low levels of Aβ deposition had little or no signs of inflammation. Importantly, there was no increase in abnormal neurites in Aβ nasally treated animals having very low plaque numbers. Infiltration of a small number of mononuclear cells immunoreactive for antiinflammatory cytokines IL-4, IL-10, and TGFβ was detected in and around the hippocampus in mice treated with nasal Aβ, 25 μg.

A strong humoral anti-Aβ antibody induction in serum of mice treated with Aβ was revealed by several methods. Using the mouse sera as primary antibodies, we were able to show human brain AD plaque IR in 3 of 18 mice treated orally with Aβ, in 4 of 7 mice treated nasally with 5 μg Aβ, and in 8 of 9 mice treated nasally with 25 μg Aβ. This IR was abolished by absorption of the sera with Aβ peptide, indicating the specificity of the antibodies for Aβ. The immunoglobulin isotypes of the mouse serum antibodies were determined to be IgG1 and IgG2b, using isotype-specific biotinylated secondary antibodies for immunohistochemistry on human AD brains. The mouse serum antibodies have epitopes within the first 15 residues of Aβ, as revealed by absorption with serial 15-mer peptides (Aβ$_{1-15}$, Aβ$_{6-20}$, Aβ$_{11-25}$, Aβ$_{16-30}$, Aβ$_{21-35}$, Aβ$_{26-42}$) and immunohistochemistry. Only peptide 1, Aβ$_{1-15}$, was able to abolish Aβ IR from the mouse sera. An Aβ antibody ELISA was performed to quantitate the amount of Aβ antibodies; serum concentrations as high as 54.56 μg/ml were observed. None of the 18 control mice had Aβ antibody titers, as tested by immunohistochemical analysis and anti-Aβ antibody ELISA.

Our results are consistent with those of Schenk et al.,[19] using a novel route of Aβ administration, and raise the possibility that cellular immune responses may also contribute to the effects observed. Thus, our results suggest that nasal Aβ immunization can alter AD neuropathologic processes in an animal model and may be useful in the prevention and treatment of AD in humans.

REFERENCES

1. SELKOE, D.J. 1999. Translating cell biology into therapeutic advances in Alzheimer's disease. Nature **399:** A23–A31.
2. ITAGAKI, S., P.L. MCGEER, H. AKIYAMA, S. ZHU & D.J. SELKOE. 1989. Relationship of microglia and astrocytes to amyloid deposits of Alzheimer disease. J. Neuroimmunol. **24:** 173–182.
3. EIKELENBOOM, P. & F.C. STAM. 1982. Immunoglobulins and complement factors in senile plaques: an immunoperoxidase study. Acta Neuropathol. **57:** 239–242.
4. ROGERS, J., N.R. COOPER, S. WEBSTER, et al. 1992. Complement activation by β-amyloid in Alzheimer disease. Proc. Natl. Acad. Sci. USA **89:** 10016–10020.
5. DICKSON, D.W., S.C. LEE, L.A. MATTIACE, S.-H.C. YEN & C.F. BROSNAN. 1993. Microglia and cytokines in neurological disease, with special reference to AIDS and Alzheimer's disease. Glia **26:** 816–834.
6. ABRAHAM C.R., D.J. SELKOE & H. POTTER. 1988. Immunochemical identification of the serine protease inhibitor a$_1$-antichymotrypsin in the brain amyloid deposits of Alzheimer's disease. Cell **52:** 487–501.
7. KALARIA, R.N., P.G. GALLOWAY & G. PERRY. 1991. Widespread serum amyloid P immunoreactivity in cortical amyloid deposits and the neurofibrillary pathology of Alzheimer's disease and other degenerative disorders. Neuropathol. Appl. Neurobiol. **17:** 189–201.
8. PEPYS, M.B., G.A. TENNENT, D.R. BOOTH, et al. 1996. Molecular mechanisms of fibrillogenesis and the protective role of amyloid P component: two possible avenues for therapy. Ciba Found. Symp. **199:** 73–81; discussion 81–79.
9. DICKSON, D.W. 1997. The pathogenesis of senile plaques. J. Neuropathol. Exp. Neurol. **56:** 321–339.
10. CHEN, Y., V.K. KUCHROO, J.-I. INOBE, D.A. HAFLER & H.L. WEINER. 1994. Regulatory T-cell clones induced by oral tolerance: suppression of autoimmune encephalomyelitis. Science **265:** 1237–1240.
11. BITAR, D.M. & C.C. WHITACRE. 1988. Suppression of experimental autoimmune encephalomyelitis by the oral administration of myelin basic protein. Cell Immunol. **112:** 364–370.
12. HIGGINS, P. & H.L. WEINER. 1988. Suppression of experimental autoimmune encephalomyelitis by oral administration of myelin basic protein and its fragments. J. Immunol. **140:** 440–445.
13. METZLER, B. & D.C. WRAITH. 1993. Inhibition of experimental autoimmune encephalomyelitis by inhalation but not oral administration of the encephalitogenic peptide: influence of MHC binding affinity. Int. Immunol. **5:** 1159–1165.

14. MA, C.-G., G-X. ZHANG, B-G. XIAO, J. LINK, T. OLSSON & H. LINK. 1995. Suppression of experimental autoimmune myasthenia gravis by nasal administration of acetylcholine receptor. J. Neuroimmunol. **58:** 51–60.
15. OKUMURA, S., K. MCINTOSH & D.B. DRACHMAN. 1994. Oral administration of acetylcholine receptor: effects on experimental myasthenia gravis. Ann. Neurol. **36:** 704–713.
16. GAMES, D., D. ADAMS, R. ALESSANDRINI, *et al.* 1995. Alzheimer-type neuropathology in transgenic mice overexpressing V717F β-amyloid precursor protein. Nature **373:** 523–527.
17. MASLIAH, E., A. SISK, M. MALLORY, L. MUCKE, D. SCHENK & D. GAMES. 1996. Comparison of neurodegenerative pathology in transgenic mice overexpressing V717F β-amyloid precursor protein and Alzheimer's disease. J. Neurosci. **16:** 5795–5811.
18. JOHNSON-WOOD, K., M. LEE, R. MOTTER, *et al.* 1997. Amyloid precursor protein processing and Aβ42 deposition in a transgenic mouse model of Alzheimer disease. Proc. Natl. Acad. Sci. USA **94:** 1550–1555.
19. SCHENK, D., R. BARBOUR, W. DUNN, *et al.* 1999. Immunization with amyloid-β attenuates Alzheimer-disease-like pathology in the PDAPP mouse. Nature **400:** 173–177.13.

Cytidine (5′)Diphosphocholine Modulates Dopamine K+-evoked Release in Striatum Measured by Microdialysis

J. AGUT,[a,c] J.A. ORTIZ,[a] AND R.J. WURTMAN[b]

[a]Centro de Investigación Grupo Ferrer, Barcelona 08028, Spain

[b]Department of Brain and Cognitive Sciences, Massachusetts Institute of Technology, Cambridge, Massachusetts 02139, USA

ABSTRACT: Experiments were performed to determine whether exogenous cytidine (5′)diphosphocholine (CDP-choline) could modify the release of dopamine (DA) in the striatum. Rats were divided into two groups, receiving either a standard diet (UAR 004) or the same diet supplemented with CDP-choline (250 mg/kg day) for 28 days. On the last day the dialysis probes were inserted in the striatum, and DA, homovanillic acid (HVA), and 3,4-dihydroxyphenylacetic acid (DOPAC) efflux were measured in the dialysis stream basally and during K+ depolarization (80 mM K+). Basal DA, HVA, and DOPAC did not show any difference between treated and untreated groups. Depolarization with K+ increased DA levels by up to 3,000% in the control group and by up to 4,770% in the CDP-choline–treated group ($p < 0.05$), and reduced extracellular HVA and DOPAC concentration by up to 45 and 35%, respectively, both in the untreated and CDP-choline–treated groups. These results show that long-term treatment with CDP-choline increases the K+ induced release of DA and suggest, in accordance with previous research, that by providing exogenous choline and cytidine, CDP-choline modulates dopaminergic transmission.

Functional integrity of neural cell membranes is necessary not only for cell survival and growth, but also for neurotransmitter release and communication between neurons. We have described that exogenous administration of CDP-choline increases phospholipid brain levels.[1,2] We, and others,[3,4] have also described that CDP-choline administration increases striatum levels of DA and DA metabolites, but it is not known whether these latter effects are associated with changes in the release of neurotransmitters by neurons. In the present study, we investigated whether chronic administration of CDP-choline could affect the evoked dopamine release by K+ depolarization measured by microdialysis in awake rat.

MATERIALS AND METHODS

Two groups of nine male Sprague-Dawley rats, weighing 60–70 g at the beginning of treatment, were housed in conventional cages and given free access to food

[c]Address for correspondence to: Dr. J.A. Agut, Centro de Investigación, Grupo Ferrer, Juan de Sada, 32, 08028 Barcelona, Spain. Tel.: 34-93-339-20-21; fax: 34-93-411-27-64
e-mail: agut.research@ferrer-grupo.com

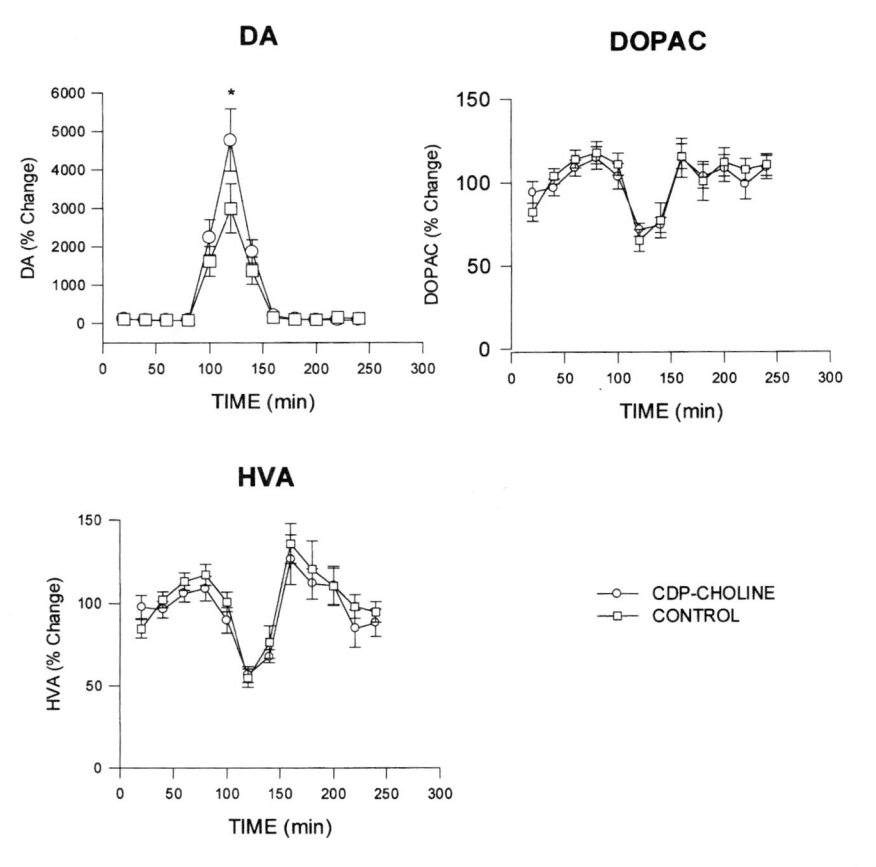

FIGURE 1. Effect of CDP-choline treatment (250 mg/kg·day for 28 days) on K^+-stimulated DA release in the striatum. * Significantly different from control values ($p < 0.05$).

(A 04 U.A.R., France) and water. One group received 250 mg/kg of body weight/day of CDP-choline incorporated into the diet for 28 days, and the other group, used as a control, received a standard diet. On day 21 animals were anesthetized with chloral hydrate 400 mg/kg i.p., an orifice was drilled in the cranium, and a probe holder was inserted on the meninges without damaging them. Three anchor bolts were fixed at the skull, the complex (bolts and probe holder) was coated with dental cement, and the skin sutured. On day 28, a probe (CMA/12.4 mm; Carnegre Medicine, Stockholm, Sweden) was inserted (AP: +0.8, LAT: +63.2, V: −7.5 [5]) in the striatum, and Ringer's solution (120 mM NaCl, 3 mM KCl, 1.2 mM $MgCl_2$, 1.2 mM $CaCl_2$, 25 mM $NaCO_3$, 0.4 mm KH_2PO_4, and 1.2 g of glucose, pH = 7.2–7.4 with flow gas 5% CO_2 and 95% O_2) was perfused at a flow rate of 1.5 µl/min. In the case of elevated K^+Cl (80 mM), the Cl^- concentration was balanced with an appropriate decrease in NaCl concentration. Twelve fractions from each rat were collected (four baseline, two K$^+$-depolarized, and six baseline-return every 20 min over 30 μl of 0.1 M HClO$_4$), and DA, HVA and DOPAC were analyzed by high-performance liquid chromatography. DA and metabolites were separated using a thermostatized (40°C) hypersil BDS-C18 100 × 2.1 mm, 3 μm column, using 50 mM sodium dihydrogen phosphate (pH: 3 with H$_3$PO$_4$), 5 mM, 0.1 mM EDTA.2Na, 0.25 mM sodium octyl sulfate, and 10% of methanol as the mobile phase (flow rate at 0.2 ml/min), and then measured by electrochemical detection (HP detector model 1049 A 0.65 V, response time 4 s).

Individual time points of the two time-effect curves were compared using the U Mann-Whitney test. The level of significance was set at $p < 0.05$.

RESULTS

Consistent with studies using dialysis probes similar to those used in the present study, stable baseline DA, HVA, and DOPAC levels were obtained 1 h after probe implantation in striatum and were maintained for at least 4 h after the start of the experiment. Basal DA, HVA, and DOPAC levels did not show any difference between the treated and untreated groups. Depolarization induced by K$^+$, 80 mM, increased DA dialysate levels by up to 3,000% (2,999.12 ± 643.40) in the control and by up to 4,770% (4,773.46 ± 807.44, $p < 0.05$) in the CDP-choline treated group, and reduced extracellular HVA and DOPAC concentration by up to 45 and 35% respectively, in the untreated and CDP-choline treated groups (FIG. 1).

DISCUSSION

In accordance with previous work,[6] an elevated K$^+$ concentration in the microdialysis perfusion fluid increased dopamine release and reduced DOPAC and HVA concentrations. This effect may be related to a K$^+$-induced inhibition of neuronal DA uptake and an enhanced vesicular uptake.[6,7] CDP-choline administration, at a dose and time period that are able also to increase phospholipid brain levels, had no action on spontaneous DA release or DOPAC and HVA extracellular levels, but increased the K$^+$-induced release of DA, without affecting the levels of DA metabolites. These results suggest that, by providing exogenous choline and cytidine, CDP-choline can affect membrane composition and modulate neural transmission.

REFERENCES

1. AGUT, J., I. LÓPEZ-COVIELLA, J.A. ORTIZ & R.J. WURTMAN. 1993. Oral cytidine 5'-diphosphate choline administration to rats increases brain phospholipid levels. Ann. N. Y. Acad. Sci. **695:** 318–320.
2. LÓPEZ-COVIELLA, I., J. AGUT, V. SAVCI, J.A. ORTIZ & R.J. WURTMAN. 1995. Evidence that 5'-cytidinediphosphocholine can affect brain phospholipid composition by increasing choline and cytidine plasma levels. J. Neurochem. **65:** 889–894
3. MARTINET, M., P. FONTULPT & H. PACHECO. 1981. Activation of soluble striatal tyrosine hydroxylase in the rat brain after CDP-choline administration. Biochem. Pharmacol. **30:** 539–541.

4. AGUT, J., I.L.G. COVIELLA & R.J. WURTMAN. 1984. Cytidine (5′) diphosphocholine enhances the ability of haloperidol to increase dopamine metabolites in the striatum of the rat and to diminish stereotyped behavior induced by apomorphine. Neuropharmacology **23:** 1403–1406.
5. PATXIMOS, G. & C. WATSON. 1982. The Rat Brain in Stereotaxic Coordinates. Academic Press. New York.
6. BADOER, E., H. WURTH, D. TURCK, *et al.* 1989. The K^+-induced increases in noradrenaline and dopamine release are accompanied by reductions in the release of their intraneuronal metabolites from the rat anterior hypothalamus. An *in vivo* brain microdialysis study. Naunyn-Schmiedeberg's Arch. Pharmacol. **339:** 54–59.
7. UNGELL, A.L. & K.H. GRAEFE. 1987. Failure of K^+ to affect the potency of inhibitors on the neuronal noradrenaline carrier in the rat vas deferens. Naunyn-Schmiedeberg's Arch. Pharmacol. **335:** 250–254.

Index of Contributors